Oncology Nursing Society

Core Curriculum for *Oncology Nursing*

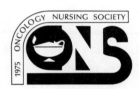

Editor
Constance R. Ziegfeld, RN, MS, OCN

Section Editors
Joanne T. Cossman, RN, MPH
Susan C. McMillan, RN, PhD
Roberta A. Strohl, RN, MN

W.B. Saunders Company
Philadelphia   Sydney
London   Tokyo
Toronto   Hong Kong

W. B. SAUNDERS COMPANY
Harcourt Brace Jovanovich, Inc.

The Curtis Center
Independence Square West
Philadelphia, PA 19106

Library of Congress Cataloging-in-Publication Data

Core curriculum for oncology nursing.

At head of title: Oncology Nursing Society.
Includes index.
1. Cancer—Nursing. 2. Cancer. I. Ziegfeld,
Constance R. II. Oncology Nursing Society.
[DNLM: 1. Curriculum. 2. Oncologic Nursing.
WY 18 C7968]
RC266.C67 1987   616.99′4′0024613   87-4800
ISBN 0-7216-2060-4

Editor: Michael Brown
Developmental Editor: Frances T. Mues
Designer: W. B. Saunders Staff
Production Manager: William Preston
Manuscript Editor: Susan Short
Illustration Coordinator: Lisa Lambert
Indexes: Nancy Weaver and Nelle Garrecht

Core Curriculum for Oncology Nursing   ISBN   0-7216-2060-4

Last digit is the print number: 9   8   7   6   5   4

Contributors

Minerva Applegate, RN, EdD
Professor of Nursing, University of South Florida College of Nursing, Tampa, Florida.
Informed Consent
Legal Issues

Anne E. Belcher, RN, PhD
Director, Masters Program in Oncology Nursing, Memorial Sloan-Kettering Cancer Center and Columbia University School of Nursing, New York, New York.
Communicating with the Patient and Family/Significant Others

Catherine M. Bender, RN, MN
Assistant Professor, Medical-Surgical Nursing, Coordinator, Oncology Program, University of Pittsburgh, Pittsburgh, Pennsylvania.
Chemotherapy

Jennifer Bucholtz, RN, MSN
Clinical Specialist, Radiation Oncology, Johns Hopkins Oncology Center, Baltimore, Maryland.
Radiation Therapy

Jody Burns, RN, CFNP, MSN
Division Administrator, Nursing, Berkshire Medical Center, Pittsfield, Massachusetts.
Identification of and Referral to Resources

Jane Clark, RN, MN, OCN
Clinical Nurse Specialist, Assistant Professor, Emory University, Atlanta, Georgia.
Nursing Management of Outcomes of Disease, Psychological Response, Treatment, and Complications

Marcia Clark, RN, MS
Nursing Coordinator, Department of Medical Oncology, Rhode Island Hospital, Providence, Rhode Island.
Cancer Economics

Margaret J. Crowley, RN, BSN, MS Ed
Formerly Adjunct Assistant Professor, Widener University, Graduate School of Nursing, Oncology Program, Chester, Pennsylvania.
Patterns of Occurrence
Risk Factors

Mary Cunningham, RN, BSN, OCN
The Texas System Cancer Center, M.D. Anderson Hospital and Tumor Institute, Houston, Texas.
Risk Factors and Coping Skills for the Oncology Nurse

Ruth Bope Dangel, RN, MN, OCN
Formerly Oncology Clinical Nurse Specialist, Riverside Methodist Hospital, Columbus, Ohio.
Historical Perspectives

Marilyn Davis, RN, MS, OCN
Instructor, School of Medicine, University of Colorado Health Sciences Center, Denver, Colorado.
Assessing and Diagnosing Cancer

Ann Marie Dozier, RN, MSN
Associate Clinical Chief for Obstetric and Gynecologic Nursing, University of Rochester, Strong Memorial Hospital, Rochester, New York.
Gynecologic Cancers

Nina Entrekin, RN, MN, OCN

Associate Professor, University of South Florida College of Nursing; Nurse Clinician, Comprehensive Breast Cancer, H. Lee Moffit Cancer Center and Research Institute, Tampa, Florida.
Breast Cancer

Joanne Peter Findley, RN, MS

Formerly Oncology Clinical Nurse Specialist, The Alexandria Hospital, Alexandria, Virginia.
Nursing Management of Common Oncologic Emergencies

Kathleen Flynn, RN, MS

Associate Professor, Surgical Clinical Nurse Specialist, Yale University School of Nursing, New Haven, Connecticut.
Historical Perspectives

Arlene Gordon, RN, MSN

Formerly Clinical Instructor, Johns Hopkins Oncology Center, Baltimore, Maryland.
Nutrition

Diane Gordon, RN, MPH

Director, Cancer Program, Provident Hospital, Portland, Oregon.
Staging: A Classification System for Cancer

Nancy Kane, RN, MSN

Clinical Nurse Specialist, Medical College of Virginia Hospitals, Richmond, Virginia.
Unproven Methods of Cancer Treatment

Lori Landis, RN, MN

Lawrenceville, Georgia.
Nursing Management of Outcomes of Disease, Psychological Response, Treatment, and Complications

Julena Lind, RN, MN

Director of Education, Center for Health Information, Education and Research, California Medical Center, Los Angeles, California.
Lung Cancer
Prostate Cancer
Colorectal Cancer

Alice Longman, RN, EdD

Associate Professor of Nursing, The University of Arizona College of Nursing, Tucson, Arizona.
Skin Cancer

Nancy Lovejoy, RN, DSN

Assistant Professor, Department of Physiological Nursing, University of California at San Francisco, San Francisco, California.
Alterations in Cell Biology
The Process of Carcinogenesis
The Role of the Immune System
Tumor Classification

Maryellen Maguire, RN, BSN

Leukemia Nurse Specialist, Dana Farber Cancer Institute, Boston, Massachusetts.
Leukemia

Deborah K. Mayer, RN, MSN, CRNP, OCN

Assistant Professor and Oncology Clinical Specialist, Massachusetts General Hospital, Institute of Health Professions, Boston, Massachusetts.
Investigational Cancer Treatment Modalities

Rose McGee, RN, PhD

Professor of Nursing and A.C.S. Professor of Oncology Nursing, Emory University, Atlanta, Georgia.
Nursing Management of Outcomes of Disease, Psychological Response, Treatment, and Complications

Barbara Burns McGrath, RN, MA

Formerly Lecturer, Cancer Specialty, Yale University School of Nursing, New Haven, Connecticut.
Terminology

Christine A. Miaskowski, RN, MS

Clinical Nurse Specialist, Jack D. Weiler Hospital of the Albert Einstein College of Medicine, Bronx, New York.
Outcome Standards for Cancer Nursing Practice

Deborah Stephens Mills, RN, MSN

Nursing Consultant to Oncology Service, Holston Valley Hospital and Medical Center, Kingsport, Tennessee.
Care Settings

Pamela S. Peters, RN, MPH

Formerly Education Director, Oncology Nursing Society, Pittsburgh, Pennsylvania.
Cancer Incidence and Trends

Barbara K. Redman, RN, PhD

Washington, D.C.
Teaching the Patient and Family or Significant Other

Susan Rokita, RN, MS

Oncology Clinical Nurse Specialist, Thomas Jefferson University Hospital, Philadelphia, Pennsylvania.
Preventive Measures

Regina M. Shannon-Bodnar, RN, MS, MSN

Clinical Nurse Specialist, University of Maryland Cancer Center, Baltimore, Maryland.
Legal Issues

Roberta Strohl, RN, MN

Clinical Specialist, Radiation Oncology, University of Maryland at Baltimore, Baltimore, Maryland.
Goals and Principles of Treatment
Investigational Cancer Treatment Modalities

Thomas J. Szopa, RN, MS, ET

Clinical Nurse Specialist, Elliot Hospital, Manchester, New Hampshire.
Surgery

Linda Tenenbaum, RN, MSN, OCN

Instructor, Nursing and Continuing Education, Broward Community College, Fort Lauderdale, Florida.
Nursing Administration of Chemotherapy

Amy Valentine, RN, MS

Associate Professor, University of Vermont School of Nursing, Burlington, Vermont.
Early Detection Measures

Connie M. Yuska, RN, MS

Clinical Nurse Manager, Northwestern Memorial Hospital, Chicago, Illinois.
Head and Neck Cancer

Preface

The purpose of this publication is to outline general nursing knowledge about the adult with cancer and to help the registered nurse synthesize, integrate, and apply these principles in the care of people with cancer.

The *Core Curriculum for Oncology Nursing* consists of contributions from oncology nurses with expertise and credentials in oncology education, clinical practice, and administration. The core curriculum content outline, developed by the Core Curriculum Task Force of the ONS Education Committee in 1984, serves as the basis for this publication, the ONS videotape series, and the development of items for inclusion in the Oncology Nursing Certification Examination. Content was carefully developed in order to ensure broad applicability and appropriate depth of information. The text is a reference for both the beginning and the experienced oncology nurse. It is an adjunct in clinical care and in preparation for the certification examination. The nurse providing direct care will find information relevant to essential issues of patient management. Content reflects the needs of practitioners in both general and specific practice settings. Educators may utilize this content as a framework for academic courses or continuing education.

The narrative outline format has been chosen to facilitate location and review of concise but complete information. Study questions are included to assist the reader in evaluating or improving understanding of content. Bibliographies are up to date and complete, and should be used as a supplement to expand on the details that were omitted from this publication because of their level of complexity or available space.

The dynamic nature of oncology care requires the nurse to enhance knowledge and interest with supplemental references. It is expected that this publication will be periodically revised to reflect the state of the art and incorporate the input of readers.

Editor

CONSTANCE R. ZIEGFELD, RN, MS, OCN
Assistant Director of Nursing
Johns Hopkins Oncology Center
Baltimore, Maryland

Section Editors

JOANNE T. COSSMAN, RN, MPH
Director of Provider Services
Community Health Care Plan, Inc.
New Haven, Connecticut

SUSAN McMILLAN, RN, PhD
Associate Professor
University of South Florida
Tampa, Florida

ROBERTA STROHL, RN, MN
Clinical Specialist, Radiation Oncology
University of Maryland
Baltimore, Maryland

Contents

SECTION SIX:
Treatment of Cancer
  Section Editor: ROBERTA STROHL, RN, MN

21
Goals and Principles of Treatment 195
ROBERTA STROHL, RN, MN

22
Surgery 199
THOMAS J. SZOPA, RN, MS, ET

23
Radiation Therapy 207
JENNIFER BUCHOLTZ, RN, MSN

24
Chemotherapy 225
CATHERINE M. BENDER, RN, MN

25
Investigational Cancer Treatment Modalities 237
DEBORAH K. MAYER, RN, MSN, CRNP, OCN and
ROBERTA STROHL, RN, MN

39
Legal Issues 405
MINERVA APPLEGATE, RN, EdD and REGINA M. SHANNON-BODNAR, RN, MS, MSN

40
Cancer Economics 415
MARCIA CLARK, RN, MS

SECTION ONE

Pathophysiology of Cancer

Section Editor
SUSAN MCMILLAN RN, PhD

1

Alterations in Cell Biology

NANCY LOVEJOY, DSN

ANATOMICAL ALTERATIONS

A. Abnormal cell size and shape.
B. Abnormal *mitosis*—process of cell division.
C. Cell membrane changes including:
   1. Increased numbers of *microvilli*—outward extending folds of membrane.
   2. Decreased numbers of membrane *microfilaments*—bundles of actin fibers and other cytoskeletal elements that anchor cell receptors and limit the fluidity of the cell membrane.
D. Cytoplasmic changes.
E. Cell organelle changes including:
   1. Fewer, smaller, and denser *mitochondria*—rod-like bodies that are the sites of cellular respiration or energy production.
   2. Hypertrophic or hypotrophic *Golgi apparatus*—organelles that are involved in the secretion of protein.
   3. Larger *vacuoles*—membranes containing cellular secretions (mucins) or debris picked up by cell.
   4. Abnormal *centrioles*—sets of microtubules involved in cell division.
F. Nuclear changes including:
   1. Thickened membranes.
   2. Enlarged *nuclei*—membrane-bound structures containing granules and nucleoli. Cancer cells have high nucleus:cytoplasm ratios.
   3. Variable shapes and sizes.
   4. *Aneuploidy*—abnormal numbers of chromosomes.
   5. Abnormal chromosome arrangements including:
      a. *Translocations*—an exchange of genes (nucleotide sequences) between chromosome pairs (Fig. 1–1).
      b. *Deletions*—loss of genes from chromosomes.
      c. *Additions*—the addition of extra genes to DNA strands.
   6. Granular, clumped, hypochromatic *chromatin*, a single strand of DNA, and DNA-binding proteins at metaphase.

3

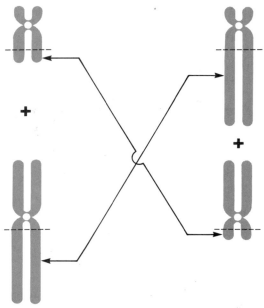

Figure 1–1. Reciprocal chromosome translocation. (Redrawn from Alberts, B., Bray, D., Lewis, J., et al.: Molecular Biology of the Cell. New York, Garland Publishing, Inc., 1983.)

BIOCHEMICAL ALTERATIONS

A. The extent of a cell's biochemical deviation from normal is a function of the degree of differentiation of the cancer cell.
  1. The less differentiated (less normal looking) the cancer cell, the more deviant the biochemical profile.
  2. Undifferentiated cancer cells tend to have biochemical profiles that resemble fetal or immature cells.
B. As cancer cells become more undifferentiated, they:
  1. Require lower concentrations of growth factors in order to reproduce. *Growth factors* are hormones that regulate growth of selected tissues. Examples of growth factors are:
    a. Nerve growth factor.
    b. Angiogenesis factor.
    c. Epidermal growth factor.
    d. Somatomedians.
  2. Utilize higher rates of anaerobic glycolysis, making them less dependent on oxygen.
  3. Lose complex cell surface glycolipids, which may interfere with:
    a. Cell-to-cell communication.
    b. Cell-to-substrate communication.
  4. Lose extracellular *fibronectin*, an adhesive, which may explain increased mobility of cancer cells.
  5. Lose *cAMP* (cyclic adenine monophosphate), a glycoprotein that controls intracellular reaction rates.
  6. Lose high molecular weight surface glycoproteins, causing loss of cell-to-cell:

    a. Cohesiveness.

    b. Adhesiveness.

    c. Density-dependent growth.

7. Produce increased numbers of cell surface enzymes (which aid in invasion and metastases).

8. Produce *autogenic* (self-stimulating) growth factors including:

    a. Tumor angiogenesis factor (TAF).

    b. Sarcoma growth factor.

    c. Platelet-derived growth factor.

9. Produce greater amounts of *prostaglandins* (PG)—fatty acid derivatives that act as local chemical signals.

    a. PG are thought to play a role in:

        (1) Escape of tumor cells from immune surveillance.

        (2) Establishment of tumor metastases.

    b. PG of special interest are:

        (1) PGE—which suppresses T cell proliferation, immunity, humoral immunity, and natural killer cells.

        (2) PGE_2—which acts synergistically with chemical carcinogens and inhibits natural killer cell activity.

        (3) PGD—which stimulates tumor angiogenesis factor.

ALTERATIONS IN CELLULAR DIFFERENTIATION

A. *Differentiation* is the process by which cells achieve specific structural and functional characteristics.

B. A *differentiated cell* is one that:

    1. Does not divide again under normal circumstances.

    2. Performs a selected function.

    3. Has a specific structure.

C. Differentiated cells may be unipotent or pluripotent.

    1. A *unipotent* cell has only one structure and function. Examples are:

        a. Neurons—cells that are capable of ideation.

        b. Pancreatic cells—cells that are capable of producing insulin or digestive enzymes.

    2. A *pluripotent* or *stem cell* is capable of becoming more than one type of cell. Stem cells are found in the:

        a. Bone marrow.

        b. Skin.

        c. Gastrointestinal tract.

D. *Dedifferentiation* refers to the process by which cells lose characteristics of normal cells.

E. Dedifferentiation may result from:

    1. Abnormal differentiation of committed, but immature stem cells in tissue.

    2. Conversion of *mature* (nondividing) cells to proliferating cells that become increasingly immature because of changes in the way genes are *transcribed* (copied). Changes in gene transcription may result from several events, including:

        a. *Somatic mutation*—alterations in certain nucleotide sequences in DNA due to random events.

        b. *Genetic recombinations*—the splitting and resplicing of specific gene se-

quences into different parts of the genome due to random events or chromosome fragility.
   c. *Gene amplification*—the appearance of extra copies of genes.
   d. Changes in local gradients of nutrients and ions.
F. Biologic properties of dedifferentiated cells include:
   1. Cell immortality in culture.
   2. Loss of contact inhibition.
   3. Alterations in antigen expression.
   4. Cloning efficiency.

ALTERATIONS IN CELLULAR KINETICS

A. *Cellular kinetics* refers to the growth and division of cells. Phases of cell cycle growth and division are shown in Figure 1–2.
B. Terms used to describe cellular kinetics include:
   1. *Cell cycle time* (Tc), which refers to the time between successive episodes of mitosis (the usual Tc of normal or neoplastic cells is 1 to 5 days).
   2. *Birth rate of cells*, which refers to the proportion of cells in mitosis divided by duration of mitosis.

$$\text{Birthrate of cells} = \frac{\text{Proportion of cells in mitosis}}{\text{Duration of mitosis}}$$

   a. *Proliferating cells* are cells that will subsequently divide. There are two types of proliferating cells: nonclonogenic and clonogenic cells.
      (1) *Clonogenic cells* have unlimited proliferation potential.
         (a) Highly anaplastic (undifferentiated) neoplasms have a high proportion of clonogenic cells.
         (b) Well-differentiated neoplasms have a low proportion of clonogenic cells.
      (2) *Nonclonogenic* cells will undergo mitosis 5 to 6 times before dying.
   b. *Growth fraction* is the ratio of the total number of cells to the number of proliferating cells.

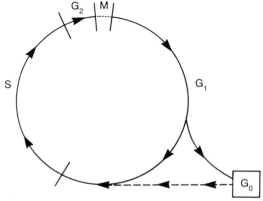

Figure 1–2. The cell cycle. G_1 is the period of interphase. G_0 is a side extension of interphase. S is the period of DNA synthesis. G_2 is the beginning of mitosis. M is the mitotic interval. (Redrawn from Pitot, H.: Fundamentals of Oncology. New York, Marcel Dekker, Inc., 1981.)

C. Terms used to describe the cellular kinetics of neoplastic cells are:
   1. *Tumor volume-doubling time*—the time within which the existing rate of neoplastic cell production yields a number of cells equal to the original neoplastic cell population. The average volume-doubling time of most solid tumors is about 2 months.
   2. *Potential volume-doubling time*—the time within which the neoplastic cell population would double if all cells were conserved and if newly produced cells retained the proliferative characteristics of original cells.
   3. *Actual tumor volume-doubling time*—the time within which the neoplastic cell population doubles.
D. Actual tumor volume-doubling time differs from potential volume-doubling time because of several factors, including:
   1. Variations in proliferative to resting cell (G_0) ratios.
      a. Most tumors have proliferative to resting cell ratios of $3:10$ to $6:10$.
      b. Slowly growing tumors have proliferative to resting cell ratios of $1:10$.
   2. Variations in vascularization.
      a. Vascularization brings necessary nutrients and removes wastes, facilitating growth.
      b. Cells near the periphery of tumors or neovasculature (tumor-induced vessels) grow faster than cells in other parts of the tumor.
   3. Extent of *tumor necrosis* (dead cells). The outward diffusion of cytotoxic products of necrotic cell breakdown increases all deaths.
   4. Variations in tumor antigen expression.
      a. Tumor antigens that resemble "self" (cell HLA or blood group antigens) allow tumors to escape the immune surveillance and grow.
      b. Soluble antigens may block the cellular immune system and facilitate growth.
   5. Treatment:
      a. Temporarily arrests cells in the G_2 phase of the cell cycle.
      b. May cause cell death after 1 to 2 cell divisions.
      c. May be followed by a high birth rate of neoplastic cells, possibly due to treatment-induced suppression of immune surveillance mechanisms.
   6. Variations in hormone levels.
      a. Many neoplasms that arise in target organs of hormones require these hormones for growth.
      b. Reduction in hormone levels reduces tumor growth.
E. Growth increases exponentially in new neoplasms.
F. Growth decreases in a Gompertzian fashion (Fig. 1–3) with increased tumor volume owing to:
   1. Decreases in the fraction of proliferating cells.
   2. Increases in the rate of cell death.
G. Smallest clinically detectable mass is 1 gm or 10^9 cells.
H. Tumor masses are usually 10 gm or 10^{10} cells at detection.
I. Tumor masses 1 cm in diameter have undergone about 30 doubling times.

STUDY QUESTIONS

1. Describe alterations in cell biology (i.e., membranes, cytoplasm, organelles, nuclei) that distinguish neoplastic cells from normal cells.

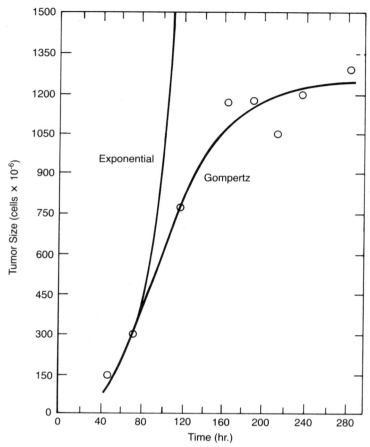

Figure 1–3. The potential (exponential) and actual (Gompertz) growth curves of neoplastic cells. (Redrawn from Pitot, H.: Fundamentals of Oncology. New York, Marcel Dekker, Inc., 1981.)

2. Identify biochemical alterations of neoplastic cells that may contribute to their unregulated growth.
3. Discuss factors that influence tumor cell kinetics.

Bibliography

Alberts, B., Bray, D., Lewis, J., et al.: Molecular Biology of the Cell. New York, Garland Publishing, Inc., 1983.

Goodwin, J.: Prostaglandins and host defense in cancer. Medical Clinics of North America, 65(4): 829–843, 1981.

Pitot, H.: Fundamentals of Oncology. New York, Marcel Dekker, 1981.

Ruddon, R. W.: Cancer Biology. New York, Oxford University Press, 1981.

Steel, G. G.: Cytokinetics of neoplasia. *In* Holland, J. F. and Frei, E. (eds.): Cancer Medicine. Philadelphia, Lea & Febiger, pp. 177–189, 1982.

Tannock, I. F.: Biology of tumor growth. Hospital Practice, 18:81–93, 1983.

Yunis, L.: Chromosomes and cancer. New nomenclature and future directions. Human Pathology, 12:494–502, 1981.

2

The Process of Carcinogenesis

NANCY LOVEJOY, DSN

INITIATING FACTORS OF CARCINOGENESIS

A. Ionizing radiation—imparts energy to absorbing material, removing electrons from atoms and molecules in its path.
  1. Types of ionizing radiation include:
      a. Electromagnetic radiation: x-rays and gamma rays.
      b. Particulate radiation: charged (alpha and beta particles and protons) and uncharged (neutrons) particles.
          (1) *Linear Energy Transfer* (LET) is a measure of the rate of energy loss by charged particles.
          (2) The higher the LET, the greater the likelihood of heritable (point) mutations.
  2. Sources of ionizing radiation exposure include:
      a. Diagnostic or therapeutic x-rays.
      b. Radioactive ground minerals.
      c. Cosmic radiation.
      d. Man-made radioactive materials, e.g., radioisotopes.
  3. Doses of ionizing radiation are specified in:
      a. Roentgen—amount of radiation exposure in air.
      b. Rad—amount of radiation absorbed per dose. 1 rad = 100 ergs/gram.
      c. Gray (international measure)—1 gray = 100 rads.
      d. Rem—unit of measure used to express the biologic effect of one rad of x-ray.
      e. Sievert (international measure)—1 sievert = 100 rems.
      f. Curve—amount of radioactivity in a radioactive substance. It is based on the amount of radioactivity in radium.
  4. Conditions that influence risk of carcinogenesis by ionizing radiation are poorly defined. Factors that appear to influence risk include:
      a. Characteristics of the host, such as:
          (1) Level of tissue oxygenation—well oxygenated cells are more radiosensitive.

(2) Genetic make-up—genetic disorders, particularly those associated with inefficient DNA repair mechanisms, increase risk.

(3) Age—children, fetuses, and the elderly are more sensitive than adults.

(4) Degrees of stress—a high degree of stress may inhibit cell repair mechanisms.

b. Cell cycle phase—cells in G_2, the postsynthetic phase, are more sensitive than cells in S or G_1.

c. Degree of differentiation—mature cells are least vulnerable.

d. Cellular proliferation rate—cells with high mitotic rates are more susceptible to radiation than those with lower rates.

e. Tissue type—hematopoietic and gastrointestinal tissue are very sensitive to radiation.

f. Total dose and rate of dose—the higher the cumulative dose and dose rate, the greater the likelihood of mutation.

5. Hazards of low level ionizing radiation.

a. Somatic effects.

(1) Breast neoplasia.

(2) Thyroid neoplasia.

(3) Bone sarcoma.

(4) Leukemia.

b. Genetic effects.

(1) Teratogenesis.

(2) Mutagenesis.

B. *Ultraviolet radiation* (UVL)—that portion of the electromagnetic spectrum with wavelengths between 10 nanometers (nm) and 400 nm (i.e., visible light and x-ray regions). Wavelengths between 230 to 320 nm are thought to be carcinogenic.

1. Sources of UVL include:

a. Sun.

b. Industrial sources, such as welding arcs and germicidal lights.

2. Effects of UVL on DNA include chain breaks.

3. Conditions that elevate risk of UVL-induced carcinogenesis include:

a. Inefficient DNA repair mechanisms found in people with:

(1) Xeroderma pigmentosum (XP).

(2) Red hair and freckles.

b. Immunosuppression.

c. Albinism.

d. Heat. Heat acts synergistically with UVL:

(1) Causing DNA denaturation.

(2) Inactivating DNA repair enzymes.

e. Benign papillomas.

4. UVL elevates risk of:

a. Melanoma.

b. Basal cell epithelioma.

C. *Chemical carcinogens*—elements and compounds that mutate DNA.

1. Chemical carcinogens include:

a. Aromatic hydrocarbons—soot, pitch, coal tar, benzene.

b. Aromatic amines—phenacetin, benzidine.

c. Alkylating agents—melphalan, busulfan, cyclophosphamide, ether.

d. Organic compounds—vinyl chloride, isopropyl oil.

      e. Tobacco products—cigarette smoke, chewing tobacco.

      f. Inorganic compounds—chromates, nickel carbonyl, asbestos.

      g. Plant products—senecio alkaloids found in herbal medicines and teas.

      h. Hormones—estrogens, diethylstilbesterol.

  2. Mode of action.

      a. Direct-acting chemical carcinogens form reactive ions that mutate DNA.

         (1) Direct-acting chemical carcinogens do not require metabolic activation by the host.

         (2) Examples of direct-acting chemical carcinogens are nitrogen mustard and busulfan.

      b. *Procarcinogens* mutate DNA only after metabolic activation.

         (1) Most chemical carcinogens are procarcinogens.

         (2) Procarcinogens must be activated by carcinogen-activating enzymes attached to the endoplasmic reticulum of cells.

         (3) Metabolic activation is influenced by several factors, including sex and diet. Carcinogenic activity of procarcinogens is, therefore, only expressed under certain limited conditions.

         (4) Examples of procarcinogens are soots, coal tar products, cigarette smoke.

      c. Solid state carcinogens.

         (1) Mechanism of carcinogenic action is not known.

         (2) Usually affect only mesenchymal cells, that is, bone, fat, muscle, blood cells.

         (3) Examples of solid state carcinogens are metal foils and asbestos.

      d. Inorganic carcinogens.

         (1) Selectively alter fidelity of DNA replication.

         (2) Examples of inorganic carcinogens are nickel carbonyl and arsenic salts.

  3. Risks—exposure to chemical carcinogens elevates the risk of all the major human cancers.

D. Viruses associated with cancer include:

  1. *Slow-acting cancer viruses*—transform in vitro cell cultures in 6 to 12 months. Examples of slow-acting DNA viruses are Adenoviruses, Papovaviruses, Herpes viruses.

  2. *Fast-acting cancer viruses*—transform in vitro cell cultures within days or weeks of exposure. Examples of fast-acting viruses are:

      a. Human T cell Lymphoma-leukemia Virus (HTLV).

      b. Japanese Adult T cell Leukemia Virus.

  3. Cancer viruses infect DNA, resulting in cell mutation.

  4. Cancer viruses exhibit *tissue specificity*, that is, they infect tissue selectively. Examples are:

      a. Epstein-Barr virus which infects lymph tissue, resulting in Burkitt's lymphoma.

      b. Hepatitis B virus which infects hepatocellular cells, resulting in hepatocellular cancer.

  5. Factors modifying the effects of viral carcinogenesis are:

      a. Age—the very young and old are more susceptible.

      b. Immunocompetence—many viruses are oncogenic only if the host becomes infected prenatally or perinatally.

E. *Oncogenes*—genes that regulate proliferative processes. The normal gene pool has about 100 carefully conserved oncogenes, i.e., oncogenes that have been inherited, unchanged for thousands of years.

1. Human oncogenes are located on chromosomes 1, 6, 8, 9, 11, 12, 15, 20, 22, and X.
2. Normally, oncogenes are only expressed at significant levels during embryogenesis.
3. Following embryogenesis, oncogenes are expressed in one of three patterns:
   a. Continuous low level expression (about 1 to 10 copies per cell).
   b. Discontinuous expression.
   c. No expression (silent genes).
4. Oncogene expression may be altered by:
   a. *Insertional mutation*—the inclusion of a virus upstream from the oncogene.
   b. Chromosome rearrangements due to inherited fragility or radiation exposures place the oncogene under the influence of a *gene enhancer*, a gene that amplifies transcription.
   c. Chemical carcinogens that alter oncogene structures.
   d. Radiation that mutates oncogenes.
5. Alterations in oncogene expression, resulting in abnormal amounts of oncogene proteins, may:
   a. Enhance the expression of other genes and oncogenes.
   b. Disrupt normal cell growth, progressively transforming cells.
6. Oncogene protein levels may soon be used to diagnose and make treatment decisions about cancer.

TRANSFORMATION

A. *Transformation* is a multistep process by which cells exposed to initiating factors become progressively dedifferentiated, assuming biologic properties associated with neoplasia.
B. Molecular mechanisms involved in transformation are poorly understood.
C. Oncogenic theories suggest that:
   1. Transformation is initiated by agents that either augment cellular oncogene activity (quantitative theory) or change oncogene function (qualitative theory).
   2. Oncogene products involved in transformation include:
      a. Phosphorylating kinases (enzymes) that regulate cell shape and proliferation rates.
      b. Growth factor activators that mimic normal growth factors, such as epidermal growth factor.
      c. *GTP* (guanosine triphosphate-binding proteins)
         (1) These proteins may activate quiescent genes by uncoupling GTP.
         (2) Uncoupled GTP may allow cells to continuously transmit signals from hormones, such as adrenalin, to the interior cell.
      d. Nuclear proteins that act conjointly to immortalize DNA replication (i.e., make it a continuous process).
   3. In actuality, there is probably more than one way to transform a cell. Disruption at any point of the regulatory network that spans from the cell surface to the nucleus probably can initiate transformation.

PROMOTING FACTORS

A. *Promoting factors* are substances that enhance cell transformation by altering the expression of genetic information.
B. Promoting factors have the following biologic properties:
1. Cannot mutate DNA by themselves.
2. Exert an effect only after an initiating factor has irreversibly altered DNA.
3. Require prolonged exposure prior to influencing the cell.
4. May be reversed at early stages of transformation.
5. Do not bind covalently to DNA and other cell macromolecules.

REVERSING FACTORS

A. *Reversing factors* are agents that inhibit the effects of promoting factors.
1. Stimulate metabolic pathways in the cell that destroy carcinogens.
2. Alter the initiating potency of chemical carcinogens.
B. Factors that reverse transformation include:
1. Drugs that:
a. Inhibit RNA synthesis, such as Actinomycin D.
b. Enhance carcinogen-deactivating enzyme systems, such as ethoxyquin.
2. Enzymes that protect cells from peroxides, such as superoxide dismutase and glutathione transferases.
3. Dietary factors including:
a. Vitamin E (tocopherol) which traps oxygen radicals.
b. Beta-carotene which protects body fat and lipid membranes from peroxidation.
c. Vitamin C (ascorbic acid) which may prevent the formation of endogenous nitrosamines (that is, nitrosamines made from secondary and tertiary amines).
d. Vitamin A (retinoids) which is essential for normal differentiation.
e. Indoles (found in brussel sprouts, cabbage, turnips, and broccoli) which detoxify carcinogens.
f. Antioxidant food additives, such as Butylated hydroxytoluene (BHT), which may enhance activity of enzymes involved in the metabolism and detoxification of chemical carcinogens.

CARCINOGENESIS

A. *Carcinogenesis*—the process by which normal cells become transformed into neoplastic cells.
B. Carcinogenesis is thought to involve two or more steps.
1. One theory is that:
a. A *first event*, i.e., exposure to an initiating factor, immortalizes the cells, making them capable of indefinite survival.
b. A *second event*, i.e., exposure to additional transforming factors or to promoting factors, activates cell oncogenes, facilitating transformation.
2. Another suggestion is that:
a. Initiation occurs after a single brief exposure to an initiating agent. Initiation is:
(1) Irreversible.

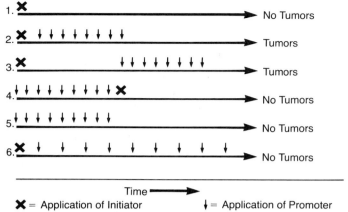

Figure 2–1. Exposure to transforming and promoting agents resulting in carcinogenesis. (Redrawn from Pitot, H.: Fundamentals of Oncology. New York, Marcel Dekker, Inc., 1981.)

    (2) Requires only brief exposure.

    (3) Must be inherited by daughter cells.

  b. Promotion requires at least two processes:

    (1) Cell proliferation that propagates the initiated damage.

    (2) Prolonged exposure to promoting agents (or transforming factors).

  c. Reversing factors can arrest promotion, but cannot reverse the effects of the initiating event.

  d. Exposures to initiating and promoting factors that may cause chemical carcinogenesis are shown in Figure 2–1.

 3. A third opinion concurs with the second, but suggests that inherited genetic disorders constitute a "first event."

  a. Examples of genetic disorders associated with increased cancer risk are shown in Table 2–1.

  b. Cancers progressing from autosomal dominant genetic defects tend to be characterized by:

    (1) Bilateral expression.

    (2) Multiple primary neoplasms.

PROCESS OF INVASION AND METASTASES

A. *Invasion* is the capacity of a neoplasm to encroach upon tissue and destroy its normal anatomic boundaries. Invasion results from:

Table 2–1. HEREDITARY DISORDERS THAT PROMOTE
THE INCIDENCE OF NEOPLASIA*

Autosomal Dominant Disorders	Autosomal Recessive Disorders
Familial Polyposis Coli	Xeroderma Pigmentosum
Gardner's Syndrome	Bloom's Syndrome
Pheochromocytoma	Fanconi's Aplastic Anemia
Neurofibromatosis	Ataxia-Telangiectasia
Retinoblastoma	Wiskott-Aldrich Syndrome

   * Adapted from Pitot, H. C.: Fundamentals of Oncology, p. 65. Copyright 1981 by Marcel Dekker, Inc., New York.

1. Pressure exerted by increasing tumor size.
2. Enzymatic destruction of tissue.
B. *Metastases* are tumor implants that are discontinuous with the *primary* (parent) tumor.
   1. Metastases are the major cause of death from neoplasms.
   2. Factors that may increase the likelihood of metastases include:
      a. Primary tumor of long duration.
      b. High mitotic rate.
      c. Trauma, including biopsy and tumor massage.
      d. Dead tumor cells.
      e. Dead normal cells.
      f. Heat.
      g. Radiation.
      h. Chemotherapeutic agents.
   3. Factors that may decrease the probability of metastases are those which reduce adherence to endothelial cells, retard intravascular coagulation, or kill tumor cells. Examples include:
      a. Aspirin.
      b. Heparin.
      c. Warfarin or Dicumarol.
      d. Fibrinolytic agents (plasmin).
      e. Radiation.
      f. Chemotherapeutic agents.
      g. Ascites.
      h. Large primary tumors (which seem to exert negative feedback on metastases).
C. Metastases occur by means of active and passive mechanisms including:
   1. *Seeding* which refers to tumor spread throughout a natural body cavity, such as the peritoneal cavity.
   2. *Transplantation* which refers to mechanical transport of tumor fragments by instruments or gloved hands.
   3. *Lymphatic spread* which refers to the systematic permeation of lymphatic channels draining the affected site. Skip areas occur only if nodes are obstructed by:
      a. Prior radiation.
      b. Chronic inflammatory changes.
      c. Quantities of neoplastic cells.
   4. *Hematogenous spread* which refers to the dissemination of tumor cells through arteries or veins. Steps in this multistaged event include:
      a. The development of a clone of neoplastic cells with *high metastatic potential*, that is, cells with low antigenicity, high mitotic rates and cloning efficiency.
      b. Vascularization of the primary tumor is induced by *tumor angiogenesis factor* (TAF), which is released from neoplastic cells.
      c. Migration of metastatic cells to the tumor periphery.
      d. Penetration of extracellular matrix of the tumor by lysosomal enzymes, collagenases, and other factors.
      e. Penetration of vessels by tumor cells:
         (1) Migration through epithelial junctions (gaps) in thin-walled capillaries, venules, lymph vessels, or neovasculature (tumor-induced vasculature).

(2) Intravasation of arteries. *Intravasation* is an active process involving:
  (a) *Adhesion*—the binding of neoplastic cell receptors to the basement membrane of endothelial cells.
  (b) *Retraction*—the drawing back of endothelial cells in response to substances emitted by the neoplastic cell, leaving the basement membrane exposed (see Fig. 2–2).
  (c) *Matrix degradation*—digestion of the basement membrane by neoplastic enzymes.
f. Release of neoplastic cells into lymph fluid or blood.
  (1) Single neoplastic cells entering arterial bloodstream usually die within 24 hours because of:
    (a) Immune surveillance mechanisms.
    (b) Microenvironmental factors that cause neoplastic cells to differentiate.
    (c) Oxygen concentrations.
    (d) Bloodstream turbulence and shear forces.
  (2) Clumps of neoplastic cells (6 to 7 cells) that become encapsulated with polymerized fibrin or platelet aggregates are more likely to survive. However, certain hematologic neoplastic cells, such as lymphoma cells, do not form fibrin capsules.
g. Arrest of neoplastic cells. Neoplastic cells may stop in predilected lymph, venule or capillary beds because of:
  (1) *Mechanical entrapment*—impaction of the tumor clumps or cells in vessels too small to permit circulation.
  (2) *Tissue chemotactic factors*—factors that cause cells to migrate to specific tissues.
  (3) Preference for epithelium surfaces of specific organs.
h. Egress of neoplastic cells from vessels by:
  (1) Migration through endothelial junctions.
  (2) *Extravasation*, which refers to the process by which neoplastic cells exit arteries (Fig. 2–2), involves:
    (a) Epithelial or neoplastic proteases that dissolve fibrin clots which surround tumor clumps.
    (b) Adhesion to endothelium of an artery.
    (c) Penetration through the basement membrane.
    (d) Retraction of epithelium cells.
    (e) Matrix degradation by tumor enzymes.
i. Metastatic vascularization.
  (1) Metastatic cells emit TAF (tumor angiogenesis factor).
  (2) Neovasculature is formed as soon as 72 hours after tissue penetration.
  (3) Until neovascularization, growth is limited to 10^6 cells.
j. Metastatic invasion.
  (1) Metastases invade normal tissue by emitting *autocrine* or self-stimulating migration factors that degrade certain cell structures.
  (2) Cell degradation products act as chemotactic factors, causing tumors to grow in directed patterns.
D. The most common sites of metastases are:
  1. Lung.
  2. Liver.

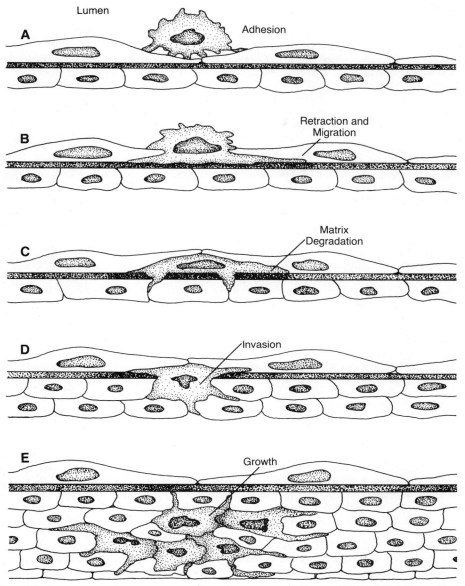

Figure 2–2. *Extravasation of arteries. (Redrawn from Nicolson, G.: Cell surfaces and cancer metastasis. Hospital Practice 17:84, 1982.)*

    3. Central nervous system.
    4. Bone.

STUDY QUESTIONS

1. Describe mechanisms by which radiation, chemical carcinogens, viruses, and oncogenes initiate carcinogenesis.
2. Discuss reasons why cells exposed to initiating factors may not become transformed into neoplastic cells.
3. Describe the process of metastatic spread.

Bibliography

Ames, B.: Dietary carcinogens and anticarcinogens. Science, 221:1256–1264, 1983.

Bishop, L.: Oncogenes. Scientific American, 246:80–92, 1982.

Bolande, R. P. and Vekemans, M. J. J.: Genetic models of carcinogenesis. Human Pathology, 14: 658–662, 1983.

Cline, M. J., Slamon, D. J. and Lipsick, J. S.: Oncogenes: Implications for the diagnosis and treatment of cancer. Annals of Internal Medicine, 101:223–233, 1984.

Committee on Diet, Nutrition, and Cancer of the National Academy of Sciences: Report: Diet, nutrition, and cancer. Journal National Cancer Institute, 70:1153–1170, 1983.

Cooper, G. M.: The 1984 Walter Hubert Lecture. Activation of transforming genes in neoplasms. British Journal of Cancer, 5:137–142, 1984.

Duffy, B. L.: Ultraviolet Radiation in Medicine. Bristol, Adam Hilger Ltd., 1982.

Folkman, J.: Tumor invasion of metastasis. In Holland, J. F. and Frei, E. (eds.): Cancer Medicine. Philadelphia, Lea & Febiger, 1982.

Glickman, B. W.: DNA repair and its relationship to the origins of human cancer. In Cleton, F. J. and Simons, J. W. I. M. (eds.): Genetic Origins of Tumor Cells. Boston, M. Nijhoff Publishers, pp. 25–52, 1980.

Hunter, T.: The proteins of oncogenes. Scientific American, 251(2):70–79, 1984.

Knudson, A. G.: Mutation and cancer: Statistical study of retinoblastoma. Proceedings National Academy of Sciences, 68:820–823, 1971.

Lyon, J.: Radiation exposure and cancer. Hospital Practice 19:159–163, 166, 168–173, 1984.

Nicolson, G. L.: Cell surfaces and cancer metastasis. Hospital Practice, 17:75–86, 1982.

Pitot, H.: Fundamentals of Oncology. New York, Marcel Dekker, Inc., 1981.

Pizzarello, O. J. and Witcofski, R. L.: Basic Radiation Biology. Philadelphia, Lea & Febiger, 1975.

Poste, G. and Fidler, I. J.: The pathogenesis of cancer metastasis. Nature, 283:139–145, 1980.

Robbins, S. L., Cotran, R. and Kumar, V.: Pathologic Basis of Disease. Philadelphia, W. B. Saunders Company, 1984.

Schwartz, R. A. and Klein, E.: Ultraviolet light-induced carcinogenesis. In Holland, J. F. and Frei, E. (eds.): Cancer Medicine. Philadelphia, Lea & Febiger, pp. 109–118, 1982.

Upton, A. C.: Radiation. In Holland, J. F. and Frei, E. (eds.): Cancer Medicine. Philadelphia, Lea & Febiger, pp. 96–108, 1982.

Upton, A. C.: The biologic effects of low level ionizing radiation. Scientific American, 246:41–49, 1982.

Varmus, H. E.: Viruses, genes, and cancer. Cancer, 55:2324–2328, 1985.

Vesell, E. S.: Complex dynamically interacting host factors that affect the disposition of drugs and carcinogens. In Bartsch, H. and Armstrong, B. (eds.): Host Factors in Human Carcinogenesis. IARC Scientific Publications No. 39. Lyon: International Agency for Research on Cancer, pp. 427–434, 1982.

Wattenberg, L. W.: Inhibitors of chemical carcinogens. In Demopoulos, H. B. and Mehlman, M. A. (eds.): Cancer and the Environment. Park Forest South, Illinois, Pathotox Publishers, Inc., pp. 35–52, 1980.

Weinberg, R. A.: A molecular basis of cancer. Scientific American, 249:126–142, 1983.

Weisburger, J. H. and Williams, G. M.: Chemical carcinogenesis. In Demopoulos, H. B. and Mehlman, M. A. (eds.): Cancer and the Environment. Park Forest South, Illinois, Pathotox Publishers, Inc., pp. 89–101, 1980.

Wood, S., Holoyoke, D. and Yardley, J. H.: Mechanisms of metastasis production by blood-borne cancer cells. In Begg, R. W., Ham, A., Leblond, C. P., et al. (eds.): Canadian Cancer Conference. New York, Academic Press, pp. 167–223, 1961.

Wood, S., Jr. and Strauli, P.: Tumor invasion and metastasis. In Holland, J. F. and Frei, E. (eds.): Cancer Medicine. Philadelphia, Lea & Febiger, pp. 140–151, 1973.

3

The Role of the Immune System

NANCY LOVEJOY, DSN

IMMUNOLOGIC SURVEILLANCE

A. Immunologic surveillance theory assumes that:
   1. The immune system can recognize tumor antigens.
   2. Tumor cells must reach certain threshold concentrations before the immune system recognizes and reacts to tumor antigens.
   3. Immune surveillance becomes less efficient with aging. Therefore, the probability that the immune system will fail to recognize neoplastic cells increases with age.
   4. Immune surveillance is inefficient in the very young.

TUMOR ANTIGENICITY

A. During carcinogenesis, *tissue-specific antigens* (sometimes called differentiation antigens), blood group antigens, and histocompatibility antigens undergo:
   1. Functional changes.
   2. Density shifts, that is, antigens migrate towards each other, forming patches of antigens.
B. Tumors express novel antigens including:
   1. *Fetal antigens* refer to antigens that are normally expressed in significant quantities only during intrauterine or early postnatal life. Examples of fetal antigens are:
      a. Serum alpha-fetoprotein (AFP) which is elevated with hepatocellular and testicular neoplasms.
      b. Carcinoembryonic antigen (CEA) which is elevated with colorectal, breast, lung, and gynecologic cancers.
      c. Elevated fetal antigen levels:
         (1) At diagnosis they are predictive of:
            (a) Decreased survival time.

19

   (b) Poor response rates.
   (c) Increased risk for recurrent disease.
   (2) Following treatment they are predictive of recurrent or progressive disease in apparently disease-free patients.
   (3) Drop in the terminal phase of illness.
2. *Placental antigens* refer to antigens that are normally produced by the placenta.
   a. Examples are human chorionic gonadotropin (HCG) and human placental lactogen (HCL).
   b. Placental antigens are usually associated with gynecologic cancers.
3. *Tumor-specific transplantation antigens* (TSTA) refer to antigens that develop as a result of exposure to transforming factors (chemical carcinogens, oncogenic viruses, or radiation).
   a. Virally induced TSTA are *virus-specific*, that is, neoplasms induced by specific viruses express the same antigens.
   b. Physically induced TSTA (chemical carcinogens, radiation) may or may not express the same antigens.
      (1) Chemically induced TSTA are often "private" to the specific tumor.
      (2) The strength of chemically induced tumor antigens is dependent on the dose and strength of the chemical carcinogen.
4. *T-antigens* are tumor antigens caused by DNA oncogenic viruses.

MECHANISMS OF ESCAPE FROM IMMUNOLOGIC SURVEILLANCE

A. Neoplastic invasion of bone and lymph tissue, resulting in decreased supplies of lymphocytes.
B. The expression of novel surface antigens resembling *self antigens*, that is, antigens that normally appear on the cell surface.
C. Shedding of soluble tumor antigens which bind antibody. These antigen-antibody complexes suppress lymphocyte, macrophage, and natural killer cell activity.
D. Reduction in the number of surface antigens, resulting in weakened antigenicity.
E. Production of tumor suppression factors, such as prostaglandins and fibrin degradation products, which inhibit stimulation of lymphocytes.
F. Formation of a fibrin coat around tumor clusters protects encapsulated cells from immune surveillance.
G. Previous exposure to carcinogenic agents during the fetal or neonatal period causes the immune surveillance system to recognize tumor antigens as self antigens.
H. Tolerance caused by continued recurrence of tumor cells, resulting in exhaustion of the reactive immunologic clone.
I. *Inefficient tumor burden,* that is, the tumor is too small to excite immunologic recognition.

STUDY QUESTIONS

1. Explain mechanisms by which neoplastic cells escape immune surveillance.
2. Describe changes in cell antigens that may be markers of neoplastic cells.

Bibliography

Benjamini, E., Rennick, D. M. and Sell, S.: Tumor immunology. *In* Stites, D. P. (ed.): Basic and Clinical Immunology. Los Altos, CA, Lange Medical Publications, pp. 223–240, 1984.

Pitot, H.: Fundamentals of Oncology. New York, Marcel Dekker, Inc., 1981.

Ruddon, R. W.: Cancer Biology. New York, Oxford University Press, 1981.

4

Tumor Classifications

NANCY LOVEJOY, DSN

PRECANCEROUS CONDITIONS

A. *Hypertrophy* refers to an abnormal increase in cell size. Hypertrophy occurs in cells that are stimulated but cannot divide, such as cardiac tissue.

B. *Hyperplasia* refers to an abnormal increase in the number of cells that are normally found in a tissue type.

C. *Metaplasia* refers to a reversible process involving the replacement of one adult cell type by another adult cell type not normally found in an organ site.
   1. Metaplasia is initiated by chronic irritation, inflammation, vitamin deficiency, or other pathologic process.
   2. An example of metaplasia is replacement of columnar epithelial cells in respiratory passages of smokers by squamous cell epethelium.
   3. Metaplasia is usually reversed once the initiating stimulus is removed.

D. *Dysplasia* refers to a process involving the replacement of one mature cell type with a less mature cell type. Dysplasia may be reversed, persist, or progress (be transformed) to neoplasia (cancer).

E. *Anaplasia* refers to cellular disorganization commonly found in dysplasia, but not as extensively as in neoplasia.
   1. *Positional anaplasia* refers to the fact that the nuclei of adjacent cells are altered in relation to one another (Fig. 4–1).
   2. *Cytologic anaplasia* refers to marked variation in cell features, including nuclear size, staining characteristics, nucleolar size, and nucleus:cytoplasm ratios (Fig. 4–1).

CANCEROUS CONDITIONS

A. *Neoplasia* refers to a relatively autonomous growth of tissue.

B. *Cancer* is the common term for all malignant neoplasias.

C. *Tumor* refers to an abnormal growth of cells, either malignant or nonmalignant.

23

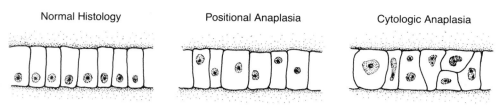

Normal Histology   Positional Anaplasia   Cytologic Anaplasia

Figure 4–1. *Normal histology, positional anaplasia, and cytologic anaplasia. (Redrawn from Pitot, H.: Fundamentals of Oncology. New York, Marcel Dekker, Inc., 1981.)*

NEOPLASTIC CLASSIFICATION SYSTEMS

A. Characteristics that distinguish malignant neoplasms from benign neoplasms are described by the Biologic Classification System (Table 4–1).
B. Neoplastic tissue is described by the Histogenetic Classification System. In this system, tumors are named from Latin and Greek terms (Table 4–2).
  1. Benign tumors often end in the suffix "oma," the Greek root for tumor.
    a. *Papillomas* or *polyps* are benign epithelial neoplasms that produce finger-like or warty projections from epithelial surfaces.
    b. *Cystomas* and *cystadenomas* are large cystic masses in the ovary.
  2. Malignant tumors usually have the suffix "sarcoma" or "carcinoma."
    a. *Sarcomas* are tumors that originate in connective tissue, that is, bone, cartilege, muscle, fibrous tissue. Prefixes describing specific connective tissue sarcomas include:
      (1) *"Osteo"* which describes sarcomas arising in the bone.
      (2) *"Chondro"* which describes sarcomas arising from the cartilage.
      (3) *"Lipo"* which describes sarcomas of fat.
      (4) *"Rhabdo"* which describes sarcomas of skeletal muscle.
      (5) *"Leiomyo"* which describes sarcomas of smooth muscle.

Table 4–1. CHARACTERISTICS OF BENIGN AND MALIGNANT NEOPLASMS*

Benign	Malignant
Encapsulated with Fibrous Tissue	Nonencapsulated
Noninvasive	Invasive
Highly Differentiated	Poorly Differentiated
Rare Mitoses	Relatively Common Mitoses
Slow Growth	Rapid Growth
Little or No *Positional Anaplasia*	Positional Anaplasia to Varying Degrees
Little or No *Cytologic Anaplasia*	Cytologic Anaplasia to Varying Degrees
No Metastases	Metastases
Contact Inhibition	Decreased Contact Inhibition
No Agglutination by Plant Lectins	Increased Susceptibility to Agglutination by Plant Lectins

* Adapted from Pitot, H. C.: Fundamentals of Oncology, 1981, p. 23. Copyright by Marcel Dekker, Inc., New York.

Table 4–2. BODY TISSUES AND THE TUMORS THAT ARISE
FROM THEM

Tissue	Benign Tumors	Malignant Tumors
Connective Tissue	*———oma*	*sarcomas*
Adult Fibrous Tissue	Fibroma	Fibrosarcoma
Embryonic (Myxomatous) Fibrous Tissue	Myxoma	Myxosarcoma
Fat	Lipoma	Liposarcoma
Cartilage	Chondroma	Chondrosarcoma
Bone	Osteoma	Osteogenic Sarcoma
Notochord		Chordoma
Connective Tissue, Probably Fibrous	Fibrous Histiocytoma	Malignant Fibrous Histiocytoma
Endothelium and Mesothelium		
Blood vessels	Hemangioma, Hemangiopericytoma	Hemangiosarcoma, Angiosarcoma
Lymph vessels	Lymphangioma	Lymphangiosarcoma
Mesothelium	—	Mesothelioma
Blood and Lymphoid Cells		
Hematopoietic Cells	"Preleukemias," "myeloproliferative disorders"	Leukemia of Various Types, Aleukemic Leukemia
Lymphoid Tissue	Lymphoid Hyperplasia	Malignant Lymphoma, Lymphosarcoma
	Plasmacytosis	Plasmacytoma, Multiple Myeloma
	—	Hodgkin's Disease
Muscle	*———oma*	*sarcomas*
Smooth Muscle	Leiomyoma	Leiomyosarcoma
Striated Muscle	Rhabdomyoma	Rhabdomyosarcoma
Epithelial Tissues	*———oma*	*Carcinomas*
Stratified Squamous	Papilloma	Squamous Cell Carcinoma, Epidermoid Carcinoma
	Seborrheic Keratosis and Some Skin Adnexal Tumors	Basal Cell Carcinoma and Some Malignant Skin Adnexal Tumors
Glandular Epithelium	Adenoma (May be Either Papillary or Cystic, Giving Rise to Terms Such as Papillary Adenoma or Cystadenoma and Papillary Adenocarcinoma or Cystadenocarcinoma.)	Adenocarcinoma
Liver	Hepatic Adenoma	Hepatoma, Hepatocellular Carcinoma
Kidney	Renal Tubular Adenoma	Renal Cell Carcinoma, Hypernephroma
Bile Duct	Bile Duct Adenoma	Cholangiocarcinoma
Transitional Epithelium	Transitional Cell Papilloma	Transitional Cell Carcinoma
Placenta	Hydatidiform Mole	Choriocarcinoma
Testis	—	Seminoma, Embryonal Cell Carcinoma

Table 4–2. BODY TISSUES AND THE TUMORS THAT ARISE
FROM THEM (*continued*)

Tissue *Connective Tissue*	Benign Tumors *–––oma*	Malignant Tumors *sarcomas*
Neural Tissue		
Glial Cells of Several Types	—	Glioma, Grades I-III, Anaplastic; Glioblastoma Multiforme (grade IV)
Nerve Cells	—	Neuroblastoma
	—	Medulloblastoma
	Ganglioneuroma	—
Meninges	Meningioma	Malignant Meningioma
Nerve sheath	Schwannoma, Neurilemmoma	Malignant Schwannoma
	Neurofibroma	Neurofibrosarcoma

APUD System (APUD = Amine Precursor Uptake and Decarboxylation)

The APUD system is a recently defined series of cells which have endocrine functions in that
they secrete one of a variety of small amine or polypeptide hormones. The storage forms of
these hormones in the cytoplasm are small dense-core membrane-bound granules visible by
electron microscopy. Some of these cells appear to be derived from neural crest cells which
migrate into a variety of organs.

Pituitary	Basophilic Adenoma	—
	Eosinophilic Adenoma	—
	Chromophobe Adenoma	—
Parathyroid	Parathyroid Adenoma	Parathyroid Carcinoma
Thyroid (C Cells)	C Cell Hyperplasia	Medullary Carcinoma of Thyroid
Bronchial Lining (Kulchitsky Cells)	—	Bronchial Carcinoid, Oat Cell Carcinoma
Adrenal Medulla	Pheochromocytoma	Malignant Pheochromocytoma
Pancreas	Islet Cell Adenoma, Insulinoma, Gastrinoma	Islet Cell Carcinoma
Stomach and Intestines	Carcinoid	Malignant Carcinoid
Carotid Body and Chemoreceptor System	Chemodectoma, Paraganglioma	Malignant Paraganglioma

Other Neural Crest–Derived Cells

Pigment-Producing Cells in Skin, Eyes, and Occasional Other Sites	Nevus	Melanoma
Schwann Cells of Peripheral Nervous System	(See Above)	(See Above)
Merkel Cells in Squamous Epithelium (Unknown Function)	—	Merkel Cell Neoplasm (Similar to Oat Cell Carcinoma)

Tumors Composed of More Than One Tissue Type

Breast	Fibroadenoma	Cystosarcoma Phyllodes
Renal Anlage	—	Wilm's Tumor

Gonadal Tumors

Terminology for tumors of the ovary and testis is somewhat more confusing. One general class of
tumors arises from multipotential cells that give rise to tumors containing a variety of tissue
types, often within the same tumor. These "germ cell" tumors include seminoma (called

Table 4–2. BODY TISSUES AND THE TUMORS THAT ARISE
FROM THEM (*continued*)

dysgerminoma in women), choriocarcinoma, embryonal carcinoma, endodermal sinus tumor, and teratocarcinoma. All of these are malignant. Some tumors in this category are benign, and are referred to as teratomas. However, the term teratoma is also applied to malignant tumors at times. Although all of these tumors are most common in the ovaries or testes, they also occur in extragonadal sites.

Another group of gonadal tumors arises from the connective tissue stroma. In the male these include Sertoli-Leydig cell tumors (homologous tumors in the female may be arrhenoblastoma, although most pathologists now use Sertoli-Leydig cell tumor), and in the female, granulosa-theca cell tumors, hilar cell tumors, and lipid cell tumors. Although all of these tumors technically arise from the connective tissues, they are given separate names because of the specialized nature and function of the gonadal stroma cells.

A number of epithelial tumors occur in the ovary. For most it will be easy to separate benign from malignant, because they are named in exactly the same way as other epithelial lesions. However, in some lesions, the pathologist may call a tumor "borderline" or "of low malignant potential." These terms are applied to a group of potentially malignant lesions that metastasize much less frequently than the carcinomas.

    b. *Carcinomas* are tumors that originate in the epithelium. Certain prefixes describe the type of epithelium from which sarcomas arise.
      (1) *"Adeno"* describes tumors arising from glandular epithelium (columnar).
        (a) Because all adenomas have similar histologic patterns, the organ of origin is also named.
        (b) For example, a malignant epithelial neoplasm located in the pancreas is called pancreatic adenocarcinoma.
      (2) *"Squamous"* describes tumors arising from squamous epithelium.
    c. *"Blastoma"* is a suffix used when tissue resembles embryonic structures. Examples are neuroblastoma and myoblastoma.
    d. *Mixed* tumors are those tumors containing more than one neoplastic cell type. An example of a mixed tumor is pleomorphic adenoma.
    e. *Teratomas* are a special case of mixed tumors which may be benign or malignant. These tumors arise from three germ layers: endoderm, ectoderm, and mesoderm.
      (1) *Endoderm*—the invaginated cells of the embryo that ultimately form the gastrointestinal tract and associated structures.
      (2) *Ectoderm*—the outmost layer of the embryo that forms the skin and related structures.
      (3) *Mesoderm*—cells located between endoderm and ectoderm layers of the embryo that give rise to supporting structures such as the bone, fat, muscle, blood.
    f. There are many exceptions to rules for naming benign and malignant neoplasms, particularly of nervous tissue, lymph nodes, bone marrow, and epithelium. Examples include:
      (1) Melanoma—a malignant neoplasia of melanocytes.
      (2) Hepatoma—a malignant neoplasia of the liver.

HEMATOLOGIC MALIGNANCIES

A. There are two major types of leukemias that mature from hematopoietic stem cells—myelogenous and lymphatic.
B. The prefix "lympho" is used to describe leukemia of lymphoid origin.

Table 4–3. SIMPLE CLASSIFICATION OF LEUKEMIA*

Acute Leukemia
  Lymphocytic
  Myelogenous
  Myeloblastic
  Promyelocytic
  Myelomonocytic
  Monocytic
  Erythroleukemia
  Eosinophilic
  Basophilic
  Undifferentiated (Stem Cell)
Chronic Leukemia
  Lymphocytic
  Myelocytic, Granulocytic
  Myelomonocytic
  Hairy Cell Leukemia

* From Judith Beach Campbell, J. B., Preston, R. and Smith, K. Y.: 1983, The leukemias. Nursing Clinics of North America. *18*:524, 1983.

C. The prefix "myelo" or "granulo" is used to describe leukemia of myeloid origin.
D. The suffix "blastic" is used to describe immature cells.
E. As an example, acute lymphoblastic leukemia describes a white blood cell disease involving very immature cells of lymphoid origin.
F. Classifications of leukemia are shown in Table 4–3.

STUDY QUESTIONS

1. Describe how metaplasia differs from dysplasia.
2. Explain what tissue of origin the terms "sarcoma" and "carcinoma" describe.
3. Discuss what the prefixes "lympho" and "myelo" connote with respect to leukemia.

Bibliography

Campbell, J., Preston, R. and Smith, K.: The leukemias: Definition, treatment, and nursing care. Nursing Clinics of North America, *18*:523–541, 1983.
Ferrell, L.: Pathophysiology of neoplasia. Paper presented at the University of California, San Francisco, 1984.
Pitot, H.: Fundamentals of Oncology. New York, Marcel Dekker, Inc., 1981.
Robbins, S. L., Cotran, R. and Kumar, V.: Pathologic Basis of Disease. Philadelphia, W. B. Saunders Company, 1984.

SECTION TWO

Cancer Epidemiology

Section Editor
JOANNE T. COSSMAN, RN, MPH

5

Terminology

BARBARA BURNS McGRATH, RN, MA

CANCER EPIDEMIOLOGY

A. The primary concern is with disease as it manifests in populations, rather than individuals. The primary goal is prevention; the focus is on patterns of distribution.
B. Epidemiologists monitor the indicators of cancer occurrence, interpret changes, and investigate environmental causes of cancer in humans.
C. More than one factor contributes to the occurrence of disease. Examples of concepts used by epidemiologists to study causation are:
   1. Interaction of agent, environment, and host.
   2. Predisposing factors to a disease and their complex relations with each other and with the disease.

EPIDEMIOLOGIC PURPOSES AND PROCESS

A. A major purpose of epidemiologic studies of cancer is to investigate the causes of cancer by exploring the relationship between variables.
B. Observational studies (descriptive and analytic) allow nature to take its course. Changes or differences in one characteristic are studied in relation to changes or differences in the other if any.
   1. Descriptive studies usually determine the incidence, prevalence, and mortality rates for cancer in large population groups. Common characteristics of the individuals are sought that separate ill persons from well persons: age, sex, race, location of occurrence of the disease, time trends, and geographic differences. General distribution of the disease in the population is described to generate hypotheses or to monitor changes in occurrence.
   2. Analytic studies are used to test hypotheses suggested by descriptive studies and to generate new hypotheses based on results of laboratory studies or clinical observation. The investigation usually begins with a hypothesis associating a suspected etiologic factor to a specific type of cancer. Examples of analytic studies are: correlation, case-comparison, cohort, cross-sectional, and serologic studies.

31

3. Experimental or intervention studies consider the effect on the population of manipulating environmental influences. A potential etiologic factor may be removed from the environment, or a potentially preventive or curative factor may be introduced into controlled experiments on human populations; this type of epidemiologic study is not used as frequently as observational studies.

INCIDENCE VERSUS PREVALENCE

A. Incidence—the number of new cases diagnosed during a specified period. Incidence rates are useful in comparing changing trends in the detection of new cases. They are calculated by the following formula:

$$\text{Incidence Rate} = \frac{\text{Number of new cases of cancer in a given period}}{\text{Total number in population exposed to the risk of developing cancer during that period}}$$

B. Prevalence is a measure of existing disease at a designated point in time. Prevalence rates are useful in identifying changing trends in existing disease. They are determined by the following formula:

$$\text{Prevalence Rate} = \frac{\text{Number of persons with a cancer at a specified time}}{\text{Total number in group at the specified time}}$$

AGENT

A. When a factor must be present for a disease to occur, it is called the agent of that disease.
B. An agent is considered to be necessary, but its presence is not sufficient to cause disease, because suitable conditions of the host and environment must also be present for disease to develop.

HOST

A. A person susceptible to the disease is known as the host.
B. Examples of intrinsic host factors are: genetic predisposition, age, sex, immunity, behavior.

ENVIRONMENT

A. Factors in the environment influence the existence of the agent, exposure, or susceptibility to disease.
B. Examples of extrinsic (environmental) factors are: biologic environment, social environment, physical environment.

TIME

A. The pattern of disease occurrence in time is often an informative descriptive characteristic. Short-term increases or decreases are quite apparent to observers, but long-term trends (called secular trends) are less perceptible.
B. There is a steady rate of occurrence with most common cancers. This suggests that the cancers have been determined by life-style or environmental factors acting over years or decades.

CARCINOGEN

A. Carcinogen—a cancer producing substance.
B. Examples of carcinogens: cigarette smoke, asbestos, dietary fat, alcoholic beverages, benzene, vinyl chloride, diethylstilbesterol, cyclophosphamide melphalan.

STUDY QUESTIONS

1. What is the purpose of cancer epidemiologic studies?
2. What is the difference between incidence and prevalence?
3. Is it necessary for all three variables, agent, host, and environment to be present for disease to occur?

Bibliography

DeVita, V., Hellman, S. and Rosenberg, S.: Cancer: Principles and Practice of Oncology, 2nd ed. Philadelphia, J. P. Lippincott Co., 1985.
Friedman, G.: Primer of Epidemiology, 2nd ed. New York, McGraw-Hill Book Co., 1980.
Moses, M.: Cancer and the workplace. American Journal of Nursing, *79*(11):1985–1988, 1979.

6

Cancer Incidence and Trends

PAMELA S. PETERS, RN, MPH

CANCER RANK AMONG LEADING CAUSES OF DEATH

A. Second to heart disease as overall leading cause of death in U.S.
   1. Will account for estimated 472,000 deaths in U.S. in 1986.
   2. Equals close to 1/2 the number of deaths due to heart disease.
B. Variations in rank by sex and age.
   1. Among top four leading causes of death for both sexes and all age groups in U.S.
   2. Ranks fourth for males aged 15–34, preceded by accidents, homicide, and suicide.
   3. Ranks first for females aged 35–54.
   4. Preceded by accidents as second leading cause of death among children and young adults aged 0–34.
C. Historic variations in cancer rank.
   1. Rank has risen as deaths due to infectious diseases have decreased.
   2. In 1900, 40% of all deaths were due to 11 major infectious diseases; decreased to 6% by 1973.
   3. Three major chronic conditions (heart disease, cancer, and stroke) accounted for 16% of deaths in 1900 and 58% in 1973.
   4. Better diagnostic techniques and reporting influence statistics.

INCIDENCE OF CANCER IN U.S.

A. 930,000 estimated new cases during 1986.
B. Estimated incidence by site and sex for major cancer sites is illustrated in Table 6–1.
C. Age-adjusted incidence rates per 100,000 population for both sexes, all races, is 331.5.
D. Occurs less frequently in women (304.1 per 100,000) than men (379.3 per 100,000).
E. Primarily disease of elderly; 51% of all cases diagnosed in those 65 and older.
   1. Median age at diagnosis is 63.5 years for women and 66.9 years for men.

Table 6–1. 1986 ESTIMATED CANCER INCIDENCE BY
SITE AND SEX*†

Site	Total	Males	Females
Lung	149,000	100,000	49,000
Colon and Rectum	140,000	67,000	73,000
Breast (Female)	123,900	—	123,900
Prostate Gland	90,000	90,000	—
Urinary Tract	60,500	41,700	18,800
Uterus	50,000	—	50,000
Lymph Tissues	44,500	22,800	21,700
Oral Areas	29,500	19,800	9,700
Pancreas	25,500	13,000	12,500
Leukemias	25,600	14,000	11,600
Skin	23,000	12,000	11,000
All Others	194,100	84,700	83,800
Total	930,000	465,000	465,000

* Adapted from CA-A Cancer Journal for Clinicians, New York, American Cancer Society, Vol 36, No 1, 1986, p. 16.
† Excludes nonmelanoma skin cancer and carcinoma in situ.

   2. Prior to age 50, incidence is higher in women; after 60, dramatic increase in incidence occurs in males.
F. Rare in children (0–14); 6,550 estimated new cases in 1986.
G. Among Americans born in 1985, one third will eventually develop invasive cancer.
H. Age-adjusted rate of carcinoma in situ for 100,000 population is 26.7; 5.1 in males and 47.5 in females. Combining invasive and in situ lesions increases overall incidence by 1.3% for males and 15.6% for females.
I. Invasive cancers exclude carcinoma in situ and nonmelanoma skin cancers.
J. Age-adjusted rate—cancer risk increases significantly with age. As the proportion of older individuals increases in any population, so does the overall number of cancers. Data are age adjusted mathematically to compare statistics over time in a given population or to compare statistics among countries with different age proportions.

HISTORIC TRENDS IN CANCER INCIDENCE

A. Age—between 1973 and 1979 changes in four age groups show greatest increase among adults 65–74 years; less increase among the 45–64 age group; stable rates in 15–44 year olds; decrease among children 0–14.
B. Sex—incidence rates among males increased, while rates for females decreased between 1973 and 1981.
C. Race—incidence increased more among blacks (27%) than whites (12%) during the past several decades; differences are attributed to economic, environmental, and social factors.
D. Changes in incidence per 100,000 population for select sites between 1969–1977.
   1. Melanoma nearly doubled among whites.
   2. Breast cancer increased sharply for both races, most frequently among whites.

3. Cancer of uterine cervix decreased markedly for both races, but remains two times higher in blacks.
4. Endometrial cancer incidence increased most markedly among white women.
5. Ovarian cancer decreased slightly for both races.
6. Prostate cancer increased more in blacks.
7. Bladder and kidney cancer increased for all sex-race groups.
8. Leukemia decreased for all sex-race groups.
9. Stomach cancer declined among men and white women, but increased among black women.
10. Colon cancer increased markedly for black males and slightly for other sex-race groups.
11. Cancer of the rectum decreased slightly in black males and increased gradually in other sex-race groups.
12. Pancreatic cancer decreased slightly among white men, remained constant among white women, and increased significantly among blacks.
13. Lung cancer has shown a marked increase in women.

E. Hypotheses on incidence changes.
   1. Increased awareness of public and medical community resulting in earlier detection of slow-growing tumors.
   2. Special federal programs and funding such as the National Cancer Act of 1971.
   3. Warnings of risks associated with chemicals and drugs, resulting in decreased exposure as with estrogen and uterine corpus cancer.
   4. Increase in performance of self-examinations such as Breast Self Exam. Practice resulted in peak incidence during mid-1970's.

CANCER MORTALITY IN U.S.

A. Estimated cancer deaths for 1986 are 472,000; age-adjusted death rate per 100,000 is 196.
B. Average life expectancy decreases by 16 years after diagnosis of cancer.
C. Cancer deaths do not always reflect incidence.
   1. Sex—men die more frequently than women; 1 of 5 women and 1 of 4 men born in 1985 will eventually die of cancer.
   2. Age—cancer deaths occur most often in older age groups. Chances of eventual cancer death are not uniformly predominant in any age group; rates change with advancing age and with changes in other causes of death. Death rates for children and young adults declined markedly since 1964 and are leveling off. Slight declines have been seen for 45–64 age group; rates are constant for persons 65–74, and increases have been seen in the 75+ age group.
   3. Site—deaths by cancer site are illustrated in Table 6–2. Sites with poorest prognoses include lung, esophagus, and pancreas; sites with most favorable prognoses include testis and uterine corpus.
   4. Stage at diagnosis—mortality rates increase with advanced stage of disease at diagnosis. Variances between survival rates for localized (Stage I) cancers versus cancers with regional or distant spread range from 16% (esophagus) to 65% (ovary).
   5. Geography—variations reflect environmental differences, personal habits, life styles, and occupational exposures. Mortality rates are highest in

Table 6–2. 1986 ESTIMATED CANCER MORTALITY BY SITE AND SEX*

Site	Total	Males	Females
Lung	130,000	89,000	41,100
Colon and Rectum	60,000	29,100	30,900
Breast (Female)	40,200	—	40,200
Prostate Gland	26,100	26,100	—
Pancreas	24,000	12,300	11,700
Lymph Tissues	23,700	12,300	11,400
Urinary Tract	19,800	12,800	7,000
Leukemias	17,400	9,600	7,800
Uterus	9,700	—	9,700
Oral Areas	9,400	6,350	3,050
Skin	7,500	4,500	3,000
All Others	104,200	51,450	52,650
Total	472,000	253,500	218,500

* Adapted from CA-A Cancer Journal for Clinicians, New York, American Cancer Society, Vol 36, No 1, 1986, p. 17.

industrialized regions; lowest deaths per 100,000 population are in Alaska (87) and highest in District of Columbia (281).

D. International Patterns—mortality rate varies by level of economic development of country. Developed countries (¼ total world population) have avverage death rate of 150 per 100,000 population, whereas mortality rates in underdeveloped countries are close to one half this rate.

HISTORIC TRENDS IN CANCER MORTALITY

A. Number of cancer deaths per 100,000 population has increased by 11% during the past four decades.
B. Age-adjusted death rates per 100,000 population in U.S. show gradual rise; in 1950–1959 there were 158.3; in 1960–1969 there were 162.4; and in 1970–1979 there were 169.0.
C. Probability of eventually dying of cancer is generally increasing among all sex-race groups and is greatest for males.
D. Greatest increase seen in lung cancer, consistent with smoking patterns; increase among men from 5 deaths per 100,000 in 1930 to almost 70 in 1977. By 1986 deaths from lung cancer are expected to exceed those from breast cancer in women.
E. Cancer mortality among children declined from 8.3 per 100,000 in 1950 to 4.2 per 100,000 in 1981.

SURVIVAL RATES IN U.S.

A. Over five million Americans are cancer survivors; three million were diagnosed over 5 years ago.
B. Survival rates vary with age, sex, race, site, and stage at diagnosis.
  1. Age—except for breast and colon cancers, survival rates decrease as age increases.

2. Sex—survival rates among women are higher than among men owing to differences in tumor site distribution.
3. Race—whites have higher survival rates than blacks; more whites are diagnosed with localized lesions.
4. Stage at Diagnosis—persons diagnosed with widespread metastatic disease have poor survival rates.

C. Historic trends in survival rates.
1. Steady increase in survival rates for all sex-race groups.
2. Five year survival improved from 1:5 in 1930, 1:4 in 1940, 1:3 in 1960 to 3:8 in 1985. When normal life expectancy is taken into consideration, 49% of all persons diagnosed with cancer in 1985 will be alive 5 years after diagnosis.
3. Five year survival rates between 1950–1954 and 1977–1981 have increased for cancer of the lung (7%), colon and rectum (12%), prostate (28%), breast (15%), and uterus (18%).
4. Improvements in survival reflect improvements in patient management, diagnosis and treatment, promotion and acceptance of early detection measures, availability and use of medical care.

STUDY QUESTIONS

1. Describe cancer's rank among other leading causes of death by patients' age and sex.
2. Describe the impact of age, sex, race, site, and stage of disease on cancer incidence, mortality, and survival.
3. Discuss the historic variations that have occurred in cancer incidence, mortality, and survival.
4. Explain hypotheses that account for historic trends in cancer incidence, mortality, and survival.

Bibliography

Cancer Facts & Figures, 1986. New York, American Cancer Society, 1986.

Cancer statistics, 1986. Ca-A Cancer Journal for Clinicians, *36*(1):16, 1986.

Marino, L. B.: The Nature and scope of the cancer problem. *In* Marino, L. B. (ed.): Cancer Nursing. St. Louis, C.V. Mosby Company, pp. 20–34, 1981.

Muir, C. S. and Nectoux, J.: International patterns of cancer. *In* Schottenfeld, D. and Fraumeni, J. (eds.): Cancer Epidemiology and Prevention. Philadelphia, W.B. Saunders Company, pp. 119–137, 1982.

Myers, M. H. and Hankey, B. F.: Cancer patient survival of cancer. *In* Schottenfeld, D. and Fraumeni, J. (eds.): Cancer Epidemiology and Prevention. Philadelphia, W.B. Saunders Company, pp. 166–178, 1982.

Page, H. S. and Asire, A. J.: Cancer Rates and Risks, 3rd ed. (DHHS, Public Health Service, NIH Publication No. 85–691). Bethesda, MD, NIH, April 1985.

Pollack, E. S.: Tracking cancer trends: Incidence and survival. Hospital Practice, *19*(8):99–116, 1984.

Seidman, H., Mushinski, M. H., Gelb, S., and Silverberg, E.: Probabilities of eventually developing or dying of cancer—U.S. 1985. Ca-A Cancer Journal for Clinicians, *35*(1):36–56, 1985.

Young, J. L., Jr. and Pollack, E. S.: Incidence of cancer in the United States. *In* Schottenfeld, D. and Fraumeni, J. (eds.): Cancer Epidemiology and Prevention. Philadelphia, W.B. Saunders Company, pp. 138–165, 1982.

7

Patterns of Occurrence

MARGARET J. CROWLEY, RN, BSN, MS Ed

INTERNATIONAL PATTERNS

A. Cancer incidence of all sites is fairly constant among countries. There is a three- to fourfold difference between populations with the highest and the lowest rates. That the incidence in both advanced and underdeveloped countries is within the three- to fourfold spectrum suggests that cancer is not only a disease of industrialized nations.

B. Wordwide incidence of childhood cancers is remarkably similar—leukemia has the highest rate. The highest rate of childhood cancers is observed among the youngest age group. The short latency period suggests that childhood cancer involves a different process from that of adult cancer, which involves cumulative exposure to environmental factors.

C. Cancer *site* incidence between countries is the most notable difference—10- to 30- fold.
   1. Epidemiologic studies suggest site differences are associated with behavioral, cultural, and dietary factors.
   2. Racial or ethnic differences are *generally* not significant; however, skin cancer occurs more frequently in whites. Incidence of lymphoproliferative diseases may be decreased in Chinese or Japanese persons.
   3. Immigrant studies demonstrate that incidence of cancer by site changes in migrants to incidence found in the new county. Cancer rate for black Americans is closer to that for white Americans than to the African rate. Japanese in Hawaii have a rate closer to that for caucasians in Hawaii than for Japanese in Japan.

D. Specific examples of differences in cancer incidence by site include:
   1. Skin cancer—highest rate in fair-skinned Australians.
   2. Nasopharyngeal cancer—highest among Chinese and those of Chinese ancestry.
   3. Liver cancer—high in China, Africa, Southeast Asia; *rare* in U.S. and Europe.
   4. Breast cancer—high in U.S. and Europe; low in Japan.

5. Prostate cancer—high in Europe and U.S.; low in Japan and China.
6. Colon and rectum cancer—high in North America, New Zealand, United Kingdom; low in Africa, China, Japan.

UNITED STATES PATTERNS OF INCIDENCE

A. Surveillance, Epidemiology and End Results Program (SEER) established in 1973 by National Cancer Institute—ongoing study of cancer incidence and survival in U.S.
   1. Ten percent (10%) of U.S. population represented from variety of areas— San Francisco-Oakland area; metropolitan Detroit, Connecticut, Hawaii, Iowa, New Mexico, Utah, Puerto Rico, New Orleans, Seattle (1974), Atlanta (1975), New Jersey (1985)
   2. Deliberate oversampling of certain ethnic minorities allows for comparisons of data among ethnic groups. The sampling includes:
      a. 47% of all Japanese-Americans.
      b. 36% of all Chinese-Americans.
      c. 15% of all American-Indians.
      d. 9% of all Blacks.
      e. 9% of all Hispanics.
   3. This sampling may not provide good representation of national cancer patterns for blacks.
B. Age differences—Pattern of cancer occurrence low in childhood, high over age 60.

Ethnic Differences

A. Hispanics versus Anglo-Americans. Hispanics have lower incidence rates for males and females for all sites combined. Hispanics have higher incidence of stomach, uterine cervix, and gallbladder cancers (may be related to diet, sexual activity, availability medical care). Lower incidence of colon, breast, and lung cancers (may be related to diet, reproductive history, cigarette use).
B. Blacks versus Whites. Blacks have higher overall incidence and mortality rates. Specific sites with higher incidence rates include: lung, colon and rectum, prostate, and esophagus (may be related to lack of health care, increased exposure to carcinogens, lack of information). Notable also, black women have shown a decrease in uterine cervix cancer, but their rate is still double that for whites. Rate for endometrial cancer in blacks is half of that for whites (may be related to sexual activity, reproductive history).

Cultural Differences

A. Cultural differences are related to differences in behavior, dietary habits, reproductive habits, alcohol and tobacco use.
B. Religious influences—Seventh-Day Adventists and Mormons of Utah and California have lower incidence rates for respiratory, gastrointestinal, and genital cancers. Related to avoidance of alcohol, coffee, and tobacco and to dietary habits.
C. Lifestyle influences—Rural southern women show an increase in oral and pharyngeal cancers secondary to use of snuff, even without the use of alcohol or cigarettes.

Gender Differences

A. Females have higher overall incidence of cancer.
B. Females have higher 5-year survival rate for all ages.
C. Difference in male/female lung cancer incidence has been great, with the rate for males high and that for females low. The difference between the rates is rapidly decreasing owing to increased smoking by women.

Geographic Differences

A. Suggest environmental factors that may be involved in etiology of cancer.
B. Urban cancer incidence is higher for lung, breast, and esophagus than is rural incidence.
C. Coastal area of the South demonstrates an increase in lung cancer in males (occupational exposure to asbestos in shipyards).
D. Breast cancer showed a northeastern predominance for post-menopausal women (environmental factors). Pre-menopausal breast cancer has a uniform distribution throughout country (genetic and reproductive factors predominate).
E. Colon cancer had a 50% lower incidence in the South than in Northeastern and North Central parts of country. (Studies currently in process to see what might be related to pattern.)

STUDY QUESTIONS

1. Describe the differences between worldwide cancer incidence for *all sites* and worldwide *site-specific* cancer incidence.
2. Identify the change in cancer incidence demonstrated in immigrant studies.
3. Identify two factors that have been associated with geographic differences in cancer incidence in the U.S.

Bibliography

Blot, W. J., Fraumeni, J. F., Jr.: Geographic epidemiology of cancer in the United States. *In* Schottenfield, D. and Fraumeni, J. F., Jr. (eds.): Cancer Epidemiology and Prevention. Philadelphia, W. B. Saunders Company, pp. 179–193, 1982.

Doll, R. and Peto, R.: The Causes of Cancer. New York, Oxford University Press, 1981.

Fraumeni, J. Jr.: The Face of Cancer in the United States. Hospital Practice, 18(12):81–96, 1983.

Higginson, J.: The Face of Cancer Worldwide. Hospital Practice, 18(110):145–157, 1983.

Newell, G. R.: Epidemiology of Cancer. *In* Devita V. T., Jr., Hellman, S., and Rosenberg, S. A. (eds.): Cancer: Principles and Practice of Oncology, 2nd ed. Philadelphia, J. B. Lippincott, Co., pp. 152–183, 1985.

Pollack, E. S.: Tracking Cancer Trends: Incidence and Survival. Hospital Practice, 19(8):99–102, 111–112, 1984.

Silverberg, B. S.: Cancer Statistics, 1985. New York, American Cancer Society, 1985.

Woods, N. F. and Woods, J. S.: Epidemiology and the Study of Cancer. *In* Marino, L. B. (ed.): Cancer Nursing. St. Louis, C. V. Mosby, pp. 139–172, 1981.

8

Risk Factors

MARGARET J. CROWLEY, RN, BSN, MS Ed

VIRAL RISK FACTORS

A. Criteria for virus implication:
   1. Infection with virus precedes development of cancer.
   2. Viral nucleic acid exists in freshly isolated tumor cells.
   3. Virus transforms cells in tissue culture.
   4. Viruses of same taxonomic group produce tumors that occur naturally in animals.
   5. Supporting epidemiologic evidence exists.
   6. Immunization of high-risk individuals results in reduction in incidence of the neoplasm.
B. Specific viral associations.
   1. Herpes simplex epidemiologically linked with squamous cell carcinomas of the oral pharynx.
   2. Herpes simplex, type 2, epidemiologically linked to cervical carcinoma.
   3. Epstein-Barr virus, strong evidence—epidemiologic evidence, viral markers, antigen in tumor cells, high total antibodies—associated with Burkett's lymphoma and nasopharyngeal carcinoma.
   4. Cytomegalovirus weak, but possible link to Kaposi's sarcoma.
   5. Hepatitis B viruses associated with primary liver cancer.
   6. Retroviruses produce an oncogene in animals that may be activated during cellular proliferation. Study is being done in this area.

CHEMICAL RISK FACTORS

A. Identification of carcinogens:
   1. Epidemiologic studies identify carcinogens such as by-products of tobacco.
   2. Laboratory studies demonstrated development of cancer with exposure to a substance in animals, usually rats and mice.
   3. Molecular structure analysis and examination of basic chemical and physical properties of substances may suggest potential carcinogen for study.

45

Table 8–1. OCCUPATIONAL CANCER HAZARDS*

Agent	Cancer Site or Type	Type of Workers Exposed
Acrylonitrile	Lung, colon	Manufacturers of apparel, carpeting, blankets, draperies, synthetic furs, and wigs
4-aminobiphenyl	Bladder	Chemical workers
Arsenic and certain arsenic compounds	Lung, skin, scrotum, lymphatic system, hemangiosarcoma of the liver	Workers in the metallurgical industries, sheep-dip workers, pesticide production workers, copper smelter workers, vineyard workers, insecticide makers and sprayers, tanners, miners (gold miners)
Asbestos	Lung, larynx, GI tract, pleural and peritoneal mesothelioma	Asbestos factory workers, textile workers, rubber-tire manufacturing industry workers, miners, insulation workers, shipyard workers
Auramine and the manufacture of auramine	Bladder	Dyestuffs manufacturers, rubber workers, textile dyers, paint manufacturers
Benzene	Leukemia	Rubber-tire manufacturing industry workers, painters, shoe manufacturing workers, rubber cement workers, glue and varnish workers, distillers, shoemakers, plastics workers, chemical workers
Benzidine	Bladder, pancreas	Dyeworkers, chemical workers
Beryllium and certain beryllium compounds	Lung	Beryllium workers, electronics workers, missile parts producers
Bis(chloromethyl)ether (BCME)	Lung	Workers in plants producing anion-exchange resins (chemical workers)
Cadmium and certain cadmium compounds	Lung, prostate	Cadmium production workers, metallurgical workers, electroplating industry workers, chemical workers, jewelry workers, nuclear workers, pigment workers, battery workers
Carbon tetrachloride	Liver	Plastics workers, dry cleaners
Chloromethyl methyl ether (CMME)	Lung	Chemical workers, workers in plants producing ion-exchange resin
Chromium and certain chromium compounds	Lung, nasal sinuses	Chromate-producing industry workers, acetylene and aniline workers, bleachers, glass, pottery, pigment, and linoleum workers
Coal tar pitch volatiles	Lung, scrotum	Steel industry workers, aluminum potroom workers, foundry workers
Coke oven emissions	Lung, kidney, prostate	Steel industry workers, coke plant workers
Dimethyl sulphate	Lung	Chemical workers, drug makers, dyemakers
Epichlorohydrin	Lung, leukemia	Chemical workers

Table 8–1. OCCUPATIONAL CANCER HAZARDS* (*continued*)

Agent	Cancer Site or Type	Type of Workers Exposed
Ethylene oxide	Leukemia, stomach	Hospital workers, research lab workers, beekeepers, fumigators
Hematite and underground hematite mining	Lung	Miners
Isopropyl oils and the manufacture of isopropyl oils	Paranasal sinuses	Isopropyl oil workers
Mustard gas	Respiratory tract	Production workers
2-naphthylamine	Bladder, pancreas	Dye workers, rubber-tire manufacturing industry workers, chemical workers, manufacturers of coal gas, nickel refiners, copper smelters, electrolysis workers
Nickel (certain compounds) and nickel refining	Nasal cavity, lung, larynx	Nickel refiners
Polychlorinated biphenyls (PCBs)	Melanoma	PCBs workers
Radiation, ionizing	Skin, pancreas, brain, stomach, breast, salivary glands, thyroid, GI tract, bronchus, lymphoid tissue, leukemia, multiple myeloma	Uranium miners, radiologists, radiographers, luminous dial painters
Radiation, ultraviolet	Skin	Farmers, sailors, arc welders
Soots, tars, mineral oils	Skin, lung, bladder, GI tract	Construction workers, roofers, chimney sweeps, machinists
Thorium dioxide	Liver, kidney, larynx, leukemia	Chemical workers, steelworkers, ceramic makers, incandescent lamp makers, nuclear reactor workers, gas mantle makers, metal refiners, vacuum tube makers
Vinyl chloride	Liver, brain, lung, hematolymphopoietic system, breast	Plastics factory workers, vinyl chloride polymerization plant workers
Agent(s) not identified	Pancreas	Chemists
	Stomach	Coal miners
	Brain, stomach	Petrochemical industry
	Hematolymphopoietic system	Rubber industry workers
	Bladder	Printing pressmen
	Eye, kidney, lung	Chemical workers
	Leukemia, brain	Farmers
	Colon, brain	Pattern and model makers
	Esophagus, stomach, lung	Oil refinery workers

* From Office of Technology Assessment: Occupational Cancer Hazards. Boulder, Colorado, Westview Press, Inc., 1982.

    4. Tests for mutagenicity such as Ames test (measures capacity to cause genetic change in bacteria) are used to screen substances for further study.
  B. Occupational cancer hazards are listed in Table 8–1.
  C. Medical exposures—iatrogenic exposure to cancer-producing agents includes: chemotherapy, hormone treatment, therapy with immunosuppresive agents.
    1. Alkylating agents are associated with bladder and bone marrow cancers.

2. Immunosuppressive drugs are associated with cancer of the reticuloen-dothelial system.
3. Estrogen exposure in the adult is associated with cancer of endometrium; in the fetus, exposure is associated with development of vaginal cancer when the individual reaches young adulthood.
4. Anabolic steroids are associated with liver cancer.
5. Contraceptives are also associated with liver and possibly breast cancer in those women already at high risk (Table 8–2).

D. Societal exposure—variety of substances used by a society may be carcinogenic.
1. Tobacco is leading carcinogen in our time that can be eliminated or avoided. It is associated with cancers of lung, mouth, pharynx, larynx, or esophagus, as well as bladder and pancreas and possibly kidney, stomach, and liver. The risk of lung cancer 10 times greater by middle age for regular smokers vs lifelong nonsmokers.
2. Alcohol—This carcinogen interacts with tobacco and each enhances the other. Increased incidence of cancers of the mouth and pharynx with large amounts of alcohol.

DIETARY RISK FACTORS

A. Factors that increase risk:
1. Obesity—Weight 40% above average increases the risk of colon, breast, prostate, gallbladder, ovary, and uterine cancers.
2. High fat—Intake of more than 30% calories from fat is a factor in breast, colon, and prostate cancer.
3. Preservatives and seasonings—Persons who frequently eat cured and smoked and highly seasoned foods demonstrate higher incidence of cancer of esophagus and stomach.
4. Alcohol—See above.
5. Carcinogens produced in cooking—Potentially but not proven hazardous chemicals are produced when meat or fish is broiled, charcoal broiled, and smoked.
6. Food additives—Additives such as saccharin and nitrites may be implicated. No definitive conclusion.

B. Factors that decrease risk:
1. High fiber intake—Foods such as whole grain cereals, fruits, and vegetables may reduce risk of colon cancer.
2. Vitamins A and C—Diet including foods rich in these vitamins may lower risk for cancer of larynx, esophagus, and lung.
3. Cruciferous vegetables (cabbage, broccoli, brussels sprouts, and cauliflower) may play roles in cancer prevention. Researchers are currently investigating this area.

Hereditary Risk Factors (See also oncogene theory, Chapter 2)

A. Individuals with a genetic predisposition to cancer even in the absence of environmental variations.
1. Children who develop cancers such as retinoblastoma, neuroblastoma, and Wilm's tumor.

Table 8–2. ESTABLISHED HUMAN CARCINOGENIC AGENTS*†

Agent or Circumstance	Occupational	Medical	Social	Site of Cancer
Aflatoxin			+	Liver
Alcoholic drinks			+	Mouth, pharynx, larynx, esophagus, liver
Alkylating agents:				
Cyclophosphamide		+		Bladder
Melphalan		+		Marrow
Aromatic amines:				
4-Aminodiphenyl	+			Bladder
Benzidine	+			Bladder
2-Naphthylamine	+			Bladder
Arsenic	+	+		Skin, lung
Asbestos	+			Lung, pleura, peritoneum
Benzene	+			Marrow
Bis(chloromethyl) ether	+			Lung
Busulphan		+		Marrow
Cadmium	+			Prostate
Chewing betel, tobacco, lime			+	Mouth
Chromium	+			Lung
Chlornaphazine		+		Bladder
Furniture manufacture (hardwood)	+			Nasal sinuses
Immunosuppressive drugs		+		Reticuloendothelial system
Ionizing radiations	+	+		Marrow and probably all other sites
Isopropyl alcohol manufacture	+			Nasal sinuses
Leather goods manufacture	+			Nasal sinuses
Mustard gas	+			Larynx, lung
Nickel	+			Nasal sinuses, lung
Estrogens:				
Unopposed		+		Endometrium
Transplacental (DES)		+		Vagina
Overnutrition (causing obesity)			+	Endometrium, gallbladder
Phenacetin		+		Kidney (pelvis)
Polycyclic hydrocarbons	+	+		Skin, scrotum, lung
Reproductive history:				
Late age at 1st pregnancy			+	Breast
Zero or low parity			+	Ovary
Parasites:				
Schistosoma haematobium			+	Bladder
Chlonorchis sinensis			+	Liver (cholangioma)
Sexual promiscuity			+	Cervix uteri
Steroids:				
Anabolic (oxymetholone)		+		Liver
Contraceptives		+		Liver (hamartoma)
Tobacco smoking			+	Mouth, pharynx, larynx, lung, esophagus, bladder
UV light	+		+	Skin, lip
Vinyl chloride	+			Liver (angiosarcoma)
Virus (hepatitis B)			+	Liver (hepatoma)

  * From Doll, R. and Peto, R.: The Causes of Cancer. New York, Oxford University Press, 1981.

  † A plus sign indicates that evidence of carcinogenicity was obtained.

Note: Occupational exposure to phenoxyacid/chlorophenal herbicides (or their impurities) is a reasonably well established cause of soft tissue sarcomas or perhaps lymphomas.

2. Adults with polyposis of colon develop colon cancer.
B. Individuals with predisposition imposed by environmental variation in the absence of genetic variation.
   1. Accounts for the majority of cancers.
   2. See definition of environmental factors (Chapter 5).
C. Individuals with predisposition imposed by both genetic and environmental factors.
   1. Xeroderma pigmentosum (rare)—defect in DNA repair mechanism such that individual exposed to ultraviolet light develops skin tumors and internal tumors.
   2. Daughters of breast cancer patients (especially if mother had pre-menopausal bilateral cancer) have increased suseptability to breast cancer.
   3. Lightly pigmented individuals (e.g., Celtic ancestry) have increased risk of skin cancer caused by exposure to sun.

RADIATION EXPOSURE

A. Ultraviolet radiation.
   1. Component of sunlight that is associated with skin cancer. Risk increases with length of exposure and fairness of the skin.
   2. Principle cause of basal cell carcinoma of face and neck in light-skinned persons.
   3. Associated with lip cancers, squamous cell carcinoma, and melanoma.
B. Ionizing radiation.
   1. Low-dose exposure—medical (50% of general public exposure) and natural background exposure (45%). Very difficult to establish dose-response relationship. Developing fetus and children most susceptible.
   2. High-dose exposure—accidental (A-bomb in Hiroshima and Nagasaki) and occupational exposure (uranium mines, radiologists, radium watch dial painters).
   3. Specific studies of A-bomb survivors indicate increased incidence of leukemia, and cancers of breast, thyroid, lungs, and digestive organs.

SEXUAL DEVELOPMENT, REPRODUCTIVE PATTERNS, AND SEXUAL PRACTICE

A. Early menarche (before 13) and late menopause (after 55) are associated with increased incidence of breast cancer.
B. Undescended testicles are associated with an increased incidence of testicular cancer.
C. Birth of first child after age 30 *increases* the risk of breast cancer, whereas the birth of a first child before age 20 *decreases* risk.
D. Nulliparity increases the risk of cancer of breast, endometrium, and ovary.
E. Sexual practices may increase risk of cancer of uterine cervix. Factors include increased number of sexual partners and earlier age of sexual activity.

HORMONAL RISK FACTORS (See also Medical

Exposures and Reproductive Patterns)

A. There is little evidence that hormones are themselves carcinogenic.

B. Hormones most likely act to sensitize the cell to a carcinogen, promote the carcinogenic process, and may modify the growth of an established tumor.

MECHANICAL RISK FACTORS—There is no evidence
for mechanical irritation as a cause of cancer.

STUDY QUESTIONS

1. Identify three viruses that have been linked with an increase in cancer incidence.
2. Describe two methods of identifying potential carcinogens.
3. Describe the role of heredity in cancer.

Bibliography

American Cancer Society: 1985 Cancer Facts and Figures. New York, American Cancer Society, 1985.

Borden, E. C.: Infectious Carcinogenesis: Virus and Human Neoplasia. *In* Kahn, S. B., Love, R. R., Sherman, C., and Chakravorty, P. (eds.): Concepts in Cancer Medicine. New York, Grune and Stratton, pp. 89–100, 1983.

Doll, R. and Peto, R.: The Causes of Cancer. New York, Oxford University Press, 1981.

Jordan, V. C.: Hormones. *In* Kahn, S. B., Love, R. R., Sherman, C., and Chakravorty, R. (eds.): Concepts in Cancer Medicine. New York, Grune and Stratton, pp. 177–186, 1983.

Knudson, A. G.: Genetic predisposition to cancer. *In* Hiatt, H. H., Watson, J. D., and Winston, J. A. (eds.): Origins of Human Cancer. Cold Spring Harbor, New York, Cold Spring Harbor Laboratory, pp. 45–52, 1977.

Office of Technology Assessment: Cancer Risk: Assessing and Reducing the Dangers in Our Society. Boulder, Colorado, Westview Press, Inc., 1981.

Schottenfield, D. and Fraumen, J. F.: Cancer Epidemiology and Prevention. Philadelphia, W. B. Saunders Company, 1982.

SECTION THREE

Cancer Prevention and Detection

Section Editor
JOANNE T. COSSMAN, RN, MPH

9

Preventive Measures

SUSAN ROKITA, RN, MS

OPTIMAL DIETARY PATTERNS

A. Assessment.
  1. 60–90% of all cancers are thought to be related to environmental factors.
  2. Diet is implicated as a risk factor in cancer development.
  3. Dietary patterns must be assessed during the health history in order to identify high-risk individuals and to institute preventive measures.
  4. The exact relationship between diet and cancer development is not completely understood, but dietary risk factors are thought to include:
     a. Obesity.
     b. Vitamin deficiencies (A, C, and E).
     c. Intake of specific food substances.
     d. Consumption of carcinogenic substances.
B. Recommendations.
  1. Avoid obesity.
     a. Cancer Prevention Study I (CPS I) by the American Cancer Society (1960–1972) found a greatly increased incidence among the obese for cancer of the uterus, gallbladder, kidney, stomach, colon, and breast.
     b. According to the CPS I, among individuals 40% or more overweight, there was a 55% increased risk for cancer incidence among females and a 33% increased risk for cancer incidence among males.
     c. Animal studies indicate that maintenance of near ideal body weight with nutritionally adequate diets has prolonged animal lifespans and reduced cancer incidence.
     d. Weight reduction measures are necessary to decrease this cancer risk factor.
  2. Decrease total fat intake in diet.
     a. Animal and human studies imply that high levels of fat in the diet increase the likelihood of developing cancers of the breast, colon, and prostate.
     b. Both saturated and unsaturated fats have been shown to enhance tumor growth by supplying promotional stimuli directly to colonic

mucosa or by causing hormonal imbalances that support both breast and prostatic cancers.

   c. The National Academy of Sciences recommends that fats in the diet should comprise only 30% or less of total calories consumed.

   d. Alterations in food habits of most individuals are necessary to reduce consumption of fats and oils; fat reduction leads to a lower caloric intake.

3. Increase total fiber in diet.

   a. Epidemiologic studies indicate that colon cancer is lower among individuals whose diet is chiefly unrefined, high fiber foods such as whole grains, fruits, and vegetables.

   b. High fiber diets are thought to decrease transit time of fecal material through the bowel, thus decreasing contact time of carcinogenic matter with the bowel mucosa.

   c. Adding high fiber foods such as cereal grains to one's diet may substitute for other foods high in fat content and decrease total caloric intake, which is a beneficial secondary gain.

4. Increase vitamin A in the diet.

   a. Vitamin A and its synthetic chemical derivative, retinoids, are necessary for epithelial growth and differentiation. Retinoids are thought to play a major role in normal cellular differentiation among noncancerous, pre-malignant and malignant cells.

   b. Studies in humans indicate that individuals with a diet high in vitamin A have a reduced incidence of cancers of the larynx, esophagus, and lung.

   c. High doses of vitamin A or long-term vitamin A therapy can be toxic. Serious side effects involve the skin and mucous membranes (cheilitis, conjunctivitis, exfoliation), hepatotoxicity, and central nervous system disorders (pseudotumor cerebri, headache).

   d. Foods rich in vitamin A include some fruits and the dark green and deep yellow vegetables (carrots, tomatoes, spinach, apricots, peaches, and cantaloupe).

5. Increase vitamin C in the diet.

   a. It is believed that vitamin C aids in tumor encapsulation by maintaining collagen formation, inhibiting nitrosamine production from nitrites and nitrates, and aiding the formation of immunoglobulins and the functioning of lymphocytes in fighting malignancy.

   b. Studies in humans are conflicting and inconclusive; however, some indicate a longer survival time with high levels of vitamin C consumption. Low levels of vitamin C intake have been associated with an increased incidence of cancer, especially of the stomach and esophagus.

   c. Toxicity with vitamin C supplementation is rare—nausea, vomiting, diarrhea, and skin rashes may be seen.

   d. Foods rich in vitamin C include fruits and vegetables such as strawberries, citrus fruits, currants, cabbage, tomatoes, walnuts, and rose hips.

6. Increase vitamin E in the diet.

   a. Animal studies have shown that vitamin E inhibits growth of gliomas, neuroblastomas, melanomas, and leukemias. Human testing is inconclusive and no consistent relationship between vitamin

E levels and cancer has been found. Phase I and II clinical trials are continuing.

    b. Toxicities of vitamin E therapy are rare, but may include thrombophlebitis, pulmonary embolism, elevated cholesterol levels, hypertension, breast tumors, and gynecomastia.

    c. Vitamin E is found in vegetable oils (soybean, corn, cottonseed, and sunflowerseed), alfalfa, and lettuce leaves.

  7. Increase cruciferous foods in the diet.

    a. Cruciferous vegetables, belonging to the mustard family, include cabbage, broccoli, Brussels sprouts, kohlrabi, and cauliflower.

    b. Epidemiologic studies indicate that the ingestion of cruciferous vegetables is associated with decreased incidence of gastrointestinal and respiratory cancers. Studies are continuing.

  8. Decrease alcohol consumption.

    a. Increased alcohol consumption, especially combined with tobacco use, increases the risk for cancers of the oral cavity, larynx, and esophagus.

    b. Excessive alcohol consumption also leads to cirrhosis, which is a risk factor for liver cancer.

    c. Alcoholic beverages should be drunk only in moderation if at all.

  9. Avoid salt-cured, smoked, or nitrate-cured foods.

    a. Conventional smoking of foods (especially meats and fish) may lead to GI absorption of tars containing numerous carcinogens. Industries are beginning to use a "liquid smoke," which is thought to be less dangerous.

    b. Although limited, evidence exists that associates salt-cured or pickled foods with a higher incidence of stomach and esophageal cancers.

    c. Increase intake of baked, roasted, boiled, steamed, or stewed foods; decrease intake of broiled or grilled foods.

    d. Nitrates and nitrites (added as food preservatives) enhance nitrosamine formation in foods and are thought to be implicated in the development of gastric and esophageal cancers. These preservatives have been reduced in foods by order of the U.S. Department of Agriculture.

  10. Avoid aflatoxin consumption.

    a. Aflatoxins are poisons produced from molds (mycotoxins) of peanuts, corn, and milk products during harvesting, processing, and storage. Mycotoxins are implicated in the development of cancers of the liver, kidney, trachea, and subcutaneous tissues.

    b. Store these foods in dry containers. If mold develops, discard.

C. Areas of concern and caution.

  1. Food additives.

    a. Substances added to foods for coloring or preservation have been found to be carcinogenic in animals; however, there is no clear association with cancer in humans.

    b. Without documented evidence of human cancer risk, recommendations cannot be made, and regulations are presently not enforced by the Food and Drug Administration.

  2. Artificial sweeteners.

    a. Saccharin at high levels has been documented to cause bladder cancer in rats. Moderate use in humans has not clearly demonstrated an increase in bladder cancer; however, the long-term effects cannot be predicted.

b. Newer artificial sweeteners are now on the market; however, their long-term effects are not known.

3. Coffee intake.

a. Some human studies have associated high coffee intake and incidence of pancreatic cancer, whereas others do not substantiate these findings.

b. No studies to date have associated caffeine intake and cancer incidence.

c. Without conclusive data, recommendations cannot be made regarding coffee and caffeine consumption.

MINIMIZATION OF EXPOSURE TO CARCINOGENS

A. Avoid smoking.

1. Smoking is thought to be responsible for 75% of all lung cancers in the United States and is associated with the incidence of cancers of the head and neck, esophagus, pancreas, kidney, and bladder.

2. Smoking history must be assessed during the health history, and data must include years smoked, number of cigarettes smoked per day, and depth of inhalation.

3. Smoking low tar and nicotine cigarettes may decrease the hazard of smoking only slightly, since the chemicals contained within these brands may also be hazardous.

4. Smoking combined with alcohol, asbestos, and radiation exposure produces a synergistic effect in terms of cancer risk, and the incidence rate dramatically increases.

5. Passive smokers (nonsmokers exposed to cigarette smoke on a regular basis) may also be at higher risk for cancer development.

6. Antismoking campaigns and support groups are necessary to help smokers stop smoking.

B. Avoid oral tobacco use.

1. Studies from India and the United States indicate a high incidence of oral cancer among oral tobacco users.

2. The use of oral tobacco is rising among U.S. teenagers, which may lead to a future rise in oral cancer incidence.

3. Education of the public and health professionals regarding the hazards of oral tobacco use is necessary, along with programs to aid people in stopping oral tobacco use.

C. Avoid exposure to fibers.

1. Avoid asbestos exposure.

a. Individuals exposed to asbestos fibers have a higher incidence of mesotheliomas of the lung pleura and abdominal peritoneum.

b. The combination of asbestos exposure and smoking multiplies the hazardous effects of these carcinogens in the body.

c. Asbestos fibers can be found in products used for fireproofing, insulating, soundproofing, and decorating, as well as in piping, brake linings, and protective clothing.

        d. Enforcement of work safety regulations, which include the use of masks, respirators, coveralls, gloves, etc., are mandatory for protection.

   2. Avoid dust exposure.

        a. Workers in the furniture industry, shoe and boot industry, and woodworking industry are exposed to large quantities of dust in their workplace, which increases risk of cancer of the nasal cavity.

        b. Institution of and compliance with protective safety regulations in these industries are essential.

D. Avoid chemical exposure.

   1. Avoid exposure to arsenical pesticides and insecticides.

      Arsenic has been identified as a chemical agent associated with increased incidence of lung, skin, and possibly breast cancers.

   2. Avoid exposure to chromium.

      Chromium workers worldwide have higher incidence rates of cancers of the lung, nasal cavity, and larynx.

   3. Avoid exposure to nickel.

      Workers in the nickel industry show a higher incidence rate of cancers of the nasal cavity, paranasal sinuses, and lungs. Smoking acts synergistically with nickel exposure in these individuals.

   4. Avoid exposure to Bis (Chloromethyl) ether.

      Factory workers exposed to ether, even in low concentrations, have displayed high rates of lung cancer.

   5. Avoid exposure to vinyl chloride.

      Exposure to vinyl chloride has been associated with cancer of the skin, bones, lungs, and breast and with lymphomas and melanomas in animals. Angiosarcomas of the liver in humans have been associated with vinyl chloride exposure, and increased incidence is expected to continue.

   6. Avoid exposure to aromatic hydrocarbons.

      Steel industry workers are exposed to hydrocarbons in coal and petroleum soot, the byproducts of undercombustion of coal, wood, and oil, and pitch and tar residues. This exposure has been associated with an increased incidence in lung cancer.

   7. Avoid exposure to benzpyrene.

      Benzpyrene found in soot and coal tar, shale oil, and petroleum oil has been implicated in the incidence of cancers of the skin, lungs, bladder, and scrotum.

   8. Avoid exposure to aromatic amines.

      Aromatic amines are a group of chemicals used in the dye, rubber, and leather industries. The most common and hazardous of the amines include 2-Naphthylamine, benzidine, 1-naphthglamine, and 4-aminobiphenyl. All have been implicated in the incidence of bladder cancer.

   9. Avoid benzene exposure.

      The industrial chemical benzene used as a solvent and fuel has been associated with leukemias and aplastic anemias among exposed individuals.

   10. Avoid exposure to cytotoxic chemicals.

        a. Patients who have received cytotoxic drugs, especially the alkylating agents, display a higher incidence of cancer of the bladder and leukemias.

b. Health care personnel exposed to these agents during preparation, administration, and disposal must follow environmental safety precautions to prevent the inhalation, ingestion, and skin absorption of these agents.

11. Avoid estrogen use.

    a. Estrogens have been implicated in cancer development when used in three groups of women: post-menopausal women, women taking oral contraceptives, and women with threatened abortions.

    b. Post-menopausal women who are prescribed estrogen replacement therapy may possibly have an increased risk of endometrial cancer; however, data remain inconclusive.

    c. Data also remain inconclusive regarding estrogen use in oral contraceptives. Some research indicates a higher risk in these women for liver and breast tumors. Benefit versus risk ratio remains unclear.

    d. Large doses of diethylstilbestrol (DES), prescribed to stop threatened abortions, have been implicated in a high incidence of clear cell adenocarcinoma of the vagina in daughters of women who take the drug.

E. Avoid radiation exposure.

1. Most information regarding the effects of radiation exposure comes from the survivors of the atomic bombing of Hiroshima and those living near nuclear testing sites. A higher incidence of leukemia has been found among these individuals.

2. Ionizing radiation exposure to patients and medical staff can also occur with diagnostic procedures utilizing x-rays and radiation therapy for such conditions as ankylosing spondylitis and thymus enlargement. Increased incidence of cancers of the thyroid and liver and increased evidence of leukemia result. Bone cancer increases have also been found among radium watch dial painters.

3. Protection and minimization of exposure to ionizing radiation is imperative. Hazards can be reduced if medical personnel use discretion in ordering diagnostic tests and radiation treatments, and if exposed individuals receive frequent monitoring.

4. Health care professionals exposed to radiation in their occupational environment need to take safety precautions to ensure minimal exposure.

F. Avoid excessive exposure to sunlight.

1. The leading cause of all types of skin cancer is sunlight exposure. Skin cancers occur more frequently in areas where the sun shines longer and exposure is greater. Skin cancers occur more frequently among fair-skinned, blue- and green-eyed individuals. Skin cancers are also more prevalent among those who are exposed to sunlight frequently such as farmers, sunbathers, and construction workers.

2. Avoidance of overexposure to sunlight is recommended for all individuals, especially those more prone to skin damage. Individuals may also reduce the ultraviolet radiation from sunlight by reducing their exposure during the hours of 10 AM to 2 PM daily, when 60% of these rays reach the earth's surface. Protection from harmful effects of sunlight exposure can be achieved by using a protective sun screen whenever prolonged sun exposure is expected.

REST AND EXERCISE PATTERNS

A. Psychological benefits of exercise.
 1. Induces relaxation.
 2. Serves as release for mental strain.
 3. Relieves tension and anxiety.
 4. Aids in restful sleep.
 5. Increases sense of self-sufficiency.
 6. Enhances self concept.
 7. Reduces depression.
 8. Increases mental clarity.
B. Physiologic benefits.
 1. Establishes and maintains adequate muscle tone.
   a. Important for adequate blood flow.
   b. Strengthens heart muscle, which decreases resting heart rate and increases efficiency of heart muscle.
   c. Tones and strengthens diaphragm, which is essential for adequate ventilatory patterns.
 2. Aids in digestive processes of gastrointestinal system.
 3. Aids in appetite control, which is necessary to reduce obesity.
 4. Aids in the utilization of stored fat, thereby decreasing obesity.
 5. Enhances gaseous exchange in lungs, enhances efficiency of lung tissue.
C. Relationship of exercise, stress, and cancer incidence.
 1. Chronic stress has been associated with reduced efficacy of the immune system, which is responsible for the destruction of malignant cells as they develop.
 2. Regular exercise provides an outlet to channel stress and anxiety and may stimulate the function of the body's immune system, thus enhancing the recognition and destruction of malignancies.
 3. Animal studies indicate decreased tumor growth in laboratory animals regularly exercised as opposed to animals that are not exercised.
D. Recommendations for exercise patterns.
 1. No exercise programs should be initiated without physical examination by a qualified physician; special attention should be given to any existing physical limitations.
 2. Regular exercise programs, when physically appropriate, should be initiated and utilized on a continual basis. Utilizing an exercise "buddy system" helps to ensure regular participation of program members.
 3. Aerobic exercise (which utilizes oxygen) is recommended over anaerobic exercise (which does not utilize oxygen), since only aerobic exercise burns away fat stores and helps to reduce obesity.
E. Rest, relaxation and recreation as wellness-promoting factors.
 1. Time set aside for daily rest and recreation is essential.
 2. True relaxation exists when the body is in a state of restfulness, with a resulting decrease in pulse, respiratory rate, and brain wave activity.
 3. True rest interrupts the stress response and allows stress levels to return to normal. Similarly, recreation should enhance relaxation and should increase the energy level in order to be beneficial.
 4. Use of relaxation techniques, guided imagery, and meditation all counter the stimulation of the sympathetic nervous system resulting from stress and enhance wellness within the body.

METHODS TO FACILITATE COPING

A. Stress and health.
   1. Individuals try to maintain a steady state of equilibrium (homeostasis) in their internal and external environments.
   2. Stressors, which can be physical, psychological, or social, upset this equilibrium and require responses from the organism to restore homeostasis.
   3. The General Adaptation Syndrome (GAS) for stress adaptation is as follows:
      a. The Alarm Reaction—The organism reacts to a stressor. Resistance to stressors is lowered, and if the stressor is severe enough, death can result before adaptation can occur.
      b. Stage of Resistance—The organism begins adapting to a stressor through defense activation; resistance is higher. The length of this stage is variable and depends on the organic level of adaptability and severity of the stressor involved.
      c. Stage of Exhaustion—The organism is no longer able to adapt, energy sources are depleted, the alarm reaction repeats without resolution, death ensues.
   4. The GAS indicates that organisms have finite adaptational energies; when under prolonged stress, the organism may wear down, organ systems may fail to function, and diseases may result—including cancers.
   5. Should the organism's immune system, which thwarts cancer development, wear down and fail to function secondarily to exhaustion from stressors, neoplasia can theoretically occur.
   6. Some psychosocial stressors are thought to be contributing factors in cancer development. These include:
      a. Severe emotional disturbance in childhood with resultant feelings of isolation, loneliness, rejection, and the need to win affection.
      b. Strong career or interpersonal involvement in early adulthood with repression of true feelings of lowered self-esteem.
      c. A breakdown in career or interpersonal relationship brings about a return of feelings of isolation, loneliness, rejection, and despair (cancer incidence increases feelings of despair).
   7. Despite the existing controversy regarding emotions, stress, and cancer incidence, preventive measures aimed at facilitating coping mechanisms may be necessary.
   8. Coping mechanisms to reduce stress responses include:
      a. Improve problem-solving and decision-making skills.
      b. Utilize psychological defense mechanisms appropriately.
      c. Maintain sound health practices, such as:
         (1) Adequate diet.
         (2) Adequate sleep.
         (3) Avoid alcohol and drug abuse.
         (4) Adequate exercise.
         (5) Adequate recreation.
      d. Utilize introspection to develop a sense of self-awareness.
      e. Utilize self-disclosure to communicate feelings and concerns with others and minimize distress.
      f. Utilize self-regulating modalities such as relaxation techniques, bio-

feedback, self-hypnosis, meditation, and guided imagery to reduce stressors and enhance coping.
  g. Utilize professional counseling services when necessary to aid in resolution of emotional conflict.

NURSING ROLE

A. Assessment of:
  1. Weight patterns.
  2. Dietary patterns.
  3. Alcohol consumption.
  4. Tobacco use (smoking and oral use).
  5. Fiber exposure (asbestos, dust).
  6. Chemical exposure.
  7. Hormone use.
  8. Radiation exposure.
  9. Sunlight exposure.
  10. Sleep/rest pattern.
  11. Physical exercise/recreation patterns.
  12. Coping skills.
B. Educational responsibilities.
  1. Public education—primary role of health care professionals.
    a. Collaboration with existing organizations such as the Public Education Committee of the American Cancer Society, the American Lung Association, and the National Cancer Institute Office of Communications provides opportunities to address public audiences for dissemination of cancer prevention information.
    b. Incorporation of cancer prevention teaching into daily nursing practice is essential.
  2. Professional education.
    a. Health care professionals need to remain current regarding changes in recommendations for cancer prevention.
    b. Collaboration with the Professional Education Committee of the American Cancer Society aids in dissemination of current information to health care professionals.
    c. Involvement with professional nursing organizations such as the Oncology Nursing Society (ONS) aids in supporting the education and networking systems of oncology nurses.
C. Outcomes of nursing interventions.
  1. Utilization of cancer prevention information to bring about lifestyle/habit changes is very complex.
  2. In order to drastically change lifestyles, individuals must:
    a. Possess knowledge of a personal susceptibility to an illness.
    b. Perceive the risk to be great.
    c. Believe that the lifestyle change will alter their risk of illness.
  3. Nurses must provide factual information to assist individuals who desire change, without imposing their own value systems on those individuals not accepting change.
D. Consumer responsibilities.
  1. Knowledgeable oncology nurses should be active in social and political

decision-making regarding health care issues that impact on cancer prevention.
2. As individuals, our own lifestyle and habit choices serve as role models for others.

STUDY QUESTIONS

1. What dietary recommendations aid in the prevention of cancer?
2. What physical agents are thought to be carcinogenic?
3. What chemical agents are thought to be carcinogenic?
4. Describe the psychological and physical benefits of exercise.

Bibliography

American Cancer Society: Special Report. Nutrition and cancer: Cause and prevention. New York, American Cancer Society, 1984.

Bailey, J. T.: Taking charge of your stress and well-being. *In* Claus, K. E. and Bailey, J. T. (eds.): Living With Stress and Promoting Well-Being. St. Louis, C.V. Mosby Co., pp. 61–70, 1980.

Diekelmann, N.: Primary Health Care of the Well Adult. New York, McGraw-Hill Book Co., 1977.

Johnson, B. L.: Prevention and early detection. *In* Johnson, B. L. and Gross, J. (eds.): Handbook of Oncology Nursing. New York, Wiley & Sons, pp. 93–114, 1985.

Loescher, L. J. and Sauer, K. A.: Vitamin therapy for advanced cancers. Oncology Nursing Forum, *11*(6):38–45, 1984.

Lowenfels, A. B. and Anderson, M. E.: Diet and cancer. Cancer, *39*:1809–1814, 1977.

McNaull, F. W.: Carcinogenic agents in the environment. *In* McIntire, S. N. and Cioppa, A. L. (eds.): Cancer Nursing: A Developmental Approach. New York, Wiley & Sons, pp. 536–556, 1984.

Nevidjon, B. M.: Cancer and stress. *In* McIntire, S. N. and Cioppa, A. L. (eds.): Cancer Nursing: A Developmental Approach. New York, Wiley & Sons, pp. 557–571, 1984.

Patrick, P. K. S.: Burnout: Antecedents, manifestations, and self-care strategies for the nurse. *In* Marino, L. B. (ed.): Cancer Nursing. St. Louis, C.V. Mosby Co., pp. 113–135, 1981.

Selye, H.: Stress and a holistic view of health for the nursing profession. *In* Claus, K. E. and Bailey, J. T. (eds.): Living With Stress and Promoting Well-Being. St. Louis, C.V. Mosby Co., pp. 125–136, 1980.

Simonton, O. C., Matthews-Simonton, S. and Creighton, J.: Getting Well Again. New York, Bantam Books, 1978.

Squirer, C. A.: Smokeless tobacco and oral cancer: A cause for concern? Ca-A Cancer Journal for Clinicians, *34*(5):5–10, 1984.

Tauraso, N. M.: How to Benefit From Stress. Fredrick, Maryland, Hidden Valley Press, 1979.

Weisburger, J. H.: Mechanism of action of diet as a carcinogen. Cancer, *43*:1987–1995, 1979.

Wynder, E. L.: Dietary habits and cancer epidemiology. Cancer, *43*:1955–1961, 1979.

10

Early Detection Measures

AMY VALENTINE, RN, MS

RISK ASSESSMENT

A. Definition: evaluation or appraisal of an individual's or group's health status or potential for cancer.
B. Identification of risk—related directly and indirectly to lifestyle, environmental and hereditary factors, previous history of illness and injury.
C. Risk factors:
   1. Do not assure disease.
   2. Alert individuals to potential for disease.
   3. Alert individuals to factors that may be altered to reduce or eliminate potential for disease.
D. Risk factors for specific disease sites (Table 10–1).
E. Level of risk.
   1. Multiplicity of cancer occurrences increases risk.
   2. Persons at high risk require follow-up with appropriate precautionary techniques, preventive activities, and screening modalities.
F. Nursing role.
   1. Education of individuals and the public about smoking cessation, limiting alcohol intake, dietary modification, weight control, sexual practices, and limiting sun exposure.
   2. Education of high risk groups about appropriate screening tests and diagnostic procedures in their risk category.
   3. Participation in creating a safe and healthy environment in which to live and work.

SCREENING AND PREVENTION METHODS

A. Health history and physical assessment should be the initial and most vital screening tool for all cancer sites, and for identification of an individual's risk. The history and physical should:
   1. Be obtained from every person.
   2. Be complete, accurate, and documented.

Table 10–1. RISK FACTORS FOR SPECIFIC CANCER SITES

Risk Factors	Cancer Sites
Occupational exposure	Head and neck, lung
Nickel, chromium, radioisotopes, petroleum chemicals, asbestos, arsenic	
Previous history of illness, injury, irritation	
Ill-fitting dentures	Oropharynx
Chronic dermatitis, burn scars	Skin
Familial polyposis	Colon and rectum
Ulcerative colitis	Colon and rectum
Fibrocystic disease	Breast
Dyplasia of breast	Breast
Maldescent of testicle	Testicle
Herpes Type II infection	Cervix
Hormonal irregularities	Endometrium
Behaviors/Life Style	
Smoking	Lung
Chewing tobacco, snuff	Head and neck
Heavy alcohol consumption	Head and neck
Excessive sun exposure	Skin
Obesity	Endometrium
Multiple sexual partners	Cervix
Early age of coitus	Cervix
Familial history	Breast, Colon
Dietary	
High fat, low fiber	Colon and rectum
High fat	Breast, prostate
Environmental	
Air pollution	Lung
Wood smoke	Head and neck
Residence in sunbelt areas, and exposure to sun for extended periods of time	Skin

   3. Take into account all body systems, present complaint, past, personal and family history, as well as cultural, social, and economic factors.
   4. Use risk factors identified to guide further screening, testing, and establishment of suggested prevention practices.

B. Screening methods.
   1. The use of screening tests on asymptomatic populations is controversial. The epidemiologic validity, reliability, and yield of a test depend on the sensitivity of the test, the extent of screening previously done, and the degree to which the person willingly participates.
   2. Screening modalities are not without risk. Radiation exposure with mammography is one example. For specific screening test information refer to Chapter 11.

C. Self-care practices for screening and prevention include:
   1. Breast self-examination (BSE).
   2. Periodic testicular self-examination (TSE).
   3. Good personal hygiene.
   4. Skin inspection.
   5. Limiting alcohol intake.
   6. Smoking cessation.
   7. Weight control.

8. Dietary modification to limit fats and increase fiber.
9. Minimizing exposure to carcinogens in the work setting by compliance with safety standards.

D. American Cancer Society (ACS) guidelines for screening and detection (Table 10–2).

E. Methods to enhance prevention.
1. Identification of and follow-up surveillance of high-risk individuals or groups.
2. Establishment of environmental safety standards and regulation of exposure to hazardous substances.
3. Establishment of programs to inform individuals and groups of risk and precautions.

F. Nursing role in prevention.
1. Increasing skills in history-taking, physical examination, teaching, and counseling.
2. Role modeling good health practices.
3. Educating individuals and groups regarding:
   a. Health behaviors and attitudes to increase prevention.
   b. Importance of and methods of self-examination (BSE, TSE, skin, oral).
   c. Preventive and screening methods available for the high-risk individuals.
4. Incorporation of American Cancer Society guidelines into all health teaching and the clinical practice setting.

STUDY QUESTIONS

1. List three activities a nurse can do in daily practice to encourage early detection and prevention of cancer.
2. Describe individual health practices a person can do to detect skin, head and neck, and colon and rectum cancer.

Table 10–2. AMERICAN CANCER SOCIETY'S GUIDELINES FOR CANCER RELATED CHECKUPS

Test	Age	Recommendation
Papanicolaou test	Over 20; under 20 if sexually active	Every 3 yr after two initial negative tests 1 yr apart
Pelvic examination	20–40	Every 3 yr
	Over 40 or at menopause	Yearly
Endometrial tissue sample	At menopause if high risk	High risk: history of infertility, obesity, failure of ovulation, abnormal uterine bleeding, estrogen therapy
Breast self-examination	Over 20	Monthly
Breast physical examination	20–40	Every 3 yr
Mammogram	35–40	One baseline mammogram
	40–50	Every 1–2 yr
	Over 50	Yearly
Stool guiac slide test	Over 50	Yearly
Digital rectal examination	Over 50	Yearly
Sigmoidoscopic examination	Over 50	Every 3–5 yr after two initial negative examinations 1 yr apart

Bibliography

Behnam-Kahn, S. (ed.): Concepts in Cancer Medicine. New York, Grune and Stratton, 1983.

Faulkenberry, J.: Cancer prevention and detection: Lung cancer. Cancer Nursing, 8(3):185–194, 1985.

Faulkenberry, J.: Cancer prevention and detection: Colorectal cancer. Cancer Nursing, 7(5):415–424, 1984.

Frank Stromborg, M.: Nursing's contribution to case findings and the early detection of cancer. In Marionnno, L. (ed.): Cancer Nursing. St. Louis, C. V. Mosby Co., 1981.

Nash, J.: Cancer prevention and detection: Breast cancer. Cancer Nursing, 7(2):163–178, 1984.

Sandella, J.: Cancer prevention and detection: Testicular cancer. Cancer Nursing, 6(6):468–486, 1983.

Sandella, J.: Ovarian cancer. Cancer Nursing, 8(1):63–75, 1985.

Schottenfeld, D. and Fraumeni, J.: Cancer Epidemiology and Prevention. Philadelphia, W. B. Saunders Company, 1982.

White, L.: Cancer prevention and detection: Cervical cancer. Cancer Nursing, 7(4):335–345, 1984.

SECTION FOUR

Diagnosis and Staging of Cancer

Section Editor
ROBERTA STROHL, RN, MN

11

Assessing and Diagnosing Cancer

MARILYN DAVIS, RN, MS, OCN

HISTORY

A. Comprehensive data base.
1. Individual identification: Name, age, sex, race, date and place of birth, occupation, religion, next of kin, insurance coverage, referral.
2. Principal problem: brief quote in patient's or informant's own words.
3. Development of principal and pertinent secondary problems covering:
   a. Severity: location, quality, and quantity of symptom.
   b. Temporality: onset, duration, frequency, precipitators.
   c. Other: alleviating or aggravating factors.
   d. Preconceptions: what patient thinks may be going on.
4. Previous state of health:
   a. Illness.
   b. Injuries.
   c. Hospitalizations.
   d. Surgical procedures.
5. Allergies.
6. Present state of health and health practices. For the following categories, ask the patient to describe a typical 24 hour period of time.
   a. Prescription and over the counter medication pattern.
   b. Food and fluid intake.
   c. Sleep/work cycle.
   d. Elimination pattern.
   e. Habits—exercise, consumption of caffeine, alcohol, tobacco products.
7. Family medical history.
   a. State of health of immediate family members—parents, grandparents, siblings, children.
   b. If deceased, cause of death.

    c. If diagnosis of cancer in an immediate family member, specify site and outcome.

B. General review of systems.
  1. Weight—present weight, usual weight.
  2. Performance status—present level of activity, usual level of activity, weakness, fatigue, malaise.
  3. Skin and mucus membranes—color, integrity, turgor, edema, persistence of slow-growing lesions, new moles, changes in old moles, scaly patches, color of nailbeds, clubbing.
  4. Neurologic function—headache, seizures, visual disturbances, syncope, vertigo, sensory deficits.
  5. Head and neck—difficulty chewing, dysphagia, local pain, tenderness, swelling, hoarseness, otalgia, odynophagia, nasal discharge, asymmetry, adenopathy.
  6. Respiratory tract—new or persistent productive or nonproductive cough, hemoptysis, chest wall pain, dyspnea on exertion, shortness of breath.
  7. Breasts—lumps, discharge, tenderness, skin changes, axillary adenopathy, gynecomastia (male), pattern of self examination, date and result of mammogram.
  8. Cardiac function—hypertension, dyspnea, orthopnea, chest pain.
  9. Gastrointestinal tract—anorexia, early satiety, abdominal pain, nausea, vomiting, hematemesis, change in bowel pattern, melana, tenesmus, date and result of hemeoccult stool test.
  10. Gynecologic system—vaginal discharge, abnormal vaginal bleeding, pelvic pain, abdominal enlargement, date and result of Pap test, pattern of menses.
  11. Urinary tract and bladder—frequency, hesitancy, urgency, dysuria, hematuria, pelvic or flank pain or mass.
  12. Male genitalia—enlargement of testis, pain, external genitalia lesion(s), pattern of testicular self examination, date of most recent digital rectal examination of prostate.
  13. Musculoskeletal system—swelling, enlargement, pain, stiffness, redness, limitation of movement.
  14. Endocrine system—sweating, tachycardia, palpitations, flushing.
  15. Hematologic system—fever, sweating, painless lymphadenopathy, pruritus, bruising, anemia, petechia, purpura.
  16. *Note:* The degree to which the nurse performs the physical assessment depends on the practice setting and her/his skills.

PHYSICAL AND DIAGNOSTIC EXAMINATIONS

    Table 11–1 lists selected laboratory tests used in the diagnosis, management, and follow-up of cancer.

A. Skin.
  1. Inspection and assessment—color, warmth, moisture, integrity, turgor, edema.
    a. Lesions—type, size, location, distribution.
      (1) Moles—change in color, size, shape, sensation, or bleeding. Inspect soles of feet, axillae, scalp, interdigital webs, mucus mem-

Text continued on page 79

Table 11–1. SELECTED LABORATORY TESTS IN THE DIAGNOSIS, MANAGEMENT, AND FOLLOW-UP OF CANCER

In general, an isolated normal, elevated, or decreased laboratory value is not an absolute in the diagnosis and management of a specific malignancy. Rather, laboratory values add to the clinical diagnostic, management, and evaluative process. Institutional reference ranges may vary significantly with different methods and standardization modes.

Name	Specimen and Reference Range	Clinical Information*	Comments
Tumor Markers			
Acid phosphatase	Serum Total Males: 2.5–11.7 μ/L Females: 0.3–9.2 μ/L	↑ in prostatic cancer (↑ in 5% with tumor confined to prostate gland, 20% with regional extension of tumor and 80% with bone metastases)	In males, 50% of acid phosphatase is prostatic. Remainder is from liver, disintegrating platelets, and erythrocytes.
	Tartrate: Inhibited Fraction Males: 0.2–3.5 μ/L Females: 0–0.8 μ/L	↑ some primary bone malignancies, multiple myeloma	Transient rise possible after transurethral resection of prostate or biopsy. Generally not influenced by digital prostate examination. Usually falls within several weeks of institution of successful hormonal manipulation in advanced prostate cancer.
Alkaline phosphatase	Serum Adult: 4–13 μ/100 ml (King-Armstrong) 1.5–4.5 μ/100 ml (Bodawsky) 0.8–2.3 μ/100 ml (Bessey-Lowry)	↑ in metastatic cancer to bone and liver, osteogenic sarcoma, myeloma, and Hodgkin's lymphoma with bone involvement	May also be elevated in conditions of increased bone metabolism such as healing fractures, renal disease, and liver disease
Alpha Fetoprotein (AFP)	Serum <30 ng/ml	↑ in 70% of hepatocellular cancers, in choriocarcinoma, teratoma, embryonal cell tumors of testis and ovary, some pancreatic, stomach, colon, and lung tumors. Not in pure seminomas without teratomatous component	Oncofetal protein synthesized in the liver. Useful in monitoring tumor response to treatment.
Carcinoembryonic Antigen (CEA)	Plasma Nonsmokers: 0–5 ng/ml Smokers: 0–10 ng/ml	↑ in 70% of colon cancers. Also seen in lung, pancreas, stomach, breast, head and neck, and prostate malignancies. ↑ in 20% of heavy smokers	Helpful in monitoring response to therapy or indicating disease recurrence.
Chorionic Gonadatropin (beta subunit) (β-HCG)	Serum or Plasma Males and nonpregnant females: <5.0 IU/L	↑ in a hydatidiform mole, choriocarcinoma, testicular teratoma, ectopic HCG production by some cancers of the pituitary gland, stomach, pancreas, lung, colon, and liver	Serial determinations helpful in monitoring response to treatment or early detection of recurrence.

Table continued on following page

Table 11–1. SELECTED LABORATORY TESTS IN THE DIAGNOSIS, MANAGEMENT, AND FOLLOW-UP OF CANCER (*continued*)

In general, an isolated normal, elevated, or decreased laboratory value is not an absolute in the diagnosis and management of a specific malignancy. Rather, laboratory values add to the clinical diagnostic, management, and evaluative process. Institutional reference ranges may vary significantly with different methods and standardization modes.

Name	Specimen and Reference Range	Clinical Information*	Comments
Tumor Markers (continued)			
Pancreatic Oncofetal Antigen (POA)	Serum	Positive in large percentage of pancreas tumors.	
Placental alkaline phosphatase (PAP)	Serum (Regan Isoenzyme)	↑ in a variety of tumors only half of which demonstrate ↑ serum alkaline phosphatase. ↑ in 40% of seminomas	Ectopic synthesis may be of value in monitoring tumor response to treatment.
Hormones			
Adrenocorticotropic Hormone (ACTH)	Plasma Highest in morning; lowest at bedtime.	↑ in ectopic ACTH-producing tumors (lung, particularly small cell), adrenal carcinoma, adenoma	Paraneoplastic syndrome usually accompanied by hypokalemia, hyperglycemia, lethargy, confusion, nausea and vomiting with absence of classic Cushing's syndrome manifestations.
Androstendione	Serum Male: 107 ± 25 ng/dl Female: 151 ± 38 ng/dl	↑ in ectopic ACTH-producing tumors, ovarian tumors	Produced in adrenals and gonads. Precursor in biosynthesis of androgens and estrogens.
Antidiuretic Hormone (ADH)	Plasma	↑ in brain tumors (primary or secondary). ↑ in systemic malignancies with ectopic ADH production	Inappropriate secretion of ADH is paraneoplastic syndrome, occurring most frequently in small cell carcinoma of lung. Hyponatremia in the presence of excessive urinary sodium is generally found.
Calcitonin	Fasting Serum or Plasma Male: <100 pq/ml Female: <25 pq/ml	↑ in medullary carcinoma of the thyroid, some lung and breast tumors, carcinoids, colon cancer and GI malignancies	To confirm diagnosis of medullary carcinoma, calcium or pentagastric stimulation test performed.
Estrogens, Total	Serum Adult Male: 40–115 ng/L Adult Female: 61–350 ng/L	↑ in estrogen-producing ovarian tumors, some testicular tumors and adrenal cortical tumors	
Estrogen (Estradiol) Receptor Assay	0.5–1.0 gram of tissue Negative: <3.0 fmol/mg protein Borderline: 3–10 fmol/mg protein Positive: >10 fmol/mg protein	60% of breast cancers are characterized by estrogen receptors	Useful for identifying breast tumors most likely to respond to endocrine manipulation.

Table 11–1. SELECTED LABORATORY TESTS IN THE DIAGNOSIS, MANAGEMENT, AND FOLLOW-UP OF CANCER (*continued*)

In general, an isolated normal, elevated, or decreased laboratory value is not an absolute in the diagnosis and management of a specific malignancy. Rather, laboratory values add to the clinical diagnostic, management, and evaluative process. Institutional reference ranges may vary significantly with different methods and standardization modes.

Name	Specimen and Reference Range	Clinical Information*	Comments
Hormones (continued)			
Glucagon	Plasma	↓ in some pancreatic neoplasms	
Growth Hormone (hGH)	Serum or Plasma Male: <2 ng/ml Female: <10 ng/ml	↑ in ectopic secretion by some stomach and lung tumors	
Parathyroid Hormone (hPTH)	Fasting Serum	↑ squamous cell or epidermoid lung cancers and renal cell producing an ectopic hyperparathyroidism	Ectopic tumor produces PTH. May be associated with hypercalcemia.
Progesterone	Serum Male: 0.12–0.3 ng/ml Nonpregnant Female: 0–30 ng/ml	↑ in some ovarian tumors, molar pregnancy	
Progesterone Receptor Assay	1 Gram of tissue Normal: ≤5 fmol/mg protein Positive: >10 fmol/mg protein		May be useful in predicting tumors likely to respond to endocrine manipulation.
17 Ketogenic Steroids	24 hour acidified urine Male: 5–23 mg/d Female: 3–15 mg/d	↑ in adrenal adenoma and carcinoma, ectopic ACTH syndrome	
17 Keto-steroids	24 hour urine Male: 8–22 Female: 6–15	↑ in adrenal tumors, testicular tumors, interstitial cell tumors, androgenic ovarian tumors	
Testosterone	Serum Adult Male: 572 ± 135 ng/dl Nonpregnant Females: 37 ± 10 ng/dl	↑ some adrenocortical tumors, gonadotropin-producing extragonadal tumors	Fall to castration level following adequate hormonal manipulation in advanced prostatic cancer.
Blood Chemistries			
Calcium	Fasting Serum Adult: 8.4–10.2 mg/dl	↑ in 9% of malignancies with bone involvement (mainly breast, lung, and kidney). Also in multiple myeloma, lymphomas, leukemias, squamous cell carcinoma of the lung, cancer of the kidney, esophagus, pancreas, liver, and bladder	Hypercalcemia occurs in about 10% of patients with cancer, some of whom will have no bony involvement.
Cholesterol	Serum, Plasma Fasting ≥12 hrs. Adults: 140–310 mg/dl	↓ in 16% of malignancies with bone involvement. ↑ in some prostatic, liver, and pancreatic malignancies	

Table continued on following page

Table 11–1. SELECTED LABORATORY TESTS IN THE DIAGNOSIS, MANAGEMENT, AND FOLLOW-UP OF CANCER (*continued*)

In general, an isolated normal, elevated, or decreased laboratory value is not an absolute in the diagnosis and management of a specific malignancy. Rather, laboratory values add to the clinical diagnostic, management, and evaluative process. Institutional reference ranges may vary significantly with different methods and standardization modes.

Name	Specimen and Reference Range	Clinical Information*	Comments
Blood Chemistries (*continued*)			
Ferritin	Serum Male: 15–200 mg/dl Female: 12–150 mg/dl	↑ in acute myeloblastic and lymphoblastic leukemias, some Hodgkin's lymphomas, and breast cancers	Main iron storage protein in body.
Glucose	Serum Adult: 70–105 mg/dl	↑ in pheochromocytoma, glucogonama; pancreatic malignancies. May be ↑ in presence of islet cell tumor, carcinoma of the adrenal gland, and stomach, and fibrosarcoma	
Uric Acid	Serum Male: 4.2–8 mg/dl Female: 3.2–7.3 mg/dl	↑ in some disseminated malignancies. ↓ in some neoplasms including Hodgkin's lymphoma, multiple myloma, and bronchogenic carcinoma	Monitor while on cytotoxic therapy.
Enzymes			
Amylase	Serum Adult: 56–190 IU/L	↑ in some lung and ovarian tumors	
Amylase Isoenzymes	Serum	↑ in some bronchogenic or serous ovarian tumors	
Lactic Dehydrogenase (LDH) and LDH isoenzymes	Serum Ranges are highly method-dependent, i.e.: 1. Pyruvate to lactate (210–420) 2. Lactate to pyruvate (45–90)	↑ in extensive carcinomatosis and malignant processes (about 50% of cancer patients have alterations in LDH patterns). ↑ in 90% of patients with acute leukemia	LD I helpful when elevated in nonseminanatous germ cell tumors of the testis. LD II, LD III, and LD IV. With massive platelet destruction and in lymphomas and lymphocytic leukemias LD IV may be ↑ in carcinoma of the prostate.
Leucine Aminopeptidase (LAP)	Serum 14–4 U/L	↑ in 60% of patients with pancreatic carcinoma with liver metastases	
Lysozyme	Serum 4.0–13.0 mg/L	↑ in acute monocytic or myelomonocytic leukemia and chronic myeloid leukemia	

Table 11–1. SELECTED LABORATORY TESTS IN THE DIAGNOSIS, MANAGEMENT, AND FOLLOW-UP OF CANCER (*continued*)

In general, an isolated normal, elevated, or decreased laboratory value is not an absolute in the diagnosis and management of a specific malignancy. Rather, laboratory values add to the clinical diagnostic, management, and evaluative process. Institutional reference ranges may vary significantly with different methods and standardization modes.

Name	Specimen and Reference Range	Clinical Information*	Comments
Enzymes (continued)			
Serum Gamma Glutamyl Transpeptidase (SGGT)	Serum Males: 6–37 mU/ml Females: 4–24 mU/ml	↑ in some cases of renal cell carcinoma and liver metastases	Elevation may precede findings on liver scan.
Serum Glutamic Oxaloacetic Transaminase (SGOT)	Serum Adult: 5–40 U/ml	↑ in about 50% of patients with liver metastases or infiltration	
Serum Glutamic Pyruvic transaminase (SGPT)	Serum Adult: 5–35 U/ml	↑ in some liver carcinomas	
Proteins (Immunoglobulins are produced by lymphocytes and plasma cells. They are fractionated into major components by electrophoresis.)			
Immunoglobulin A (IgA)	Serum Adult: 60–330 mg/100 ml	Slight polyclonal ↑ in some malignancies of breast, and monoclonal ↑ in IgA myeloma	Approximately 15% of total immunoglobulins. Protects mucosal surfaces as first line of defense against microorganisms.
Immunoglobulin D (IgD)	Serum Adult: 0–15 mg/dl	Slight monoclonal ↑ in IgD myeloma	About 1% of immunoglobulins. Physiologic function unknown. May receive or differentiate on lymphocytic surfaces. 90% of multiple myelomas are of IgD type, and almost all patients will have Bence-Jones urinary proteins.
Immunoglobulin E (IgE)	Serum Adult: .01–.04 mg/100 ml	Slight monoclonal ↑ in IgE myeloma. Slight ↑ in certain advanced stage neoplasms	About 1% of immunoglobulins. Functions in severe allergic reactions.
Immunoglobulin G (IgG)	Serum Adult: 550–1900 mg/dl	Slight monoclonal ↑ in IgG myeloma	Accounts for 75% of total immunoglobulins. Produces antibodies to bacteria, fungi, viruses, and toxins. Occurs as second line immune response after IgM. Involved in passive immunization of the newborn.

Table continued on following page

Table 11–1. SELECTED LABORATORY TESTS IN THE DIAGNOSIS, MANAGEMENT, AND FOLLOW-UP OF CANCER (*continued*)

In general, an isolated normal, elevated, or decreased laboratory value is not an absolute in the diagnosis and management of a specific malignancy. Rather, laboratory values add to the clinical diagnostic, management, and evaluative process. Institutional reference ranges may vary significantly with different methods and standardization modes.

Name	Specimen and Reference Range	Clinical Information*	Comments
Proteins (continued)			
Immunoglobulin M (IgM)	Serum Adults: 45–145 mg/dl		Approximately 10% of immunoglobulins. First antibody to respond to bacteria and bacteria toxins.
Haptoglobin (Hp)	Serum Adult: 30–160/100 ml	May be ↑ in cancer, particularly with metastases, and in lymphomas	Produced by liver. Single result of limited value. Serial determinations suggested.
Hematology			
Leukocyte Count (White Blood Cell Count, WBC)	Whole Blood Adult Male: 3,900–10,600/ mm³ Adult Female: 3,500– 11,000/mm³	↑ in hematologic malignancies, and myeloproliferative disorders	Some expressions of leukemia show normal or ↓ WBC. Life span of leukocytes in peripheral circulation is 6–8 hours.
Differential Count	% of total WBC	↑ in a wide range of myeloproliferative disorders. May be ↑ in wide spread malignancies. ↓ in aplastic anemia, marrow replacement of tumor	Neutrophils active in phagocytosis.

Neutrophils
  Segmented
  Bands
	56%
	3%		

Lymphocytes	34%	↑ in lymphocytic leukemias. May be ↑ in Hodgkin's disease and malignancies	Antibody production.
Monocytes	4%	↑ in monocytic leukemia	Stimulate plasmacytes to produce immunoglobulins.
Eosinophils	2.5%	May be ↑ in chronic myelogenous leukemia, Hodgkin's disease, metastatic malignancies	Release granules of serotonin, histamine, and heparin. Allergic responses.
Basophils	0.5%	May be ↑ in chronic myelogenous leukemia, Hodgkin's disease	Control blood viscosity. Granules contain heparin.
Platelet Count	Whole Blood Adults: 150,000–400,000/ mm³	↑ myeloproliferative disorders. May be ↑ in advanced malignancies. May be ↓ in leukemias, tumors metastatic to bone marrow	Life span 6–10 days in peripheral circulation.

Table 11–1. SELECTED LABORATORY TESTS IN THE DIAGNOSIS,
MANAGEMENT, AND FOLLOW-UP OF CANCER (*continued*)

In general, an isolated normal, elevated, or decreased laboratory value is not an absolute in the diagnosis and management of a specific malignancy. Rather, laboratory values add to the clinical diagnostic, management, and evaluative process. Institutional reference ranges may vary significantly with different methods and standardization modes.

Name	Specimen and Reference Range	Clinical Information*	Comments
Hematology (continued)			
Hematocrit	Whole Blood Adult Males: 42–52% Adult Females: 37–47%	↑ in anemia associated with many malignant processes, leukemias	Erythrocyte life span approximately 120 days. Result may be falsely low if drawn in recumbent patient.
Hemoglobin	Whole Blood Adult Males: 13.5–17.5 gm/dl Adult Females: 12.0–16.0 gm/dl	↑ in anemia associated with many malignant processes, leukemias	Results may be falsely high in dehydration.

* ↑ = Elevated; ↓ = Decreased.

brane of skin surfaces, nail beds, in addition to face, neck, sun-exposed areas, trunk and extremities.
  (2) Purpura—petechia or ecchymosis.
  (3) Scaly patches or plaques.
  (4) Ulcerative or exophytic areas.
  b. Nails—color, clubbing.
2. Histologic confirmation—biopsy. (See Chapter 22.)
  a. Punch (large lesions).
  b. Incisional (large lesions).
  c. Excisional (small lesions).
B. Head and Neck.
  1. Inspection.
    a. Face—note any asymmetry at rest or with movement.
    b. Eyes—note:
      (1) Abnormal protrusion—unilateral or bilateral.
      (2) Scleral jaundice.
      (3) Lumps or swelling around eyes.
    c. Trachea—note:
      (1) Deviation from midline position.
      (2) Rise of larynx, trachea, and thyroid with swallowing.
  2. Palpation—tenderness, masses, nodules, enlargement.
    a. Frontal and maxillary sinuses.
    b. Nodes—presence of small, mobile, nontender nodes common; further examination is indicated if any node(s) enlarged, firm, or fixed.
      (1) Preauricular, posterior auricular, and occipital nodes drain the superficial facial and skull tissue.
      (2) Tonsillar, submental, and submaxillary nodes drain the mouth, throat, and lower facial tissues.

   (3) Cervical nodes (posterior, superficial, and deep) drain the oropharynx, nasopharynx, larynx, and superficial tissues.
   (4) Supraclavicular nodes drain regional superficial tissues as well as the abdomen, breast, thorax, and arms.
   c. Thyroid.
3. Digital examination of oral cavity and tongue.
4. Histologic confirmation by biopsy (thin needle or excisional).
   a. Indications:
      (1) Erythroplasia or leukoplakia of oral cavity.
      (2) Suspicious lesions of oral cavity, oropharynx, nasopharynx, larynx, hypopharynx, nasal cavity, paranasal sinuses, or salivary glands.
      (3) Biopsy of persistent, hard, fixed, or growing node if there is no evidence of primary tumor after triple endoscopy (nasopharyngoscopy, laryngoscopy, esophagoscopy) and radiologic work-up.
5. Laboratory investigations—CBC, chemistry profile.
6. Diagnostic procedures as clinically indicated—chest x-ray, radiographs of selected areas, CT scans or tomograms of regional area, sialogram (suspected parotid tumor), soft tissue xerogram, rhinoscopy, triple endoscopy, barium esophagram.
C. Thorax.
   1. Inspection.
      a. Rate and rhythm of breathing.
      b. Movement of chest—note abnormal retraction or bulging of interspaces or impairment of respiratory movement.
      c. Asymmetry.
   2. Palpation—tenderness, masses, cutaneous nodules, enlargements.
      a. Mediastinum.
      b. Breasts.
      c. Bilateral axillary nodes drain breasts and lungs.
      d. Supraclavicular and infraclavicular nodes drain the head, neck, and upper extremities.
   3. Percussion—note presence and location of abnormal percussion. Note:
      a. Resonance indicates an air-containing lung.
      b. Hyperresonance indicates an emphysematous lung.
      c. Dullness indicates fluid-filled or solid underlying tissue.
   4. Auscultation.
      a. Pitch, intensity, and duration.
      b. If alterations are heard, listen to the spoken voice; increased clarity suggests consolidated tissue.
      c. Breasts—check for symmetry at rest and with movement. Note the presence of:
         (1) Thickening, dimpling, or edema.
         (2) Nipple retraction, inversion, asymmetry, or discharge.
         (3) Venous prominence.
   5. Histologic confirmation.
      a. Lesions identified on a chest x-ray are investigated with serial sputum cytologies, transtracheal biopsy, bronchoscopy, mediastinoscopy, lung biopsy.
      b. Effusions are investigated with fluid cytology.

      c. Cutaneous or breast lesions are investigated with aspiration or excisional biopsy accompanied by hormone (estrogen and progesterone) receptor assays.

  6. Laboratory investigations—CBC, electrolyte, calcium, phosphorus, and alkaline phosphatase concentrations, and liver and renal function tests.

  7. Diagnostic procedures as clinically indicated—chest x-ray, CT scans or tomograms of regional area, bone scan, skeletal x-ray of suspicious areas, liver scan, mammogram, myelography, gallium scan.

D. Heart.

  1. Inspect anterior chest for thrills and heaves.

  2. Auscultation:
    a. Apical rate and rhythm.
    b. Note presence of abnormal heart sounds, murmurs.

  3. Arterial palpation—rate, rhythm, intensity:
    a. Carotid.
    b. Brachial.
    c. Femoral.
    d. Dorsalis pedis.

  4. Diagnostic procedures—EKG. Further laboratory and clinical investigations in event of baseline abnormalities.

  5. Laboratory investigations—CBC, electrolyte, calcium phosphorus, alkaline phosphatase levels, and liver and renal function tests.

  6. Diagnostic procedures as clinically indicated—chest x-ray, CT scans or tomograms of regional area, bone scan, skeletal x-ray of suspicious areas, liver scan mammogram, myelography, gallium scan.

E. Abdomen.

  1. Inspection—note:
    a. Dilated veins.
    b. Asymmetry.
    c. Organ enlargement.
    d. Masses.
    e. Ascitic fluid. If this is suspected, change the patient's position; the fluid gravitates to area of dependency.

  2. Auscultation.
    a. Presence or absence of bowel sounds.
    b. Note presence of bruits or hepatic or splenic friction rubs.

  3. Percussion.
    a. Liver—estimate lower border of liver. Advance from area of tympany at level of umbilicus upward to area of dullness (lower border of liver).
    b. Spleen—estimate edge by passing from tympany to dullness, usually approximating 10th left posterior rib at midaxillary line. Note any increased area of dullness.

  4. Palpation—tenderness, masses, borders, contour, size, and consistency.
    a. Liver.
    b. Spleen.
    c. Kidneys.
    d. Inguinal nodes.

  5. Laboratory investigations—CBC, serum iron and iron binding capacity, liver function and renal function tests, and tests for carcinoembryonic antibody (CEA), alpha fetoprotein, and alkaline phosphatase.

6. Diagnostic procedures as clinically indicated—chest x-ray, bone scan (in presence of skeletal symptoms and/or elevated alkaline phosphatase level), upper GI series, abdominal CT scan, ultrasonography, liver-spleen scan, endoscopy, KUB, laparotomy, barium enema, colonoscopy.
7. Biopsy of suspected primary or metastatic masses.

F. Male genitalia.
1. Inspection—note:
   a. Abnormal hair distribution.
   b. Masses or asymmetry.
   c. Lesions.
   d. Cutaneous nodules.
2. Palpation—tenderness, masses, consistency, contour, shape.
   a. Scrotum.
   b. Scrotal contents (testes, epididymides).
   c. Urethra.
   d. Inguinal lymph nodes.
   e. Supraclavicular lymph nodes.
   f. Breasts (if gynecomastia present).
3. Digital rectal examination.
   a. Prostate gland—masses, tenderness, firmness, size, contour.
   b. Rectum—masses, constriction, tenderness.
4. Histologic confirmation.
   a. Prostate gland—investigate with transperineal or transurethral needle biopsy or transurethral resection.
   b. Testes are investigated with inguinal orchiectomy.
   c. Cutaneous nodules or scrotal or penile lesions are investigated with needle aspiration or biopsy.
   d. Urethra is investigated with transurethral biopsy.
5. Laboratory investigations—CBC, kidney and liver function profile, calcium, alkaline phosphatase, acid phosphatase (if suspicious prostate findings) beta HCG, alpha fetoprotein, LDH (if suspicious testes findings), CEA.
6. Diagnostic procedures as clinically indicated—intravenous pyelography, CT scans, chest x-ray, chest tomography, ultrasonography (abdomen, scrotal contents, prostate, kidneys), liver scan (if hepatomegaly or elevated liver function tests), bone scan (if osseous pain or elevated alkaline phosphatase level), radiography of selected areas of bone pain or findings on bone scan.

G. Female genitalia.
1. Inspection—note:
   a. Abnormal hair distribution.
   b. Masses or asymmetry.
   c. Lesions.
2. Palpation—tenderness, masses, shape, consistency, fluid.
   a. Ovaries.
   b. Uterus.
   c. Lower abdominal region.
3. Pelvic and rectal exam (mucosal integrity and color, lesions, bleeding or discharge, constriction, masses, nodules, extent of tumor if present).
   a. External genitalia.

    b. Vagina.
    c. Cervix.
    d. Uterus and ovaries.
    e. Rectum.
  4. Histologic confirmation.
    a. Needle, excisional, or conization biopsy of any visible abnormal area.
    b. Scraping of endocervical canal and/or uterine walls.
    c. Cervical and vaginal Pap smears.
    d. Surgical exploration.
    e. Laparotomy with biopsy.
  5. Laboratory investigations—CBC, electrolytes, liver and renal function tests, calcium, alkaline phosphatase, cytologic exam of effusions.
  6. Diagnostic procedures as clinically indicated—abdominal ultrasonography and CT scans (to define areas of abnormality or adenopathy), intravenous pyelogram (to look for ureteral obstruction or deviation), liver scans (if liver function tests abnormal or liver involvement suspected), bone scan (if osseous pain or elevated alkaline phosphatase level), cystoscopy (if bladder mucosal involvement suspected), sigmoidoscopy and barium enema (for mass lesion evaluation), chest x-ray.
H. Bladder and renal units (kidneys, ureters, renal pelvis).
  1. Inspection—note:
    a. Abdominal or flank asymmetry or masses.
    b. Presence of lower extremity edema or edema of genitalia.
  2. Palpation—tenderness, masses, consistency, contour, shape.
    a. Pelvis and abdomen.
    b. Flank area.
  3. Histologic confirmation.
    a. Hypernephroma—thin needle biopsy of renal mass generally not recommended. Renal angiography and exploratory surgery may be indicated with pathologic confirmation of surgical specimen.
    b. Random bladder biopsy and biopsies of suspicious bladder mucosal irregularities or growths.
    c. Urine cytology.
  4. Laboratory investigations—CBC, renal and liver function chemistries, urinalysis (hematuria indicates need for urologic evaluation).
  5. Diagnostic procedures as clinically indicated—cystoscopy and intravenous pyelography (for unexplained hematuria, bladder irritability, unexplained flank or pelvic pain or edema), nephrotomography, renal angiography (to evaluate vascularity and vascular parasitization), liver-spleen and bone scans (in presence of osseous pain, elevated liver function tests or alkaline phosphatase), CT scans of abdomen and pelvis, chest x-ray, inferior venocavography (if large vessel tumor thrombi suspected).
I. Bone and soft tissue.
  1. Inspection—note:
    a. Skeletal or soft tissue swelling.
    b. Masses, visible bone enlargement.
    c. Lower extremity edema.
    d. Proptosis.
  2. Palpation—tenderness, masses.
    a. Any soft tissue mass or bone enlargement.

3. Histologic confirmation.
    a. Aspiration cytology or needle biopsy of soft tissue or bone mass.
    b. Open-wedge biopsy.
4. Laboratory investigations—routine blood studies.
5. Diagnostic procedures—x-ray studies of soft tissues (stippled calcification may be seen), x-ray studies of involved bones (increased density, sclerosis, or lytic area, periosteal reaction with elevated periosteum forming a triangle with bone cortex as seen in osteogenic sarcoma or spiculation of bones), CT scans (to evaluate retroperitoneum or head and neck masses), chest x-ray, lung tomograms, lymphangiography.

J. Neurologic evaluation.
1. Constellation of any of these signs and symptoms—headache, seizures, intermittent dizziness, papilledema, lateralized sensory deficits, parasthesias, ataxia, sudden sensory or motor loss, or personality changes—indicates need for complete neurologic and metabolic assessment.
2. Histologic confirmation—upon surgical resection of CNS tumors.
3. Laboratory investigations—CBC, renal and liver function, electrolytes, calcium, magnesium, serum glucose, thyroid function and other studies as clinically indicated.
4. Diagnostic procedures as clinically indicated—skull x-ray, brain CT scan, myelography, angiography, chest x-ray.

K. Hematologic evaluation.
1. Inspection—note:
    a. Pallor, petechiae, purpura.
    b. Cranial nerve dysfunction.
    c. Gingival enlargement.
    d. Hepatomegaly, splenomegaly, or lymphadenopathy.
2. Palpation—tenderness, masses, enlargement.
    a. Sternum.
    b. Liver and spleen.
    c. Tonsillar, submental, submaxillary, cervical, supraclavicular, infraclavicular, and axillary lymph nodes.
3. Histologic confirmation.
    a. Peripheral blood smear.
    b. Bone marrow examination (aspiration and biopsy).
    c. Lymph node biopsy.
4. Laboratory investigations—CBC, differentials, uric acid, calcium, phosphorus, magnesium, renal and liver function tests, coagulation studies, Coombs' tests, chromosome analyses, leukocyte alkaline phosphatase activity, serum B_{12} concentration and B_{12} binding capacity for plasma cell dyscrasias, identification and quantification of abnormal serum or urine protein indicated.
5. Diagnostic procedures as clinically indicated—chest x-ray, lung tomograms, bone scan, skeletal x-ray of painful or suspicious areas, lumbar puncture for cerebrospinal fluid examination if central nervous system abnormalities present.

STUDY QUESTIONS

1. List the information to review in taking a health history.
2. Mr. Jones is in good general health, but complains of a persistent cough and periodic dyspnea. Describe how you would evaluate his complaint.

3. Mrs. Morton is a 50-year-old woman having a routine check up. She has a significant family history of colon cancer. What assessment techniques are indicated by her history?

4. Ms. James returns for a 6-month check-up following a modified mastectomy for stage I breast cancer. List the important components of her assessment.

Bibliography

Bates, B.: A Guide to Physical Examination. Philadelphia, J.B. Lippincott, 1983.

Casciato, D. A. and Lowitz, B. B.: Manual of Bedside Oncology. Boston, Little, Brown and Company, 1983.

Wallach, J.: Interpretation of Diagnostic Tests. Boston, Little, Brown and Company, 1978.

Tietz, W. W.: Clinical Guide to Laboratory Tests. Philadelphia, W.B. Saunders Company, 1983.

Jaffe, M. S. and Kindmore, L. C.: Diagnostic and Laboratory Cards for Clinical Use. Bowie, MD., Robert J. Brady Company, 1984.

12

Staging: A Classification System for Cancer

DIANE GORDON, RN, MPH

DEFINITION

A. Staging is a method of describing and classifying the local extent or metastasis of a malignant tumor at the time of diagnosis.
B. It is also a method of quantifying the severity of disease.

OBJECTIVES OF STAGING

A. Aid the clinician in planning treatment.
B. Give some indication of prognosis.
C. Assist in the evaluation of end results.
D. Facilitate in the exchange of information between treatment centers.
E. Assist in the continuing investigation of cancer.

STAGING SYSTEMS

A. A general staging system exists for all sites; a system categorizes tumors as local, regional, or distant. Other staging systems have also been developed for gynecologic and urologic tumors, soft tissue sarcomas, and hematologic malignancies.
B. There are two major agencies concerned with the classification of malignant disease: the International Union Against Cancer (UICC) and the American Joint Committee on Cancer (AJCC). The present system of staging depends on the primary tumor, lymph node involvement, and metastatic spread (TNM classification); it was originally devised by the UICC and further developed by the AJCC. This system is a refinement of the general staging system.
C. There is a basic similarity to all staging systems—the extent of disease or how far the tumor has spread from the site of origin.

D. General Staging System.
   1. Consists of the following categories:
      a. In situ—a noninvasive or noninfiltrating neoplasm.
      b. Localized—an invasive neoplasm confined entirely to the organ of origin.
      c. Regional—an invasive neoplasm that extends directly beyond the organ of origin into surrounding tissue.
      d. Distant—a neoplasm that spreads to distant parts of the body either through direct extension or via the lymphatic or circulatory system.
E. TNM Staging System.
   1. Categorized as follows:
      a. T categories—extent of the primary tumor is commonly based on three features:
         (1) Size.
         (2) Depth of penetration.
         (3) Invasion of adjacent structures.
      b. N categories—describe the presence, extent, and location of regional lymph node metastases.
      c. M categories—describe the presence or absence of distant metastases and the degree of dissemination.
F. Model Classification System.
   1. A clinical oncotaxonomy schema has been developed for all sites to apply one standard set of TNM definitions, based upon a fixed set of criteria.
   2. A model classification schema for the TNM categories is shown in Table 12–1.

GENERAL RULES FOR STAGING

A. The purpose of staging is to quantify the anatomic extent of disease.
B. Staging requires assessment of:
   1. Primary tumor (T).
   2. Regional lymph nodes (N).
   3. Metastases (M).
C. Extent of the cancer is identified at each step of the staging process through a numeric/symbolic assignment to each of the TNM categories (Fig. 12–1).
D. The AJCC groups disease into four stages (I–IV) for the purpose of standardizing end results reporting. The exact criteria for each stage will vary with each site.
E. Host Classification.
   1. A subjective measure of performance status is necessary for ongoing evaluation of the TNM system. A baseline performance status is determined with repeated evaluations to assist in determining treatment.
      a. The most commonly employed method of assessing performance status is the Karnofsky Scale of 0 to 100. Zero represents death, and 100 represents normal activity with no complaints. The Eastern Cooperative Oncology Group (ECOG) Scale of 0–4 with 0 representing fully active and 4 representing complete disability is also commonly used.
      b. The AJCC has proposed a modification of the Karnofsky and ECOG scales as follows:

         H   The physical state (performance scale) of the patient, considering all cofactors determined at the time of stage classification and subsequent follow-up examinations.

Table 12–1. THE TNM SYSTEM*

Model Classification

T0: No evidence of a primary lesion found grossly or microscopically. Evidence of malignant change without microinvasion and without a target lesion identifiable clinically.

T1: A lesion confined to the organ of origin. It is mobile, does not invade adjacent or surrounding structures or tissues, and is often superficial.

T2: A localized lesion characterized by deep extension into adjacent structures or tissues. Invasion is into capsules, ligaments, intrinsic muscle and adjacent attached structures of similar tissue or function. There is some loss of tumor mobility, but it is not complete; therefore, fixation is not present.

T3: An advanced lesion that is confined to the region rather than to the organ of origin, whether solid or hollow. The critical criterion is fixation, which indicates invasion into a fixed structure or past a boundary. These structures are most often bone and cartilage; but invasion of the extrinsic muscle walls, serosa and skin are also included. Surrounding detached structures of different anatomy or function are in this category; however, this inclusion can be debated because of the varieties of anatomic structures.

T4: A massive lesion extending into another hollow organ causing a fistula, or into another solid organ causing a sinus. Invasions into major nerves, arteries and veins are placed in this category. Destruction of bone in addition to fixation is an advanced sign.

N0: No evidence of disease in lymph nodes.

N1: Palpable and movable lymph nodes limited to the first station. A distinction between an uninvolved and an involved palpable node needs to be made. This depends on the firmness and roundness of a node and its size, which is generally greater than 1 and often more than 2 cm—usually up to 3 cm in size and solitary.

N2: Firm to hard nodes, palpable and partially movable; they range from 3–5 cm in size. Such nodes show microscopic evidence of capsular invasion; clinically, they may be matted together. Nodes can be contralateral or bilateral.

N3: Fixation is complete. Nodes beyond the capsule with complete fixation to bone, to large blood vessels, to skin, or to nerves— usually greater than 6 cm in size.

N4: Nodes involved beyond the first station; they are in the second or distant stations. If the first two nodal stations are vertically arranged and both are involved, such double involvement is staged as N4.

NX: Nodes inaccessible to clinical evaluation.

NL: Nodes evaluated by lymphangiography. L− refers to a negative study and L+ to a positive study. An equivocal finding can be referred to as L± if equivocally positive and L∓ if equivocally negative.

N− or N+: Nodes evaluated by microscopic study and designated as negative or positive depending upon findings.

M0: No evidence of metastases.

M1: Solitary, isolated metastasis confined to one organ or anatomic site.

M2: Multiple metastatic foci confined to one organ system or one anatomic site, e.g., lungs, skeleton, liver, etc., with no functional to minimal functional impairment of system or site.

M3: Multiple organs involved anatomically, with no or minimal to moderate functional impairment of involved organs.

M4: Multiple organs involved anatomically, with moderate to severe functional impairment of involved organs.

MX: No metastatic workup done.

M: Modified to show viscera involved by letter subscript: pulmonary metastases (M_p), hepatic (M_h), osseous (M_o), skin (M_s), brain (M_b), etc.

M+: Microscopic evidence of suspected metastases, confirmed by pathologic examination.

* From Rubin, P. (ed.): Clinical Oncology: A Multidisciplinary Approach, 6th ed. New York, American Cancer Society, 1983.

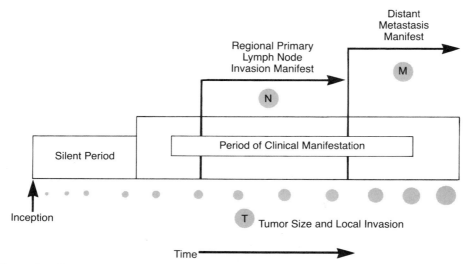

Figure 12–1. *Tumor size in relation to TNM classification. (Redrawn from Beahrs, O. H., and Meyers, M. H., (eds.): Manual for Staging of Cancer, 2nd edition, Philadelphia, J. B. Lippincott, 1983.)*

H0   Normal activity.

H1   Symptomatic and ambulatory; cares for self.

H2   Ambulatory more than 50% of time; occasionally needs assistance.

H3   Ambulatory 50% or less of time; nursing care needed.

H4   Bedridden; may need hospitalization.

SEQUENCES OF STAGING

A. Available evidence for classifying the extent of disease at different sites and at different points during the natural history and treatment should be used. Histologic confirmation of cancer is mandatory if a case is to be included in a series for evaluation.

   1. Clinical-diagnostic staging.

     a. Done prior to first definitive treatment.

     b. Generally noninvasive; relies on careful physical examination and available laboratory and radiographic studies.

     c. Includes pathologic confirmation of presence of disease and cell type.

   2. Postsurgical (pathologic) treatment staging includes pathologic review of all resected tissue.

   3. Surgical evaluative staging.

     a. Describes extent of disease after surgical exploration or biopsy.

     b. Information obtained through biopsies and histopathologic analysis is essential part of this staging procedure.

   4. Retreatment staging occurs when restaging is necessary for additional or secondary definitive treatment after a disease-free interval following first treatment.

   5. Autopsy staging is used only when cancer is first diagnosed at autopsy.

B. The stage classifications should not be changed once the extent of disease has been established. Cancers can be staged twice however; for instance, clinically staged (cTNM) and then if treated surgically, postsurgically (pathologically) staged (pTNM). This again ensures comparability of data in end results reporting.

C. Surgical staging procedures frequently performed by site:

1. Lung—Bronchoscopy and bronchial brushing, biopsy, mediastinoscopy, thoracotomy, and fine needle biopsy.
2. Esophagus—Esophagoscopy with biopsy. Exploratory laparotomy to evaluate hepatic metastasis and celiac nodes.
3. Testis and selected cases involving cervix, prostate, and bladder—Exploratory laparotomy and retroperitoneal exploration for evaluation of lymph nodes and liver.
4. Metastatic cervical lymph nodes from unknown primary source—Nasopharyngoscopy and multiple blind biopsies of nasopharynx.
5. Hodgkin's disease—For selected patients, exploratory or staging laparotomy with splenectomy, liver biopsy, and biopsy of retroperitoneal nodes is performed.
6. Melanoma—Preoperative biopsy to permit pathologists to determine depth and level of invasion.
7. Breast—When primary breast cancer is to be treated by segmental excision and radical radiotherapy in order to preserve the breast, an axillary dissection is usually done to determine if metastases have occurred.

PRINCIPLES OF STAGING A WORKUP FOR METASTATIC DISEASE

A. The most common sites of metastases are lung, liver, bone, bone marrow, adrenal glands, and brain.

B. Diagnostic procedures are necessary to determine the anatomic extent of the disease specific to each site in terms of each TNM category.

C. The rationale guiding the clinician in performing certain studies normally depends on whether the course of treatment would be altered by the results of studies.

D. Diagnostic, laboratory, and radiologic tests may detect the presence of pulmonary, skeletal, and other metastases.

1. Radiographic Procedures.
   a. Radiographs:
      (1) Site specific or full series as indicated.
      (2) Simple and frequently used routine tests to determine presence of metastases.
   b. Tomography:
      (1) Radiographic images of selected body sections that are obscured by shadows of overlying or underlying structures on routine radiography.
      (2) Higher levels of radiation than in conventional radiography and expense indicate discretion in use.
   c. Computerized Tomography (CT):
      (1) Provides cross-sectional views of soft tissue anatomy by passing multiple x-ray beams through the body at different angles and then restructuring the information in the shape of a picture using computer techniques. May be done with or without contrast agent.
      (2) Detects small lesions not seen by radiographs or tomography.

    d. Special Contrast Studies (arteriography, venography, and lymph-angiography): (see a b c).

      (1) Radiographic examination of the lymphatic or circulatory system following injection of a radiopaque iodine contrast agent.

      (2) Helpful in assessing circulatory or lymphatic system for presence of metastatic disease.

      (3) Helpful in detecting and staging lymphomas.

2. Ultrasonography.

    Series of high-frequency sound waves that can be focused, reflected, and refracted. A crystal inside the ultrasound transducer transmits an ultrasonic beam and subsequently picks up the returning sound waves or echoes. Vibrations produced by the echoes are then visually produced and displayed. Tissues of the body through and around which the sound waves travel differ in sound transmission characteristics, called acoustic impedance. The ultrasound waves are partially reflected when tissues of differing acoustic impedance come together. A high degree of difference produces a strong echo.

3. Radioisotopic Scanning Studies.

    a. Bone, liver-spleen, and brain scans.

      (1) Imaging of the targeted tissue after injection of a radioactive isotope. The isotope collects in specific concentrations at sites of abnormal metabolism. When scanned, the isotope is picked up as "hot or cold spots."

      (2) Usually done only if symptomatic or laboratory evidence arouses suspicion of metastatic disease or to rule out metastases prior to treatment.

      (3) Best screening exam for asymptomatic patients with suspected skeletal metastases; better than conventional radiography.

      (4) Increased concentration of isotope demonstrated in trauma and during healing process.

    b. Gallium imaging.

      (1) A total body scan, usually performed 24 to 48 hours after the injection of radioactive gallium; operates on same principles as other radioisotopic scanning studies.

      (2) Useful in determining unknown sites of metastatic origin, but requires confirmation with additional tests.

4. Magnetic Resonance Imaging (MRI).

    a. Provides image of section of the body in any plane, by aligning certain atoms in tissue by applying a very strong magnetic field, disturbing these atoms with a pulse of another magnetic field, measuring the radio frequency signal emitted by the atoms as they return to their previous orientation, and transforming this information into an image using computer techniques.

    b. At the present time, MRI is primarily being used for brain, spinal cord, and pelvis imaging because of difficulties with movement in other tissues.

    c. Advantages—No radiation exposure and often more sensitive than CT.

    d. Disadvantages—High cost and low availability.

5. Percutaneous liver biopsies are done only occasionally.

6. Bone marrow aspiration and biopsy are used for diseases known to originate in or spread to the bone marrow.

7. Biologic response markers are also useful in diagnosing primary tumors.
   a. CEA (Carcinoembryonic Antigen). This glycoprotein is not normally found in adults, but it is secreted by certain tumors; most characteristically seen in colorectal, pancreatic, gastric, breast, and lung cancers.
   b. HCG (Human Chorionic Gonadotropin) is most commonly found in trophoblastic neoplasms, i.e., cancer of the testis and choriocarcinoma.
   c. Alpha fetoprotein is an oncofetal protein found in hepatocellular tumors, germ cell tumors of the testis, ovary, and extragonadal sites, and occasionally in cancer of the pancreas, stomach, or biliary system.
8. Other laboratory tests, including enzyme tests such as alkaline and acid phosphatase, are also used.
9. Other tumor imaging studies are under investigation.
   a. Scintigraphy—A noninvasive nuclear imaging procedure used to determine presence of subclinical lymphatic metastasis.
   b. Labeled antibodies to carcinoembryonic antigen (CEA).
   c. Tumor-specific labeled monoclonal antibodies.
10. Nursing implications of diagnostic studies.
    a. Patient preparation:
       (1) Explanation of procedures.
       (2) Restrict food or fluids as appropriate.
       (3) Preparative procedures as indicated.
    b. Contradindications:
       (1) Radiographic studies may be contraindicated in pregnancy, or in infants or small children.
       (2) Iodinated contrast studies may be contraindicated in persons with known hypersensitivity to iodine or previous reaction to use of radioiodine contrast agents. Contrast is also contraindicated in individuals with impaired renal function.
       (3) Cost-benefit ratio must be weighed.

ANATOMIC MAPPING

A. Accurate imaging and mapping on anatomic charts and diagrams (staging checklists).
B. Follows the surgical-pathologic staging process and is used to identify macro- and micro-residuum of tumor.
C. Used extensively with Hodgkin's disease and other lymphomas and is also used with gastrointestinal tumors.

GRADING CLASSIFICATION SYSTEM

A. Histologic classification of the cancer is as important as anatomic staging in treatment planning and in predicting outcome.
B. Grading may be more important in determining prognosis than histologic type, as in soft tissue sarcomas.
C. The pathologist plays an important role in histologic classification by:
   1. Evaluating tissue within the primary site for any prognostically important tumor characteristics.

    2. Reviewing surgical specimens to determine if lines of resection are free of tumor.

    3. Evaluating regional lymph nodes for histologic confirmation of cancer.

D. Two essential features in histologic classification are histologic grade and type of tumor.

E. Cancers are usually classified as Grades I to IV, with increasing anaplasia. The following grading system is used by AJCC:

- GX—Grade cannot be assessed.
- G1—Well-differentiated.
- G2—Moderately well-differentiated.
- G3–G4—Poorly to very poorly differentiated.

F. The more differentiated a tumor is the more closely it resembles normal cells and the more favorable the prognosis.

G. Grading systems vary according to the site; one of the most common is Broders's classification used for grading squamous cell carcinomas.

STUDY QUESTIONS

1. What staging system categorizes the tumor growth as local, regional, or distant?
2. Define the intent of all staging systems.
3. How is the performance status of the patient helpful at the time of each TNM classification?
4. List the most common sites of cancer metastases.
5. Define differentiation of tumor cells.

Bibliography

Beahrs, O. H. and Myers, M. H. (eds.): Manual for Staging of Cancer, 2nd. Ed. American Joint Committee on Cancer. Philadelphia, J. B. Lippincott, 1983.

Bleiberg, H.: Improving peritoneoscopic staging of patients with solid tumors. European Journal of Cancer Clinical Oncology, 19:557–582, 1983.

Casciato, D. and Lowitz, B. (eds.): A Manual of Bedside Oncology. Boston, Little, Brown and Co., 1983.

DeCosse, J., Meijer, W. S., and Osborne, M. P.: Lymphoscintigraphy in the staging of solid tumors. Surgery Gynecology and Obstetrics, 156:384–390, 1983.

Gottschalk, A. and Zeman, R. K.: Current aspects of nuclear imaging in clinical oncology. Cancer, 47:1154–1158, 1981.

Henson, D. E.: Staging for cancer. Arch Pathol Lab Med., 109:13–16, 1985.

International Union Against Cancer (UICC): TNM Classification of Malignant Tumors. Committee of Clinical Oncology. Geneva, UICC, 1973.

Marino, L. B.: Cancer Nursing. St. Louis, C.V. Mosby Co., 1981.

Diagnostics. Nurses' Reference Library. Nursing 84 Books. Springhouse, PA, Springhouse, 1984.

Robbins, S. L., Cotran, R. S., and Kumar, V.: Pathologic Basis of Disease, 3rd ed. Philadelphia, W.B. Saunders, 1984.

Rubin, P. (ed.): Clinical Oncology: A Multidisciplinary Approach, 6th ed. New York, American Cancer Society, 1983.

Rubin, P.: A unified classification of cancers: An oncotaxonomy with symbols. Cancer, 31:963–982, 1973.

Rubin, P. and Keys, H.: The staging and classification of cancers—a unified approach. In Carter, S. K., Glatstein, E., and Livingston, R. B. (eds.). Principles of Cancer Treatment. New York, McGraw-Hill Book Co., pp. 14–25, 1982.

SECTION FIVE

Characteristics of Major Cancers

Section Editor
ROBERTA STROHL, RN, MN

13

Lung Cancer

JULENA LIND, RN, MS

RISK FACTORS

A. Tobacco smoking.
   1. Smoking is responsible for approximately 80% of lung cancer cases.
   2. At highest risk are people over 45 who have smoked two or more packs per day for 10 years or more (20 pack years).
   3. Twenty pack year people have lung cancer mortality rates 15–25 times higher than nonsmokers.
   4. The increase of lung cancer deaths in women is attributed to the increase in the number of women smoking.
      a. In 1950 the lung cancer ratio of women to men was 1:20.
      b. In 1974 the lung cancer ratio of women to men was 1:4.
      c. In 1980 the lung cancer ratio of women to men was 1:2.6.
   5. Smoking-related disorders are estimated to cost the nation about $27 billion in health care.
   6. In addition to being a carcinogen itself, tobacco smoke promotes the carcinogenic effect of other carcinogens.
B. Occupational factors.
   1. Asbestos exposure has been linked with the incidence of lung cancer (especially mesothelioma) in shipyard workers, miners, and pipe fitters.
   2. Uranium miners appear to have a particularly high incidence of small cell cancer of the lung.

SCREENING AND DETECTION

A. Screening.
   1. No good reliable early screening method.
   2. Chest x-rays combined with lung health questionnaires and sputum cytology at regular intervals have been attempted. *
   3. A 1984 study of sputum cytology screening for lung cancer concluded that cytology is not required in a screening program of chest x-rays carried out annually.

4. Cytology can contribute to the detection of localized lung cancer as an adjunct to chest x-ray in a single screening.
B. Signs and symptoms.
  1. Pulmonary manifestations.
    a. Cough.
    b. Hemoptysis.
    c. Dyspnea.
  2. Local complications (related to the growth of tumor and compression of adjacent structures):
    a. Shoulder pain.
    b. Arm pain.
    c. Superior vena cava syndrome.
  3. Metabolic complications (small cell especially):
    a. Elevated ADH (because of ADH mimic produced by the *tumor*).
    b. Elevated ACTH (because of ACTH mimic produced by the *tumor*).
C. Diagnosis.
  1. Histologic types:
    a. Epidermoid (squamous)—most common.
    b. Adenocarcinoma.
    c. Small cell (includes oat cell)—most rapidly growing.
    d. Large cell.
  2. Tests that aid in determining the size and location of the primary tumor:
    a. Chest x-ray.
    b. Lung tomogram.
    c. Bronchoscopy with brush biopsy.
    d. Needle biopsy.
  3. Tests that aid in determining the lymph node involvement.
    a. Mediastinoscopy.
    b. Scalene node biopsy.
    c. Hilar tomogram.
  4. Tests that aid in detecting distant metastases:
    a. Liver/spleen scan.
    b. Bone scan.

Table 13–1. STAGE-GROUPING IN CARCINOMA OF THE LUNG

Stage I	
TIS N0 M0	Carcinoma in situ
T1 N0 M0	A tumor that can be classified T1 without any metastasis or with
T1 N1 M0	metastasis to the lymph nodes in the ipsilateral hilar region only,
T2 N0 M0	or a tumor that can be classified T2 without any metastasis to nodes or distant metastasis.
	NOTE: TX, N1, M0 and T0, N1, M0 are also theoretically possible, but such a clinical diagnosis would be difficult if not impossible to make. If such a diagnosis is made, it should be included in Stage I.
Stage II	
T2 N1 M0	A tumor classified as T2 with metastasis to the lymph nodes in the ipsilateral hilar region only.
Stage III	
T3 with any N or M	Any tumor more extensive than T2, or any tumor with metastasis
N2 with T or M	to the lymph nodes in the mediastinum, or with distant metas-
M1 with any T or N	tasis.

Table 13–2. TNM DEFINITIONS

	T Primary Tumors
T0	No evidence of primary tumor
TX	Tumor proven by cytology but not visualized
TIS	Carcinoma in situ
T1	A tumor that is 3.0 cm or less without evidence of invasion of a lobar bronchus
T2	A tumor more than 3.0 cm in greatest diameter, or a tumor of any size which invades the visceral pleura or with its associated atelectasis or obstructive pneumonitis, extends to the hilar region; no pleural effusion
T3	A tumor of any size with direct extension into an adjacent structure, or demonstrable bronchographically to involve a main bronchus less than 2.0 cm distal to the carina; any tumor associated with atelectasis or obstructive pneumonitis of an entire lung or pleural effusion
	N Regional Lymph Nodes
N0	No demonstrable metastasis to regional lymph nodes
N1	Metastasis to lymph nodes in the peribronchial and/or the ipsilateral hilar region (including direct extension)
N2	Metastasis to lymph nodes in the mediastinum
	M Distant Metastasis
M0	No distant metastasis
M1	Distant metastasis such as in scalene, cervical, or contralateral hilar lymph nodes, brain, bones, lung, liver

      c. CT scan of the brain.

      d. Thoracentesis (to detect tumor cells in pleural fluid).

D. Staging.

    1. Stage I, II, III, IV (Table 13–1).

    2. TNM system (Table 13–2).

    3. Host performance scales which measure the physical capabilities of an individual patient are also used at the time of staging.

      a. Karnofsky scale.

      b. Zubrod scale.

METHODS OF TREATMENT

A. Surgery.

    1. Treatment of choice for cure for non–small cell cancer of the lung.

    2. Lobectomy leaves part of the lung in place. Because it is associated with lower morbidity and mortality than pneumonectomy, it is generally the preferred treatment for small tumors.

    3. Pneumonectomy removes all of the lung tissue.

    4. In the general population only about 50% of lung cancer patients are candidates for thoracotomy; only 25% are candidates for resection.

    5. Contraindications to thoracotomy include:

      a. Metastasis outside the lung.

      b. Scalene node metastasis.

      c. Metastasis to the other lung.

    6. Surgery also may be performed to palliate symptoms, such as hemoptysis.

    7. Postoperative complications include:

      a. Subcutaneous emphysema.

      b. Circulatory overload.

      c. Tension pneumothorax.

      d. Mediastinal shift.

      e. Venous thrombosis.

B. Radiotherapy.
1. Types used in lung cancer:
    a. External beam.
    b. Implants.
    c. Cranial irradiation.
2. External beam radiotherapy may be used alone for cure in those non–small cell lung cancer patients with Stage I or II disease who have lung function impairments or other conditions which preclude surgery.
3. External beam radiotherapy is often used as an adjuvant to surgery, either pre- or postoperatively. The effect on survivorship is controversial.
4. Prophylactic cranial irradiation has been used to prevent or retard the incidence of brain metastases in small cell lung cancer.
5. External beam radiotherapy has an unquestioned role in the palliation of symptoms associated with lung cancer.
    a. Can prolong the functional life of the patient and control pain.
    b. Is used to control severe cough, hemoptysis, obstructive pneumonitis, and superior vena cava syndrome.
6. Side effects of external beam radiotherapy to chest include:
    a. Fatigue.
    b. Skin reactions (7 to 10 days after treatment starts).
    c. Hair loss on chest.
    d. Dysphagia approximately 3 weeks after treatment starts because of desquamation of esophageal mucosa.
    e. Esophagitis (desquamation of esophageal mucosa).
    f. Depressed bone marrow production (sternum may get in the radiation field).
    g. Tenacious bronchial secretions.
    h. Later pneumonitis (1 to 3 months after treatment).
7. Potential side effects of cranial irradiation:
    a. Alopecia.
    b. Desquamation of portions of ear.
    c. "CNS syndrome"—memory loss for recent events, tremor, somnolence, slurred speech.

C. Chemotherapy.
1. Treatment of choice for small cell lung cancer.
    a. Has been shown to improve survival rates (12 to 18-month median survival with chemotherapy vs. 6 to 8 weeks without).
    b. Has been combined with cranial irradiation to improve survival.
    c. Combinations used include:
        (1) Cyclophosphamide-Doxorubicin-Vincristine.
        (2) Cyclophosphamide-Doxorubicin-VP - 16 - 213.
        (3) Cyclophosphamide-Lomustine-Methotrexate.
2. May be used as adjuvant therapy in non–small cell lung cancer.
    a. Has not improved survival.
    b. Disease free survival rate may be improved.
    c. Combined with surgery or radiotherapy.
    d. Combinations used include:
        (1) Cyclophosphamide-Doxorubicin-Cisplatin.
        (2) Vindesine-Vinblastine-Cisplatin.

3. Commonly used for advanced disease.
    a. Generally yield frequent but brief response rates (up to 40% in some studies).
    b. Combinations used include:
        (1) Cyclophosphamide-Doxorubicin-Methotrexate-Procarbazine.
        (2) Vindesine-Cisplatin.
        (3) Doxorubicin-5-Fluorouracil-Cisplatin.
        (4) Mitomycin-Vinblastine-Cisplatin.
4. Various types of chemotherapy agents commonly used in treating lung cancer are:
    a. Doxorubicin (Adriamycin).
    b. Bleomycin (Blenoxane).
    c. CCNU (Lomustine).
    d. Cisplatin (CDDP, Platinol).
    e. Hexamethylmelamine.
    f. M-AMSA (Amacrine).
    g. Methotrexate (Amethopterin).
    h. Procarbazine (Matulane).
    i. Vincristine (Oncovin).
    j. Vindesine (Eldisine).
    k. VP-16-213 (Etoposide).
5. Side effects of chemotherapy agents used in lung cancer (Table 13–3).

PROGNOSIS

A. Overall survival at 5 years of all lung cancer patients is less than 10%.
B. Stage I five year survival is 40–60%.
C. Stage II five year survival is approximately 12%.

NURSING CARE

A. Nursing responsibility in prevention and detection.
    1. Smoking cessation.
        a. Acts as a role model.
        b. Provides public education.
        c. Helps clients stop smoking (Table 13–4).
    2. Nursing responsibilities related to diagnostic tests:
        a. Bronchoscopy (Table 13–5).
        b. Mediastinoscopy (Table 13–6).
        c. Computerized tomography (Table 13–7).
B. Potential patient problems related to surgery:
    1. Disruption of body image.
    2. Pain related to thoracotomy.
    3. Obstruction of or failure of chest tubes.
    4. Pain, tachycardia, dyspnea related to mediastinal shift.
    5. Pain, tenderness, ischemia related to venous thrombosis.
    6. Hypoxia related to atelectasis.
C. Nursing assessment data related to surgical intervention include:
    1. Status of pulmonary function.
    2. Status of chest tubes if any.
    3. Coping mechanisms and support systems.

Table 13–3. DRUGS USED IN LUNG CANCER*

Drug Name	Administration	Metabolism	Myelosuppression	Toxicity	Special Nursing Considerations
Doxorubicin (Adriamycin)	I.V. (over 2–5 min) most common	By liver. Excreted in urine and may cause urine discoloration (pink to red in 48 hr)	Incidence is 60–80%, Nadir is d. 10–14	N&V, Alopecia, Cardiomyopathy *Severe vesicant*	Total lifetime dose not to exceed 550 mg/m^3 (or 450 mg/m^3 if radiotherapy to chest) precipitation may occur when mixed with heparin
BCNU (Carmustine)	Orally on empty stomach (3–4 hr after meals)	Absorbed from GI tract 75% excreted in urine within 4d.	Delayed. Repeated doses cause cumulative effects Nadir is 4–5 weeks and lasts 1–2 weeks	N&V	Crosses blood-brain barrier Delayed myelosuppression affects plts. more
Cisplatin (DDP, Platinol)	Several ways: 15–20 minute infusion 1 hr infusion 6–8 hr infusion 24 hr infusion	Rapidly distributed into tissues, 50% of dose is excreted in urine in 24–48 hr	Mild with moderate doses	Nephrotoxicity Ototoxicity N&V	Hydration & diuresis essential (urine output = 100–150 ml per hr) Monitor BUN, Cr. & Cr. Clearance
Cyclophosphamide (Cytoxan)	Orally (a.m. or afternoon) I.V.: doses over 500 mg give over 20–30 min in 500 cc fluid	Requires activation by liver Excreted by kidney	Leukopenia Nadir 7–14 d.	N&V Alopecia Hemorrhagic Cystitis, Antidiuretic effect	Force fluids, avoid bedtime doses, Allow 10–15 minutes for crystals to dissolve when mixing
Hexamethylmelamine (investigational)	Oral	By liver. Excreted in urine	Leukopenia & occasionally thrombocytopenia	N&V CNS disturbances Peripheral Neuropathy	Give oral med. in 3 divided doses for 21 d.
M-AMSA (investigational)	I.V. infusion in 500 cc DW in 1 hr Comes in 2 liquid vials that must be mixed	Excreted by biliary route (lesser amount through kidney)	Leukopenia is dose-limiting toxicity Nadir = 7–14 d.	N&V Phlebitis Hepatotoxicity Seizures at very high doses	Do not mix drug in saline because it may precipitate After mixing, do not refrigerate
Methotrexate (Amethopterin)	PO, I.V., SQ, Intra-arterial Intrathecal. Low dose = 30–40 mg/m^2 High dose = 100–7500 mg/m^2	Excreted in urine unchanged	Nadir = 6–9 d. after treatment	N&V Stomatitis Hepatotoxicity	Give Leucovorin rescue for high dose Follow kidney function, Mucositis = warning of toxicity. Alkalinize urine for high dose
Procarbazine (Matulane)	Oral	Absorbed from GI tract Metabolized by liver Excreted in urine Crosses blood-brain barrier	2–3 weeks after treatment stopped	N&V Myalgias, arthralgias Do not use with ETOH = headache, respiratory difficulties, flushed, scarlet face	Have patient avoid alcohol. Is MAO inhibitor. Avoid beer, yogurt, wine, cheese, bananas, herring, chicken liver
Vincristine (Oncovin)	Running I.V. or I.V. push	Rapidly cleared from plasma. Major route of excretion is bile	Rare, usually mild	Neurotoxicity: ileus, constipation, paresthesias Alopecia, jaw pain, metallic taste	Dose not to exceed 2.0 mg in adults Decrease dose in liver disease. Prophylactic bowel management Vesicant! Avoid extravasation
Vindesine	Running I.V. or I.V. push (1–3 min)	Excreted via bile	Dose related, usually moderate & transient	N&V Neurotoxicity Alopecia	Constipation may be problem; occasionally photophobia occurs
VP-16-213 (Etoposide, investigational)	Give over 30–40 min (to minimize bronchospasm & hypotension)	Excreted via bile	A dose-limiting toxicity; leukopenia, thrombocytopenia & anemia all occur	N&V Alopecia Bronchospasm Hypotension	Observe drug for clarity before use Unstable in D$_5$W Must be diluted with 20–50 volumes of NaCl

* Information compiled from: Knobf, M. K., Lewis, K., Fischer, D., Schneider, W., and Welch, D.: Cancer Chemotherapy Treatment and Care. Boston, G. K. Hall Medical Publishers, 1981.

Table 13–4. HELPING CLIENTS
STOP SMOKING

Emphasize the *choice* to *not* smoke
Encourage fluids first 3 days (decreases nicotine
   cravings)
Instruct in slow deep breathing
Decaffeinate (caffeine stimulates the craving)
Vitamin B complex may help mood swings
Instruct in exercise
Give some hand substitute for cigarettes

Table 13–5. NURSING CARE FOLLOWING BRONCHOSCOPY

Place patient flat or in semi-Fowler's position on side
Instruct patient to let saliva run from side of mouth rather than swallow
Save sputum (may have large amount)
Watch closely for laryngospasm or laryngeal edema
Instruct patient to refrain from talking or throat clearing
NPO until gag reflex returns (2–8 hrs)
Pain relief for sore throat (ice collar, and after regaining ability to swallow, lozenges, gargles)

Table 13–6. NURSING CARE RELATED TO MEDIASTINOSCOPY

Preoperative teaching: test is to evaluate lymph nodes in chest; NPO after MN; possible transient
   chest pain and sore throat following test
Postoperative care:
   Monitor V.S.
   Check dressing for bleeding
   Observe for mediastinitis (fever)
   Observe for crepitus (air leakage into subcutaneous tissue)
   Observe for pneumothorax (dyspnea, cyanosis, decreased breath sounds)
   Administer analgesics as needed

Table 13–7. NURSING CARE RELATED TO THORACIC CT SCAN

Pre-test teaching:
   Instruct patient that test is painless
   Prepare patient for large machine, clicking noises that are normal
   If contrast used, patient must fast for 4 hours
   If contrast used, prepare patient for facial flushing, sensation of warmth, nausea or salty taste
   CT scan should precede UGI (barium may obscure scan)
Post-test care:
   Watch for signs of delayed hypersensitivity (if contrast used)
   Instruct patient and family in significance of results

    4. Nutritional state.

    5. Degree of pain.

    6. Level of knowledge.

    7. Presence of venous thrombosis.

    8. Presence of mediastinal shift (Table 13–8).

D. Nursing interventions related to surgical treatment.

    1. Preoperative teaching (equipment, breathing exercises).

    2. Maintenance of chest tubes.

    3. Prevention of postoperative emboli (exercises and elastic stockings).

    4. Pain relief.

    5. Promote optimal pulmonary function (cough and deep breathing, hydration, change positions, protect remaining lung tissue).

    6. Postoperative teaching (breathing, exercises, need for cessation of smoking).

E. Potential problems associated with external beam radiation therapy to the lungs:

    1. Fatigue.

    2. Skin reactions.

    3. Hair loss on chest.

    4. Dysphagia.

    5. Esophagitis.

    6. Depressed bone marrow function.

    7. Nonproductive cough.

    8. Increased tenacity of bronchial secretions.

    9. Pneumonitis.

F. Potential problems associated with internal radiation implants:

    1. Social isolation.

    2. Skin reactions (lessened).

    3. Esophagitis.

G. Potential problems associated with prophylactic cranial irradiation:

    1. Alopecia (with dry scalp).

    2. Some desquamation of portions of ear.

    3. Otitis.

    4. Transient CNS syndrome.

H. Nursing assessment data related to radiotherapy include:

    1. Pattern of fatigue and impact on lifestyle.

    2. Degree and extent of skin reactions: itching, dryness, increased pigmentation, erythema, dry desquamation, wet desquamation.

    3. Importance of body image changes.

    4. Degree of hair loss and impact on lifestyle.

Table 13–8. SIGNS AND SYMPTOMS OF MEDIASTINAL SHIFT

Restlessness and anxiety
Dyspnea and tachypnea
Cyanosis
Tachycardia, irregular pulse, atrial dysrhythmias
Shift in point of maximal impulse of heart
Trachea deviated from midline

5. Swallowing ability ("lump" in throat on swallowing, difficulty with solid foods, pain).
6. White blood count and platelet count.
7. Mucus clearance capability (ability to generate forceful, productive cough).
8. Pulmonary function.
9. Changes in usual respiratory patterns.
10. Presence of sensory or social deprivation.
11. Presence of CNS changes.

I. Nursing interventions related to radiotherapy:
   1. Explain physiologic effects of radiotherapy.
   2. Encourage rest periods and priority setting to save energy.
   3. Skin care (see Chapter 23).
   4. Provide foods that are easily swallowed (tepid, soft, not spicy).
   5. Provide or encourage frequent oral care; encourage fluid intake.
   6. Monitor platelet and granulocyte counts.
   7. Promote better mucus clearance (hydration, diaphragmatic breathing).
   8. Postural drainage, percussion, and vibration.
   9. Teach patient or family about half-life of radioisotopes (if getting implant treatment).
   10. Advise cutting hair and buying a wig (if getting cranial irradiation).
   11. Maintain support of patient and family during treatment.

J. Nursing assessment data related to chemotherapy include:
   1. Platelet count.
   2. White blood cell count.
   3. Signs of infection.
   4. Signs of bleeding.
   5. Symptoms of nausea, number of emeses, and fluid loss.
   6. Signs of extravasation.
   7. Vital signs (BP, temperature).
   8. Signs of peripheral neuropathies (numbness, tingling in extremities, constipation).
   9. Symptoms of hematuria.
   10. Knowledge of total dose of doxorubicin.

K. Nursing interventions related to chemotherapy (see also Chapter 23):
   1. Monitor blood counts.
   2. Monitor total dose of doxorubicin.
   3. Force fluids; teach patient not to take cyclophosphamide at bedtime.
   4. Monitor bowel evacuation. Are stool softeners necessary?
   5. Promote good oral hygiene.
   6. Administer anti-emetics.
   7. Watch and instruct patient or family to watch for signs of infection (temperature, chills, cloudy urine).
   8. Support patient and family during treatment.
   9. Provide foods high in protein and calories.
   10. Explain to patients and family the side effects of treatment.

L. Nursing care related to lung cancer—rehabilitation aspects:
   1. Help family to allow patient to maintain roles and activities most important to him or her.
   2. Place emphasis on short-term goals in daily care and priority setting.
   3. Refer to community agency for respiratory program if available.

4. Instruct patient and family in the use of O_2 equipment, postural drainage, self-pacing program.
5. Teach about general strengthening exercise program.
6. Instruct patient in relaxation techniques.
7. Assist patient and family to prepare for changes in life style.
8. Keep in mind that even though prognosis may be bleak, patients retain hope.

STUDY QUESTION

Mr. Johnson is a 58-year-old married man with two teenage sons who has just been diagnosed with small cell lung cancer T2 N2 MO. Write a generic care plan that could address Mr. Johnson's potential problems. The care plan must include at least two phases of his disease progression and treatment.

For example:

      a) Diagnosis and   b) Treatment
               OR
      a) Treatment and   b) Rehabilitation
               OR
      a) Treatment and   b) Terminal illness

Bibliography

Byrne, N.: Critical care of the thoracic surgical patient. Cancer Nursing, *1*(2):135–141, 1978.

Holmes, E. M., Hill, L. D., and Gail, M.: A randomized comparison of the effects of adjuvant therapy on resected stages II and III non–small cell carcinoma of the lung. Annals of Surgery, *202*(3):335–339, 1985.

Hooker, C.: Helping patients who must stop smoking. Nursing '81, *11*:98–99, 1981.

Knobf, M. K., Lewis, K. P., Fischer, D. S., et al.: Cancer Chemotherapy—Treatment and Care. Boston, G. K. Hall Medical Publishers, 1981.

Melamed, M. R., Flehinger, B. J., Zaman, M. B., et al.: Screening for early lung cancer—results of the Memorial Sloan-Kettering Study in New York. Chest, *86*(1):44–53, 1984.

Rosenow, E. C. and Carr, D.: Bronchogenic cancer. CA Cancer Journal for Clinicians, *29*(4): 233–245, 1979.

Ruckdeschel, J. C., Caradonna, R., Paladine, W. J., et al.: Small cell anaplastic carcinoma of the lung: Changing concepts and emerging problems. CA Cancer Journal for Clinicians, *29*(2): 84–95, 1979.

Sarna, G. P., Holmes, E. C., and Petrovich, Z.: Lung cancer. *In* Haskell, C. (ed.): Cancer Treatment. Philadelphia, W. B. Saunders, pp. 197–231, 1980.

Yasko, J.: Guidelines for Cancer Care: Symptom Management. Reston VA, Reston Publishing Co, 1983.

14

Breast Cancer

NINA ENTREKIN, RN, MN

RISK FACTORS

A. Sex.
1. Most common type of cancer in women, 1 out of every 11 American women will have breast cancer at some point in her lifetime.
2. Second leading cause of cancer deaths in women.
3. 1% of breast cancer occurs in men.

B. Age.
1. Over 40 years of age.
2. Incidence increases until the age of 50 and then plateaus.

C. Personal history of breast cancer—15% develop breast cancer in the opposite breast.

D. Family history of breast cancer.
1. Risk is increased two to three times in daughters or sisters of women with breast cancer.
2. Risk may be increased seven to eight times in daughters or sisters of women with premenopausal, bilateral breast cancer.

E. Parity.
1. Risk is increased in women who have never had children.
2. Women who had first child after the age of 30 may be at even greater risk than nulliparous women.

F. Precancerous mastopathy type of fibrocystic disease.
1. Gross cystic disease.
2. Multiple intraductal papilloma.
3. Lobular neoplasia.

G. Prolonged hormonal stimulation.
1. Early menarche (before age 12).
2. Late menopause (after age 50).
3. Long-term use of exogenous estrogens for menopausal symptoms may be involved in tumor initiation.

H. Excessive ionizing radiation exposure, such as multiple fluoroscopies for tuberculosis and irradiation for mastitis.

I. Other organ cancer, particularly endometrium, ovary, or colon.

J. High dietary fat intake, particularly after menopause.

SCREENING AND DETECTION

A. Public education.

1. Promote awareness and understanding of risk factors.
   a. Interpret risk factors realistically. Two-thirds of breast cancer occurs in women who do not have a high risk profile.
   b. Women who are at high risk should have more frequent screenings.
2. Allay fears and misconceptions.
   a. Diagnosis of breast cancer does not necessarily mean loss of breast if the cancer is found at an early stage.
   b. Breast cancer is a chronic illness, not a uniformly terminal illness.
   c. Most breast lumps are benign (only 25–35% are malignant).
3. Promote awareness of warning signs and symptoms.
   a. Most common early symptom is a painless lump or thickening in the breast.
      (1) 90% discovered by the woman herself.
      (2) 50% occur in upper outer quadrant of the breast (more breast tissue is in this quadrant).
      (3) More often in left breast than in right breast.
   b. Other signs and symptoms more common in advanced disease.
      (1) Dimpling of the skin.
      (2) Nipple retraction.
      (3) Asymmetry of breasts.
      (4) Scaling of skin, often in areolar area.
      (5) Peau d'orange skin.
      (6) Serosanguinous or bloody nipple discharge.
      (7) Firm, enlarged axillary lymph nodes.
4. Teach breast self examination (BSE).
   a. All women 20 years of age and older should practice BSE monthly, although only 25–30% do.
   b. Women who receive 1:1 personal BSE instruction are more likely to practice it regularly than those instructed by other methods.
   c. Women who practice BSE monthly are more likely to find tumors at an earlier clinical stage and to survive longer than do those who do not practice BSE regularly.
5. Encourage women to have regular breast health checkups.
   a. ACS recommendations for women ages 20–40:
      (1) Exam by physician every 3 years.
      (2) BSE every month.
      (3) Baseline mammogram between ages 35–40.
   b. ACS recommendations for women ages 40 and older:
      (1) Exam by physician every year.
      (2) BSE every month.
      (3) Mammogram every 1–2 years between ages 40–49, and every year after age 50.
   c. Women at higher risk may need more frequent checkups.
   d. Screening methods are complementary and should not be substituted for each other.

B. Screening and detection methods.
  1. Mammography.
     a. Screen film mammography.
        (1) Uses molybdenum source for x-ray emission.
        (2) Moderate breast compression required to avoid motion and improve visualization.
        (3) 0.2 rad midplane breast exposure.
     b. Xeromammography.
        (1) Uses tungsten target for x-ray emission.
        (2) Uses selenium-coated aluminum plate to produce a blue and white opaque picture.
        (3) Requires less breast compression.
        (4) 0.4 rad midplane breast exposure.
     c. Both forms of mammography are equivalent, with an accuracy of 85%.
     d. In the 5-year Breast Cancer Detection Demonstration Project (BCDDP), 42% of the cancers were detected only by mammography.
  2. Ultrasonography.
     a. Uses high frequency sound waves to obtain a cross-sectional breast image, either through direct contact scanning or water bath techniques.
     b. Accurate in distinguishing between cystic and solid masses in 95% of cases.
     c. Ineffective in detecting small, nonpalpable cancers, or in distinguishing benign vs. malignant solid lesions.
  3. Thermography.
     a. Use based on finding that skin temperature may be 1–3 degrees warmer over malignant lesions due to increased vascularity.
     b. Accuracy no better than chance alone.
     c. Sensitive to breast masses greater than 2 cm rather than to early breast cancers with greatest possibility for cure.
     d. Not recommended for population screening.
  4. Computerized axial tomography (CT) scans.
     a. Accuracy of 94% in distinguishing between benign and malignant lesions.
     b. Useful in supplementing mammography to evaluate dense breasts and to search for a primary when mammogram is negative and axillary lymph node biopsy is positive.
     c. Disadvantages include radiation exposure to other parts of thorax during exam, high cost, need for IV contrast material and length of procedure.
  5. Transillumination (diaphanography).
     a. Uses an intense light to illuminate breast tissues, which are reproduced on infrared film.
     b. Accuracy of approximately 74%.
     c. Unproven value, may be useful as adjunct to physical exam when mammography is inadvisable.
  6. Magnetic resonance imaging.
     a. Uses interaction between magnetism and radiowaves to produce cross-sectional breast image.
     b. Limited availability of equipment for this new technology.
     c. May be useful in distinguishing between benign and malignant lesions in selected cases.

C. Diagnostic methods.
1. Definitive diagnosis requires biopsy and histopathologic determination of tumor.
2. Indication for biopsy is any discrete, palpable mass in breast regardless of mobility of mass, negative mammogram, length of time the mass has been present, or benign nature of previous biopsies.
3. All biopsy techniques can be done under local anesthesia on an outpatient basis.
4. Trend is for biopsy to be done as a separate procedure, apart from surgery aimed at treatment (i.e., two-step procedure).
5. Biopsy techniques.
   a. Needle aspiration biopsy.
      (1) Fine needle (21g) is passed into a localized mass and material aspirated by negative pressure applied to syringe.
      (2) Material aspirated is placed on slide, fixative applied, and sent to pathology.
      (3) If significant fluid is aspirated and lump disappears, is indicative of benign, cystic mass.
      (4) Negative pathology of solid mass may indicate need for open biopsy.
      (5) Rare complications include hematoma, infection, pneumothorax.
      (6) Accuracy of 95% when adequate material obtained with aspiration.
   b. Needle core biopsy.
      (1) Special needle with large lumen (Silverman or Tru-cut) is used to remove core of tissue.
      (2) Used when tumor is relatively large and located close to surface where biopsy unlikely to miss the tumor.
      (3) Complications and accuracy same as for needle aspiration technique.
   c. Open biopsy.
      (1) Small tumor—excisional biopsy—removal of entire lump with margin of normal tissue.
      (2) Large tumor—incisional biopsy—removal of a small portion of tumor.
      (3) Frozen section performed on tissue.
      (4) Remaining tissue of malignant samples can be sent for estrogen and progesterone receptor assay while still fresh.
      (5) Complications include hematoma, infections.
   d. Needle localization biopsy.
      (1) Used when there is suspicious mammogram but no palpable mass.
      (2) Radiologist locates suspicious area with needle, leaving in place a tiny wire with hook at the end to guide surgeon to area of biopsy. Removal of correct area is confirmed by follow-up x-ray before tissue sent to pathology.
      (3) Complications same as open biopsy.

METHODS OF TREATMENT

A. Pretreatment evaluation.
1. Medical data base established.

      a. Histologic evaluation of biopsy tissue.

      b. History and physical exam.

      c. Mammogram (bilateral).

      d. Chest x-ray.

      e. CBC and liver chemistries.

      f. Bone scan.

      g. Liver scan, if liver chemistries abnormal.

      h. Baseline biologic tumor markers.

         (1) CEA.

         (2) HCG.

         (3) Ferritin.

2. Clinical staging—TNM classification system used:

      a. Stage I: tumor less than 2 cm, axillary nodes negative.

      b. Stage II: tumor less than 5 cm, axillary nodes may be positive but are not fixed, no distant metastasis.

      c. Stage III: tumor may be greater than 5 cm, axillary nodes may be positive and fixed, supraclavicular or infraclavicular nodes may be positive, no distant metastasis.

      d. Stage IV: any combination of tumor and node involvement with evidence of distant metastasis.

3. Informed consent obtained.

      a. Legislation in some states (e.g., California, Florida, Massachusetts) mandates that physician inform woman of all breast cancer treatment options available to her. Patient has active role in decision process.

      b. No evidence that time lapse of up to 2 weeks between diagnosis and initiation of treatment has deleterious effect on survival.

B. Surgery.

1. All surgical procedures include axillary node dissection or sampling. Node status important in assessing prognosis and need for adjuvant chemotherapy.

2. All primary tumor specimens should routinely have estrogen receptor (ER) and progesterone receptor (PR) assays.

3. Radical mastectomy (Halsted) and extended radical (supraradical) mastectomy are rarely performed.

4. Trend is toward more conservative surgical procedures.

      a. Modified radical mastectomy (most widely used procedure).

         (1) Entire breast removed and, possibly, the pectoralis minor. Pectoralis major left intact.

         (2) Used for tumors of any size with goal of controlling local disease.

      b. Partial mastectomy (lumpectomy, tylectomy, quadrant excision) with irradiation.

         (1) Removal of primary tumor and some adjacent tissue with axillary sampling carried out through second incision.

         (2) Used for Stage I and II disease.

         (3) Is evidence that 5-year, disease free survival after partial mastectomy with irradiation is equal to survival after modified radical mastectomy.

         (4) Goal is control of local disease with preservation of the breast.

5. Complications of contemporary surgeries are uncommon but include infection, seroma, lymphedema, impaired shoulder mobility, and nerve injury.

C. Radiation therapy.
  1. Primary radiation.
     a. Combined with partial mastectomy to treat Stage I and II disease.
     b. Therapy is begun 3–4 weeks after surgery when incision is healed and shoulder range of motion adequate.
     c. Total 6,000 rads administered.
        (1) 4,500–5,000 rad to entire breast over 4 1/2 to 5 weeks by linear accelerator.
        (2) 1,000–1,500 rad to the tumor site by either interstitial I^{192} implants or electron beam "boost."
     d. Side effects are fatigue, skin reactions, mild discomfort, and, possibly, sore throat.
  2. Palliative radiation.
     a. Used in Stage IV disease.
     b. Provides partial to complete relief of pain due to bone metastasis.
D. Adjuvant chemotherapy.
  1. Indicated for use in disease which has progressed beyond Stage I (positive node pathology).
  2. Best results in premenopausal women with hormone-dependent (ER positive) tumors.
  3. Single agent therapy.
     a. Primarily used in elderly and possibly in patients who do not respond to combination regimens.
     b. Agents used singly include doxorubicin (adriamycin), cyclophosphamide (Cytoxan), methotrexate, 5-fluorouracil, mitomycin C, L-PAM, vinblastine (Velban), and vincristine (Oncovin).
  4. Combination drug therapy.
     a. 50–80% of patients with metastatic breast cancer experience remissions of 8–12 months duration.
     b. Six drugs in the most widely used combinations are cyclophosphamide, doxorubicin, methotrexate, 5-fluorouracil, vincristine, and prednisone.
     c. Combination regimens used to treat breast cancer.
        (1) CMF (cyclophosphamide, methotrexate, 5-fluorouracil). The mainstay of treating premenopausal women with 1–3 positive nodes.
        (2) CAF (cyclophosphamide, doxorubicin [Adriamycin], 5-fluorouracil).
        (3) CMFVP (CMF with vincristine and prednisone).
        (4) CA (cyclophosphamide and doxorubicin [Adriamycin]).
     d. Trend toward shorter courses of therapy (6 months rather than 12 months).
     e. Combinations of chemotherapy and hormones may have an increased response rate but not necessarily of an increased duration of survival.
     f. Side effects and toxicities may be more pronounced in the patient receiving concurrent irradiation to the breast (generally not given concurrently).
E. Hormonal therapy.
  1. Goal of hormonal therapy is to increase survival time.
  2. One-third of women with breast cancer respond, and postmenopausal women have more favorable responses.

3. Estrogen receptor (ER) and progesterone receptor (PR) results predict those likely to respond.
   a. 65% overall response rate in women with high positive ER results.
   b. Only 10% response rate in those with negative ER results.
   c. PR is positive in about 75% of ER + tumors; may be more accurate predictor.
      (1) If ER+ and PR+, 77% response rate.
      (2) If ER− and PR−, only 5% response.
4. Additive hormonal therapies (increase level of circulating hormone).
   a. Estrogens (65% response if ER+).
   b. Androgens (36% response if ER+).
      (1) Masculinization undesirable to patients.
      (2) Being replaced by anti-estrogens.
   c. Progestins.
   d. Glucocorticoids (47% response if ER+).
5. Ablative therapies (decrease level of circulating hormone).
   a. Castration (65% response if ER+). First line treatment in premenopausal women.
      (1) Surgical castration (oophorectomy).
      (2) Castration by radiation.
   b. Adrenalectomy (53% response if ER+).
      (1) Surgical.
      (2) Medical (aminoglutethimide used).
   c. Hypophysectomy (64% response if ER+).
   d. Anti-estrogen (53% response if ER+).
      (1) First line treatment in postmenopausal women.
      (2) Tamoxifen given with chemotherapy may increase survival rate.
6. If there has been a response to one hormonal therapy, it is likely there will be a response to another.

PROGNOSIS AND REHABILITATION

A. Factors important in long-term survival:
   1. Stage of disease:
      a. Stage I—85% 5-year survival.
      b. Stage II—66% 5-year survival.
      c. Stage III—41% 5-year survival.
      d. Stage IV—10% 5-year survival.
   2. Number of positive nodes:
      a. Negative nodes—24% recurrence at 10 years.
      b. One to three positive nodes—65% recurrence at 10 years.
      c. Four or more positive nodes—86% recurrence at 10 years.
   3. Estrogen receptor status—ER negative tumors have worse prognosis than ER positive ones.
B. Metastasis of breast cancer.
   1. Median time to recurrence is 18 months.
   2. Although the cancer is capable of spreading to any organ, common sites of metastasis are:
      a. Lymph nodes (76%).
      b. Bone (71%).
      c. Lung (69%).

      d. Liver (65%).
      e. Pleura (51%).
      f. Adrenals (49%).
      g. Skin (30%).
   3. Expected survival after distant metastasis is 18 to 36 months.
C. Lifelong follow-up care.
   1. Frequency of post-treatment evaluations:
      a. Three-month intervals for first year.
      b. Four-month intervals for second year.
      c. Six-month intervals for third year.
      d. Annually and prn after third year.
   2. Components of evaluation:
      a. Physical exam and interview.
      b. Chest x-ray.
      c. CBC, Chem 12, CEA.
      d. Repeat bone scan if CEA or Chem 12 elevated or if bone pain is reported.
      e. Repeat mammography at 6 months, 1 year, and then annually.
   3. Cosmetic restoration of breast.
      a. Patient options: no action, use of permanent external prosthesis, or reconstructive surgery.
      b. Breast reconstruction may be immediate (implant at time of modified mastectomy) or delayed (6 months to 1 year after surgery).
         (1) Is covered by most insurance carriers (as are permanent external prostheses).
         (2) Is contraindicated if disease is locally advanced, progressively metastatic, or inflammatory breast cancer.
         (3) Techniques include implants, and procedures to advance skin and muscle tissue to the chest using one of several flaps if anterior chest wall is tight and concave.
         (4) To achieve symmetry, plastic procedures may be required on remaining breast.
            (a) Reduction mammoplasty if large.
            (b) Augmentation if underdeveloped.
            (c) Mastopexy if sagging.
         (5) Nipple-areolar complex may be reconstructed.
         (6) Complications include hematoma, infection, soft tissue ischemia, seroma, contractures, extrusion of prothesis.

NURSING CARE

A. Assess:
   1. Previous knowledge and experience with breast cancer.
   2. Coping abilities and difficulties.
   3. Support systems—family, friends, co-workers, religious affiliation.
   4. Feelings about body image, sexual identity, role relationships.
B. Physiologic aspects of care:
   1. Trend toward early discharge increases the importance of preoperative discharge planning.
      a. Hospitalization often 2–3 days.
      b. Lumpectomy is done on outpatient basis in some institutions.

   c. Usually discharged with drain in place.
      (1) Teach how to empty drain reservoir, measure and record output.
      (2) Drain left in for 7–10 days or until output 30 cc/24 hrs.
   d. Teach care of incisional areas.
2. Promote functional recovery of arm and shoulder.
   a. Limited exercise first 24 hrs (squeezing ball, wrist flexion).
   b. ROM exercises begun at surgeon's discretion (2nd day to 7th day).
3. Inform of precautions to be taken with affected arm to prevent trauma and infection, which can lead to lymphedema. Potential problem is post-axillary dissection.
4. Prevent complications.
   a. Seroma, most common one, especially in obese patients. Managed with aspiration if it occurs.
   b. Hematoma usually resolves.
   c. Lymphedema, especially if axilla irradiated.
      (1) 10% develop mild to moderate edema with a circumferential measurement up to 5 cm larger than unaffected arm.
      (2) Managed with elevation, mild exercise, massage, pressure-gradient elastic sleeve.
5. Teach BSE.
6. Prepare woman for expected and normal breast sensations, which may last several years (numbness, tingling, and phantom breast sensation after mastectomy).

C. Psychosocial aspects of care.
   1. Major distress is the diagnosis of cancer itself and the loss or alteration of the breast.
   2. Breast cancer is a threat to life, self, and relationships.
   3. Common reactions are anxiety, anger, depression, denial, withdrawal.
   4. Major nursing roles are support, education, client advocacy.
   5. Spouse/significant other should be included in plan of care.
   6. Providing woman with accurate, relevant information has several outcomes.
      a. Decreases anxiety.
      b. Increases self-esteem.
      c. Facilitates decision making.
      d. Improves overall recovery and adjustment.
   7. Encourage resumption of normal activities of daily living as soon as possible.
   8. Utilize appropriate resources.
      a. Reach to Recovery.
      b. I Can Cope.
      c. AFTER (Ask a Friend to Explain Reconstruction).
      d. Other community groups.
      e. Booklets, pamphlets.

D. Sexual aspects of care.
   1. Breast cancer impacts all areas of sexuality.
      a. Gender identity.
      b. Sex role identity.
      c. Sexual preference.
      d. Sexual performance.
   2. Explore client's self-concept and importance of breast.

3. Allay fears and misconceptions about impact on sexuality.
4. Anticipate special problems of women receiving adjuvant therapy, for example, decrease in vaginal secretions if on chemotherapy.
5. Encourage or promote open communication between woman and spouse/ significant other.

STUDY QUESTIONS

1. Describe the risk factors for breast cancer.
2. Discuss the controversies in the management of breast cancer.
3. Develop a plan of care for a patient receiving surgery/chemotherapy/radiation for breast cancer.

Bibliography

American Cancer Society: Cancer statistics, 1985. CA Cancer Journal for Clinicians, *35*(1):19–35, 1985.

Fisher, B., et al.: Five-year results of a randomized clinical trial comparing total mastectomy and segmental mastectomy with or without radiation in the treatment of breast cancer. The New England Journal of Medicine, *312*:665–673, 1985.

Harris, J. R., Hellman, S., Canellos, G. P., and Fisher, B.: Cancer of the breast. *In* DeVita, V. T., Jr., Hellman, S., and Rosenberg, S. A. (eds.): Cancer: Principles and Practice of Oncology, 2nd ed. Vol. 2. Philadelphia, J. B. Lippincott Co., pp. 1119–1177, 1985.

Hassey, K. M.: Radiation therapy for breast cancer: A historic review. Seminars in Oncology Nursing, *1*:181–188, 1985.

Health and Public Policy Committee, American College of Physicians: The use of diagnostic tests for screening and evaluating breast lesions. Annals of Internal Medicine, *103*:147–151, 1985.

Knobf, M. K. T.: Primary breast cancer: Physical consequences and rehabilitation. Seminars in Oncology Nursing, *1*:214–224, 1985.

Knobf, M. K. T.: The treatment evolution. American Journal of Nursing, *84*:1110–1120, 1984.

McKhann, C. F.: The changing role of surgery in the treatment of breast cancer. Seminars in Oncology Nursing, *1*:176–180, 1985.

Morra, M. E.: Breast self-examination today: An overview of its use and its value. Seminars in Oncology Nursing, *1*:170–175, 1985.

Nail, L., Jones, L. S., Giuffre, M., and Johnson, J. E.: Sensations after mastectomy. American Journal of Nursing, *84*:1121–1123, 1984.

Nash, J. A.: Breast cancer: Screening, detection, and diagnosis. Seminars in Oncology Nursing, *1*:163–169, 1985.

Onion, P.: Prognosis with pregnancy. American Journal of Nursing, *84*:1126–1128, 1984.

Schwarz-Appelbaum, J., Dedrick, J., Jusenius, K., and Kirchner, C. W.: Nursing care plans: Sexuality and treatment of breast cancer. Oncology Nursing Forum, *11*(6):16–24, 1984.

Vogel, C. L.: Systemic therapy of breast cancer—1985. Seminars in Oncology Nursing, *1*:189–194, 1985.

Wissing, V. S.: The hormone factor. American Journal of Nursing, *84*:1117–1119, 1984.

15

Skin Cancer

ALICE LONGMAN, RN, Ed D

RISK FACTORS

A. Nonmelanoma skin cancers (basal cell and squamous cell carcinoma) (Fig. 15–1).
  1. Exogenous.
    a. Ultraviolet radiation from sunlight (UV-B spectral range, 290–320 nanometer range).
    b. Exposure to ionizing radiation (radiologists and uranium miners).
    c. Arsenic.
    d. Petroleum including coal, tar, pitch, and creosote preparations.
    e. Scars following injuries, e.g., burns.
  2. Endogenous.
    a. Fair or freckled complexion.
    b. Red, blonde, or light brown hair.
    c. Light-colored eyes.
    d. Xeroderma pigmentosum/albinism.
    e. Immunologic deficiency or suppression, e.g., lymphoproliferative carcinoma, renal transplant.
  3. Premalignant states or lesions.
    a. Actinic and senile keratosis.
    b. Seborrheic keratosis.
    c. Arsenic keratosis.
    d. Bowen's disease.
B. Melanoma (see Fig. 15–1).
  1. Exogenous.
    a. Ultraviolet radiation from sunlight.
    b. Poor tolerance of sunlight.
    c. Heavy exposure to sunlight.
  2. Endogenous.
    a. Acquired nevi (common acquired nevi and dysplastic nevi).
    b. Dysplastic nevus syndrome (familial and sporadic).

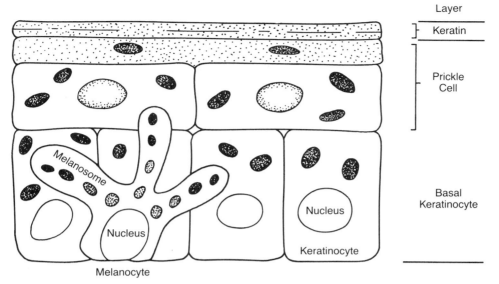

Figure 15–1. Schematic drawing of the epidermis. Keratin is the outermost layer of skin. The inner layer of epidermis has basal keratinocytes (skin cells) and melanocytes (pigment cells). The pigment is packaged in units called melanosomes, which are transferred into the keratinocytes. Skin color is determined by the total quantity of melanin in all layers of skin. Melanomas arise from melanocytes (pigment cells). (Courtesy of James J. Nordlund, M.D., and The Skin Cancer Foundation. Redrawn from Berkman, S.: The skin remembers, Cancer News 39 (2):2, 1985.)

SCREENING AND DETECTION

A. Early signs of skin cancer:
  1. Nonmelanoma.
    a. Sore that does not heal.
    b. Persistent lump or swelling.
    c. Changes in skin markings—size, color, surface, shape, surrounding skin, sensation, elevation.
  2. Melanoma.
    a. Size (enlargement).
    b. Color (especially red or black).
    c. Surface (scaliness, oozing, flakiness).
    d. Shape or outline (irregular notched border).
    e. Surrounding skin (redness, swelling).
    f. New sensations (itchy, tender, painful, lumpy).
    g. Appearance of a new raised area in a mole (especially if the mole is black).
    h. Appearance of new moles.
B. Skin assessment (Table 15–1):
  1. Skin exposure to sunlight.
    a. Time of day during exposure.
    b. Geographic area of residence(s) or recreation.
    c. Altitude and overcast weather conditions.
    d. Time of year exposed to the sun.
    e. Length of exposure(s).

Table 15–1. HOW TO DETERMINE SKIN TYPE AND
PHOTOPROTECTION NEEDS*

A skin type is determined by assessing the patient's history of reaction to noonday sun in June following a period of minimal solar exposure. Exposure to 20–30 minutes of natural sunlight in June at sea level equals 15–25 ml/cm^2 of UVB.

Skin Type	UVB/MED ml/cm	Pigmentation/Erythema History	Genetic History
I	10–20	Very poor ability to tan, burns easily and severely, then peels.	Very fair skin, freckling evident Blue, green, grey eye color Blond, red, or brown hair Unexposed skin is white
II	20–30	Tans minimally or lightly following exposure, usually burns easily resulting in a painful burn.	Fair skin, unexposed skin is white Blue, green, gray, or brown eye color Blond, red, or brown hair
III	30–40	Tans gradually following exposure, burns moderately.	"Average" Unexposed skin is white Hair and eye color usually brown
IV	40–50	Burns minimally, tans well with initial exposure.	White or light brown skin Unexposed skin is white or light brown Dark hair and eye color (Mediterraneans, Orientals, Hispanics)
V	50–60	Tans easily and profusely, rarely burns.	Brown skin, unexposed skin is brown (American Indian, East Indian, Hispanics)
VI	50–60	Deeply pigmented, never burns.	Black skin, unexposed skin is black (African and American blacks, Australian and South Indian Aborigines)

* From Anders, J. E. and Leach, E. E.: Sun versus skin. American Journal of Nursing, *83*(7): 1015–1020, 1983.

2. Skin type.
   a. Pigmentation/erythema type.
   b. Genetic history.
3. Examination of the skin.
   a. Inspect and palpate all accessible skin surfaces—smooth skin, skin folds, mucosal surfaces, epidermal appendages.
   b. Assess pre-existing lesions of the skin.
   c. Inspect scalp and entire hairline; palpate scalp.
   d. Inspect face, lips, and neck including posterior neck and postauricular areas.
   e. Inspect and palpate all surfaces of upper extremities.

f. Inspect and palpate the skin of the back, buttocks, and back of legs.
g. Inspect the external genitalia.
h. Inspect and palpate the anterior surfaces of the legs and feet.
i. Inspect and palpate all hairy surfaces; include those beneath axillary, thoracic, and pubic hair.
j. Note characteristics of normal moles.

C. Clinical characteristics of nonmelanoma skin cancer (Table 15–2):
1. Basal cell carcinoma (common form of skin cancer) (Fig. 15–2).
   a. Nodulo-ulcerative basal cell carcinoma:
      (1) Elevated lesion.
      (2) Umbilicated, ulcerated center and raised margins.
      (3) Moderately firm to the touch.

Table 15–2. INCIDENCE, CLINICAL CHARACTERISTICS, AND COMMON SITES OF PRINCIPAL CUTANEOUS CANCERS*

Incidence	Clinical Characteristics	Common Sites
BASAL CELL CARCINOMA		
Most common form of skin cancer; occurs primarily in patients exposed to prolonged or intense sunlight, especially Caucasians with light eyes, light hair, and fair complexions.	*Nodulo-ulcerative basal cell cancer:* Elevated lesions with umbillicated, ulcerated centers; raised waxy or "pearly" borders; moderately firm. *Superfical basal cell cancer:* Barely elevated plaques, usually with crusted and erythematous centers and raised, thread-like pearly borders; often multiple.	Nose, eyelids, cheeks, and trunks. Uncommon on palms and soles. Metastases are extremely rare.
SQUAMOUS CELL CARCINOMA		
Less common than basal cell carcinoma; occurs primarily on areas exposed to actinic radiation and on vermilion border of lips.	Appearance varies from an elevated nodular mass to a punched-out ulcerated lesion to a fungating mass. Unlike basal cell carcinomas, squamous cell carcinomas are opaque.	75% occur on head, 15% on hands, and 10% elsewhere. Can metastasize to regional lymph nodes; in more advanced lesions, visceral (especially pulmonary) metastasis can occur.
MALIGNANT MELANOMA		
Far less common than basal or squamous cell carcinoma. Currently about 14,000 new cases per year in U.S.	Usually irregularly pigmented (black, gray, white, blue, brown, red); often less than 2.5 cm in diameter. May be flat or elevated, eroded or ulcerated; outline usually irregular, often with notch; frequently mildly symptomatic (e.g., pruritic).	Backs of men and women, legs of women, less common in areas unexposed to sun; metastasize via lymphatics and blood vessels—often first to regional lymph nodes.

* From Gumport, S. L., Harris, M. N., Roses, D. F., and Kopf, A. W.: The diagnosis and management of common skin cancers. CA Cancer Journal for Clinicians, *31*(2):79–90, 1981.

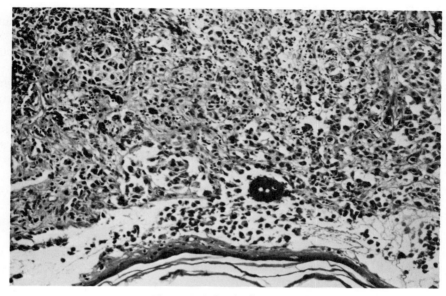

Figure 15–2. Basal cell carcinoma.

    b. Superficial basal cell carcinoma:
       (1) Superficial, sharply marginated plaque with a raised, pearly, thread-like border.
       (2) Center is usually crusted, scaly, and erythematous.
    c. Irregular local extension is the principal problem of management.
2. Squamous cell carcinoma (predominant skin cancer in skin exposed to ionizing radiation, carcinogenic chemicals, or trauma) (Fig. 15–3).
    a. Actinic keratosis is implicated in the development of squamous cell carcinoma.

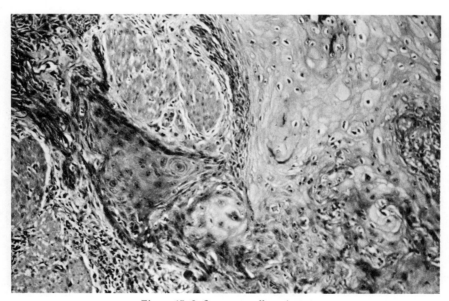

Figure 15–3. Squamous cell carcinoma.

    b. Actinic keratosis can be considered as a premalignant stage (roughly 20% progress to squamous cell carcinoma).

    c. Lesion of actinic keratosis appears slightly elevated, well-circumscribed, and erythematous with a rough and scaly surface.

    d. Bowen's disease can also be considered in situ squamous carcinoma.

    e. Lesion in Bowen's disease appears slightly elevated, well-circumscribed, scaly or crusted, and dull red.

    f. Clinical appearance of squamous cell carcinoma varies from an ulcerated infiltrating mass to an elevated, erythematous, nodular mass.

    g. Squamous cell carcinoma may metastasize to the regional lymph nodes.

D. Melanoma (approximately 50% of melanomas arise in pre-existing or congenital nevi) (Fig. 15–4):

  1. Melanoma arises from a special cell called a melanocyte, which has the ability to synthesize melanin.

  2. More likely to occur in the junctional nevus that is usually flat and smooth.

  3. Classification of melanoma:

    a. Lentigo maligna melanoma (LMN).

      (1) Large, variably pigmented, freckle-like lesions.

      (2) Develops on a benign structure called a Hutchinson's freckle.

      (3) Appears as a thickened and elevated nodule within the freckle.

      (4) Very slow to invade deeply.

    b. Superficial spreading melanoma (SSM).

      (1) Kaleidoscopic variety of colors, ranging from tan-black, brown, blue-grey to violaceous pink.

      (2) Lesion is characteristically flat to slightly elevated.

    c. Nodular melanoma (NM).

      (1) Color is a shade of blue.

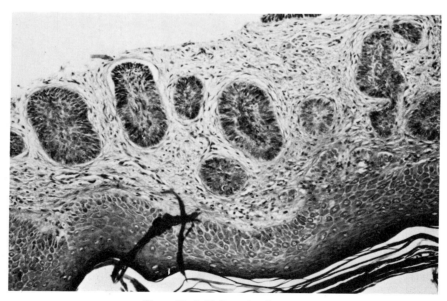

Figure 15–4. Malignant melanoma.

(2) Occasionally, there are small, dark specks at the base of the lesion.

(3) Lesion is elevated, and borders are well demarcated.

    d. Acral-lentiginous melanoma (ALM).

(1) Irregular in shape and variable change in size.

(2) Color is variegated; shades of blue and black.

(3) Lesion is smooth or ulcerated and may be raised or flat.

METHODS OF TREATMENT

A. Nonmelanoma skin cancer.
1. Definitive treatment depends on many factors: location and size of the lesion, exact histologic type of cancer, possible extension into nearby structures, presence of metastases, previous treatment used, anticipated cosmetic results, and age and general condition of the patient.
2. Accurate histologic diagnosis.
   a. Excisional biopsy with 0.5–1.0 cm margins is recommended if a lesion is small.
   b. Incisional biopsy, including 1 cm margin, is justified for larger lesions.
3. Surgery.
   a. Excision of lesion.
   b. Curettage and electrodesiccation for small lesions.
   c. Mohs' microscopically controlled surgery (surgically removes the cancer in multiple progressive layers).
   d. Cryosurgery using thermocouples.
4. Radiotherapy.
   a. If inadequate tumor margins are shown, radiotherapy can be used.
   b. Radiation is given in a highly fractionated schedule (4500 rad/3 weeks in 300 rad daily fractions) with attention to shielding.
   c. Combined approach of preoperative and postoperative radiation and surgery is often successful.
5. Chemotherapy.
   a. Topical 5-fluorouracil (5-FU).
   b. Various chemotherapeutic agents have been used for unusual skin cancers no longer manageable by surgery or irradiation by arterial infusion, local injection, or topical application.
6. Immunotherapy.
   a. Dinitrochlorobenzene (DNCB).
   b. Triethylene-immuno-benzoquinone (TEIB).
B. Melanoma.
1. Clinical and histologic staging (Table 15–3).
   a. Most important characteristic in the staging of melanoma is the vertical depth of melanotic penetration through the skin.
   b. Refinement of classification relates the prognosis of melanoma to the actual measured depth (thickness) of invasion.
   c. Clinical staging system for cutaneous melanoma:
      (1) Local.
      (2) Regional nodal disease.
      (3) Disseminated disease.
2. Accurate histologic diagnosis.
   a. Excisional biopsy yielding a specimen with a border several millimeters in diameter.

Table 15–3. CLINICAL AND MICROSTAGING CLASSIFICATION
METHODS FOR MALIGNANT MELANOMA*

Clinical Staging	Clark's Five Levels Of Cutaneous Invasion

Stage I
  Localized melanoma without metastasis to distant or regional lymph nodes
  1. Primary melanoma untreated or removed by excisional biopsy
  2. Locally recurrent melanoma within 4 cm of primary site
  3. Multiple primary melanomas
Stage II
  Metastasis limited to regional lymph nodes
  1. Primary melanoma present or removed with simultaneous metastasis
  2. Primary melanoma controlled with subsequent metastasis
  3. Locally recurrent melanoma with metastasis
  4. In-transit metastasis beyond 4 cm from primary site
  5. Unknown primary melanoma with metastasis
Stage III
  Disseminated melanoma
  1. Visceral and/or multiple lymphatic metastases
  2. Multiple cutaneous and/or subcutaneous metastases
	Level I
	  Melanoma located above the basement membrane (basal lamina) of the epidermis. These lesions are essentially in situ, are extremely rare, and present no danger.
	Level II
	  Melanoma invades through the basement membrane down to the papillary dermis.
	Level III
	  Melanoma at this level is characterized by filling and widening by melanoma cells of the papillary dermis at its interface with the reticular dermis. Characteristically, there is no invasion of the underlying reticular layer.
	Level IV
	  These lesions show melanoma penetration into the reticular dermis.
	Level V
	  Melanoma at this level is evident by its presence in the subcutaneous tissue.

* From Goldsmith, H. S.: Melanoma: An overview. CA Cancer Journal for Clinicians, *29*(4): 194–215, 1979.

    b. Step sections of the biopsy specimen at 3 mm or closer intervals throughout the specimen should be ordered.

3. Surgery.
    a. Wide, local excision leaving a 3- to 5-cm margin if it is anatomically possible.
    b. A skin graft may be required for closure.
    c. Prophylactic lymph node dissection is advocated.

4. Chemotherapy.
    a. Agents with consistent activity have been dacarbazine (DTIC) and the nitrosoureas with carmustine (BCNU) the most frequently used.
    b. Palliation may be achieved.

5. Immunotherapy.
    a. Bacille Calmette-Guérin (BCG) is the most common agent used to stimulate an immunologic response in the host.
    b. Precise role of BCG in treating melanoma is still uncertain.

6. Other.
    a. Vitamin A/retinoids.
    b. Hyperthermia.

PROGNOSIS AND REHABILITATION

A. Nonmelanoma skin cancers (basal cell and squamous cell carcinomas).
1. Basal cell carcinoma.
   a. Equally high cure rates (90–95%) with either surgery or irradiation.
   b. Metastatic ability is poor, but has the possibility of creating extensive local destruction.
   c. Free full-thickness skin graft gives an acceptable cosmetic result.
2. Squamous cell carcinoma.
   a. Equally high cure rates (75–80%) with either surgery or irradiation.
   b. Recurrence of lesion is major complication.
   c. Follow-up visits two to four times a year are important.
   d. Metastasizes to local lymph nodes and distant sites.
3. Bowen's disease. Cure rate using 5-FU is impressive (90%).
B. Melanoma.
1. Most important prognostic feature of melanoma is the size of the lesion at the time of its removal.
2. Survival rate is correlated with the depth of invasion and location of the lesion.
3. Difficult and unpredictable problem of hematogenous dissemination has not been solved.
4. Significant palliation can be achieved with use of chemotherapy and immunotherapy.
C. Special considerations.
1. Primary melanoma of the eye.
   a. Primary melanoma in the iris does well with local resection.
   b. Ciliary body and choroidal melanoma require enucleation.
   c. Success of treatment for metastatic disease from eye melanoma is uniformly poor.
2. Primary mucosal melanoma (uniformly poor prognosis).
3. Local advanced disease.
   a. Development of massive, local disease frequently in the neck, axillary, or inguinal nodal areas.
   b. Combination of radiation and hyperthermia offers palliation.
4. Metastasis to the brain warrants high-dose fraction radiation.

NURSING CARE

A. Nonmelanoma skin cancers (basal cell and squamous cell carcinomas).
1. Prevention—patient teaching.
   a. Avoidance of prolonged exposure to sunlight especially between the hours of 10 AM and 3 PM.
   b. Avoidance of sunburning and suntanning.
   c. Use of sunscreens and sunblocks.
      (1) Commercial sunscreens with a sun protection factor (SPF) of greater than 10, e.g., Presun, Probanlo, Coppertone, Super Shade.
      (2) Commercial sunblocks that have the active ingredients titanium dioxide, zinc oxide, talc, iron oxide, and kaolin.
      (3) Reapplication of sunscreens every 2–3 hours during long sun exposure.

      (4) Individuals with short hair should apply sunscreens to ears and back of neck.

      (5) Use sunscreens containing benzophenones if taking thiazides, sulfonamides, or other photosensitizing drugs.

      (6) Use of protective clothing in the sun (broad-brimmed hats, scarves, long sleeves, slacks).

      (7) Avoid use of sun lamps and tanning salons.

      (8) Avoid ultraviolet and x-ray treatments for acne and other chronic skin conditions.

2. Detection—patient teaching.
    a. History of any recent changes in lesion(s).
    b. Systematic assessment of skin (SSE) for suspicious lesions monthly.
    c. Special attention should be given to mucosal surfaces, warts and birthmarks, hairy surfaces, and soles of the feet.

3. Follow-up—patient teaching.
    a. Reinforce nonmetastatic behavior of basal cell carcinoma lesions.
    b. Need for follow-up of lesion site, periodic observation for potential reoccurrence.
    c. Sites of chronic skin damage in squamous cell carcinoma should be periodically evaluated for evidence of recurrence.

B. Melanoma.
  1. Prevention and detection.
    a. Adequate teaching for early signs and symptoms of the lesion(s).
    b. Early and prompt treatment.
  2. Treatment.
    a. Prepare patient and family for extensive surgical intervention.
    b. Open optimistic approach in discussing feelings and attitudes.
    c. Special attention to psychological impact of life-threatening cutaneous melanoma.
  3. Follow-up.
    a. Need for follow-up of lesion site, periodic observation for potential reoccurrence.
    b. High-risk individuals can reduce chances of developing melanoma.

STUDY QUESTIONS

1. Identify risk factors for the development of skin cancer.
2. Describe screening and early detection methods useful in skin cancer.
3. Describe nursing interventions for persons diagnosed and treated for skin cancer.

Bibliography

Anders, J. E. and Leach, E. E.: Sun versus skin. American Journal of Nursing, *83*(7):1015–1020, 1983.

Berkman, S.: The skin remembers. Cancer News, *39*(2):2–4, 1985.

Caldwell, E. H., McCormack, R. M., Goldsmith, L. A. and Rubin, P.: Skin Cancer. *In* Rubin, P. (ed.): Clinical Oncology for Medical Students and Physicians, 6th Ed. New York, American Cancer Society, pp. 222–229, 1983.

Fraser, M. C. and McGuire, D. B.: Skin cancer's early warning system. American Journal of Nursing, *84*(10):1232–1236, 1984.

Friedman, R. J., Rigel, D. S. and Kopf, A. W.: Early detection of malignant melanoma: The role of physician examination and self-examination of the skin. CA Cancer Journal for Clinicians, 35(3):130–151, 1985.

Goldsmith, H. S.: Melanoma: An overview. CA Cancer Journal for Clinicians, 29(4):194–215, 1979.

Gumport, S. L., Harris, M. N., Roses, D. F. and Kopf, A. W.: The Diagnosis and Management of Common Skin Cancers. CA Cancer Journal for Clinicians, 31(2):79–89, 1981.

Meyskens, F. L.: Malignant Melanoma Clinical Diagnosis Quiz. Bristol Laboratories, 8(3):2–21, St. Louis, The C.V. Mosby Co., 1984.

Page, H. S. and Asire, A. J.: Cancer Rates and Risks, 3rd Ed. N.I.H. Publication No. 85-691, U.S. Department of Health and Human Services, 1985.

Schleper, J. R.: Cancer prevention and detection: Skin cancer. Cancer Nursing, 7(1):67–84, 1984.

Stair, J. C.: Knowledge deficit related to prevention and early detection of nonmelanoma skin cancers (basal cell and squamous cell carcinoma, including Bowen's disease). *In* McNally, J. C., Stair, J. C. and Somerville, E. T. (eds.): Guidelines for Cancer Nursing Practice. Orlando, FL, Grune & Stratton, Inc., pp. 27–31, 1985.

White, L. N., Patterson, J. E., Cornelius, J. L. and Judkins, A. E.: Skin Cancer. Cancer Screening and Detection Manual for Nurses. New York, McGraw-Hill Book Co., pp. 9–15, 1979.

16

Prostate Cancer

JULENA LIND, RN, MS

RISK FACTORS

A. Age.
   1. Third most common cause of cancer deaths in men in the U.S.
   2. Over 14% of men over age 50 have cancer of prostate; incidence increases with each decade. It occurs in 50% of men over 75 years old.
   3. Some theorize that prostate cancer is normal part of the aging process, since 95% of men who die over the age of 90 have some foci of disease in their prostate at autopsy.
B. Ethnicity.
   1. Native Orientals are at low risk; however, incidence increases noticeably in those who adopt western habits, particularly dietary.
   2. The highest rate of prostatic cancer in the world is among black Americans. The disease is reportedly much lower in African blacks.
C. Environmental factors.
   1. Exposure to cadmium may lead to accumulation in the prostate and, in turn, interruption of cell growth.
   2. Transmission of virus-like particles have been investigated but not substantiated as an environmental factor.
   3. Endocrine factors may play a role. (Subcutaneous testosterone given to rats can produce prostatic cancers.)

SCREENING AND DETECTION

A. Screening.
   1. Early detection achieved through small asymptomatic nodule felt on rectal exam—50% of prostatic nodules are carcinoma. (Early detection not common.)
   2. Rectal exam as screening tool:
      a. Every year for men under 50 years old.
      b. Every 6 months for men 50 years old and older.
B. Signs and symptoms.
   1. Early signs when present include:
      a. Dysuria.

      b. Urinary hesitancy.

      c. Straining to start stream.

      d. Urgency.

  2. Later signs include:

      a. Hematuria.

      b. Chronic urinary retention with dribbling.

  3. Patients with widespread disease on presentation appear generally debilitated and older than their age:

      a. May have bone and neuritic pain secondary to osseous involvement or nerve compression.

      b. Weight loss, lethargy, and secondary disease, i.e., bronchopneumonia, may be present as a result of "chronic illness."

C. Diagnosis.

  1. Rectal examination by which the prostate may be palpated for firm, hard lesions.

  2. Biopsy.

      a. Needle—perineal or transrectal; transrectal preferred.

      b. Open—in selected cases, i.e., size of prostate demands removal.

  3. Histologic diagnosis—may be found in asymptomatic specimens removed for benign prostatic hypertrophy.

  4. Laboratory studies:

      a. Acid phosphatase—produced by prostate; any trauma to prostate can release it into blood stream.

         (1) Wait 48 hours after rectal exam or catheterization to draw acid phosphatase.

         (2) Elevated acid phosphatase in a patient suspected of having prostatic cancer can indicate metastatic disease.

      b. Prostatic acid phosphatase level can be measured by radioimmunoassay.

      c. Alkaline phosphatase.

         (1) Elevated in presence of bone metastasis.

         (2) Many patients with cancer of prostate have bone metastasis on presentation.

D. Staging.

  1. Staging work-up might include:

      a. Chest x-ray to check for hilar node, lung, and rib involvement.

      b. Excretory urogram to demonstrate obstruction caused by pelvic lymph node metastasis or direct invasion by tumor.

      c. Liver scan and brain scan.

      d. Lymphangiogram to detect presence of pelvic lymph nodes.

  2. Staging systems:

      a. Stage A: Incidental microscopic focus (not clinically palpable).

      b. Stage B: Localized, palpable nodule confined to prostate gland.

      c. Stage C: Local extension to adjacent structures.

      d. Stage D: Extrapelvic/distant metastasis.

METHODS OF TREATMENT

A. Curative treatment—primarily for Stage A and B disease.

  1. Much controversy exists over whether surgery or radiation is best utilized as primary curative treatment.

2. Stage A.
    a. If low grade (well differentiated), may leave untreated.
        (1) 15-year survivorship has been shown equal to that in the general population.
        (2) Age of patient and morbidity of treatment must be considered.
    b. High grade anaplastic tumors may respond satisfactorily to mega-voltage radiation.
3. Stage B—surgery and radiation each yield 5-year survival greater than 70%; 10-year survival greater than 50%.
    a. Surgery—radical prostatectomy for cure.
        (1) Perineal approach is generally treatment of choice.
        (2) Retropubic approach may be associated with decreased stricture formation.
        (3) Suprapubic approach.
    b. Lymph node dissection may be added to prostatectomy.
        (1) May not increase survival, but benefits have been reported.
        (2) Involves considerable morbidity.
    c. Complications associated with surgical treatment:
        (1) Impotence.
        (2) Incontinence.
        (3) Stricture formation.
    d. Radiation therapy is relatively new as cure.
        (1) Interstitial implants (temporary or permanent).
        (2) External beam therapy of 6000–7000 rads to extended field.
        (3) Reported to be associated with less impotence than with surgery.
        (4) Problems include proctitis, diarrhea, urinary frequency.
4. Large (greater than 1.5–2 cm) Stage B and Stage C lesions may receive radical curative treatment with multimodality approach:
    a. Transurethral resection of the prostate (TURP).
    b. Megavoltage radiation therapy:
        (1) 6500–7000 rads over 6–7 weeks.
        (2) Delay for 6 weeks after TURP to allow urothelial healing.
B. Palliative treatment for Stage C and D disease.
    1. Stage C is most common presenting form of prostatic cancer, approximately 45% of all prostatic cancer cases. Stage D disease accounts for approximately 40%.
    2. Radiation therapy is used for local extensions and for sites of metastasis.
        a. May be primary treatment for Stage D lesions if hormonal manipulation is ineffective or cannot be utilized.
        b. Used for palliation of pain from bone metastasis.
    3. Hormonal manipulation used primarily for palliation; prompt initiation may delay symptoms.
        a. Antiandrogens interfere with production of testosterone.
            (1) Diethylstilbestrol (DES):
                ○ Significant cardiovascular complications with higher doses such as 5 mg/day. Dose of 1mg/day seems to be as effective a treatment.
                ○ Objective responses to DES include: decreased pain, weight gain, decreased urinary symptoms, decrease in tumor size.
                ○ Relapse generally occurs within 2–3 years; usually relapsed form is hormone resistant.

      (2) Large doses of IV Stilphostrol (intravenous diethylstilbestrol) may be given in urgent situations, i.e., CNS involvement or ureteral obstruction.

  b. Orchiectomy:

      (1) Effectiveness equal to DES.

      (2) Used for patients requiring prompt response, or in patients unreliable in taking medications, or when side effects of estrogens contraindicate.

  c. Side effects associated with hormonal therapy:

      (1) Edema and cardiac failure.

      (2) Gynecomastia.

      (3) Loss of libido.

      (4) Impotence.

      (5) Thrombophlebitis.

4. Chemotherapy usually used with Stage D disease that is unresponsive or relapsed.

  a. Hormones.

  b. Many drugs have been tried including:

      (1) Doxorubicin.

      (2) Cisplatin.

      (3) Cyclophosphamide.

      (4) S-Fluorouracil.

      (5) Methotrexate.

      (6) Lomustine.

      (7) Dacarbazine.

PROGNOSIS AND REHABILITATION

A. Prognosis.

  1. Stage A (constitutes only about 5% of all cases).

    a. Low grade tumor—15-year survival closely approximates actual life expectancy.

    b. High grade tumor—prognosis may be as poor as with metastatic disease.

  2. Stage B (about 5% of cases)—10-year survival as high as 72%.

  3. Stage C (approximately 45% of cases).

    a. Average life expectancy 2–3 years.

    b. Survival at 5 years is 45%; 10 years, 26%.

  4. Stage D—the usual prognosis is 1–2 years.

B. Rehabilitation concerns.

  1. Incontinence—exercises to gain urinary control may be indicated.

  2. Impotence—counseling on subsequent surgery for penile prostheses may be indicated.

NURSING CARE

A. Potential patient problems related to radical prostatectomy for prostate cancer:

  1. Wound infection (if perineal prostatectomy).

  2. Fecal incontinence from sphincter injury.

3. Bladder spasms with pain.
4. Sexual dysfunction:
   a. Absence of emission and ejaculation as a result of removal of the seminal vesicles and transection of the vas deferens.
   b. Loss of ability to achieve erection as a result of damage to the nervous system.
5. Urinary tract infection.
6. Hematuria (common 1–4 days after surgery).
7. Clot formation (which may obstruct urinary flow).
8. Urinary incontinence (or dribbling and urgency) after catheter removed.
B. Nursing assessment data related to radical prostatectomy:
   1. Signs of wound infection (erythema, fever).
   2. Onset and duration of bladder spasms.
   3. Impact of surgery on sexual life of patient and partner.
   4. Signs of urinary tract infection (amount and color and presence of casts).
   5. Degree of hematuria and signs and symptoms of hemorrhage and shock.
   6. Patency of urinary drainage (and/or bladder irrigation system) through catheter.
   7. Amount and frequency of voiding after urethral catheter removed.
C. Nursing interventions related generally to radical prostatectomy:
   1. Pre-operative nursing interventions:
      a. Patient teaching regarding the Foley catheter, blood in urine, three-way irrigation.
      b. Enema for bowel cleansing to prevent contamination.
      c. Ted hose.
      d. Preoperative laboratory work should include coagulation studies; check results.
   2. Maintaining presence of urethral catheter (which in radical prostatectomy serves as a splint for the urethral anastomosis as well as for urinary drainage).
   3. Preventing urinary tract infection through closed catheter drainage.
   4. Maintaining adequate bladder drainage through continuous or intermittent bladder irrigation.
   5. Preventing urinary catheter obstruction (which can be caused by kinked tubing, mucous plugs, or blood clots).
   6. Administering antispasmodics to decrease discomfort of bladder spasms (should be administered concurrently with stool softeners to avoid constipation).
   7. Providing permission to discuss sexual concerns.
   8. Giving information on anatomic changes related to sexuality.
   9. Offering specific suggestions on the advantages and disadvantages of penile prostheses.
   10. Assisting the patient in managing dribbling, urgency, or urinary incontinence.
       a. Teach the patient and family that in most cases this problem will gradually improve.
       b. Teach the patient exercises to gain urinary control.
D. Nursing interventions specifically related to perineal prostatectomy:
   1. Meticulous cleansing of perineal area.
   2. Applying heat lamp treatments to perineum.
   3. Providing sitz baths.

4. Preserving skin integrity by using a T binder instead of tape to hold the dressing in place.
5. Offering a low residual diet to minimize bowel activity.
6. Avoiding rectal tubes, rectal thermometers, or enemas until wound is healed.

E. Potential patient problems related to external beam radiation therapy for prostate cancer:
1. Cystitis (1–3 weeks after start of therapy).
2. Proctitis (due to damage of intestinal lining).
3. Skin reactions—radiodermatitis (2 weeks after start of therapy).
   a. Epilation.
   b. Erythemas.
   c. Dry desquamation.
   d. Wet desquamation.
4. Radiation syndrome.
   a. Fatigue.
   b. Weakness.
   c. Anorexia.

F. Nursing assessment data related to radiotherapy for prostatic cancer:
1. Signs of cystitis (degree of urgency, frequency, and pain on urination).
2. Signs of proctitis (amount and frequency of diarrhea).
3. Degree of skin reactions.
4. Impact of fatigue on lifestyle.
5. Impact of radiotherapy on sexual life of patient and partner.

G. Nursing interventions related to radiotherapy for prostate cancer:
1. Administering bladder antispasmodics and analgesics.
2. Teaching the patient and family that drinking at least 2 liters of fluid per day will decrease discomfort associated with cystitis.
3. Administering antidiarrheal medication.
4. Teaching the patient and family to avoid a high residue diet.
5. Teaching the patient and family how to maintain skin integrity.
6. Providing nursing interventions related to sexual concerns.

H. Potential patient problems related to hormonal therapy for prostate cancer:
1. Side effects of diethylstilbestrol:
   a. Sodium retention.
   b. Hypercalcemia.
   c. Nausea.
   d. Hypertension.
   e. Feminization.
   f. Gynecomastia.
   g. Loss of libido.
   h. Impotence.
   i. Thromboembolic complications.
2. Potential problems associated with orchiectomy:
   a. Anxiety about connotation of castration.
   b. Pain.
   c. Wound infection at incision site.

I. Nursing assessment data related to hormonal therapy for prostate cancer:
1. Serum sodium and calcium levels.
2. Signs of edema.
3. Signs of hypercalcemia (polyuria, polydipsia, confusion, weakness)

4. Blood pressure changes.
5. Impact of hormonal therapy on sexual life of patient and partner.
6. Signs of pulmonary embolus.
7. Degree of anxiety regarding orchiectomy.
8. Degree and type of pain post orchiectomy.
9. Signs of wound infection.

J. Nursing interventions related to hormonal therapy for prostate cancer:
1. Administering diuretics if indicated for edema.
2. Administering drugs to control hypercalcemia if indicated (NaCl infusions, phosphate enemas, calcitonin, diuretics).
3. Teaching patient and family about the expected feminization that is a side effect of treatment.
4. Teaching the patient and family that having testicles removed in adulthood has no impact on masculinity.
5. Providing care to incision site if orchiectomy performed.

STUDY QUESTIONS

1. Identify five (5) key elements in a patient teaching plan after radical perineal prostatectomy.
2. Describe six (6) common treatment considerations for prostate cancer.
3. Write a nursing care plan for a patient undergoing radiation therapy for prostate cancer.

Bibliography

Bagshaw, M. and Ray, G.: External beam radiation therapy of prostate carcinoma. *In* Skinner, D.G. (ed.): Urological Cancer. New York, Grune & Stratton, pp. 53–71, 1983.

deKernion, J.: Cancer of the prostate. *In* Haskell, C. (ed.): Cancer Treatment. Philadelphia, W.B. Saunders Company, pp. 352–366, 1980.

Einhorn, L. H.: An overview of chemotherapeutic trials in advanced cancer of the prostate. *In* Skinner, D. G. (ed.): Urological Cancers. New York, Grune & Stratton, pp. 89–111, 1983.

Gault, P.: Prostate: a brighter outlook for patients. *In* Helping Cancer Patients Effectively. Horsham, PA, Nursing 77 Books, Intermed Communications, pp. 131–137, 1977.

Jones, A. G. and Hoeft, R. T.: Cancer of the prostate. American Journal of Nursing, *82*(5):826–828, 1982.

McCullough, D. L.: Diagnosis and staging of prostate cancer. *In* Skinner, D. and deKernion, J. (eds.): Genitourinary Cancer. Philadelphia, W.B. Saunders Company, pp. 295–310, 1978.

Paulson, D. F.: Surgical management of prostate cancer. *In* Skinner, D. G. (ed.): Urological Cancer. New York, Grune & Stratton, pp. 21–35, 1983.

Smith, D. R.: Tumors of the genitourinary tract. *In* Smith, D. R. (ed.): General Urology, 10th Ed. Los Altos, CA, Lange Medical Publications, pp. 248–299, 1981.

Speese-Swens, N. and Rutkowski, J.: Nursing care of the patient with cancer of the genitourinary system. *In* Bouchard-Kurtz, R. and Speese-Swens, N. (eds.): Nursing Care of the Cancer Patient. St. Louis, C.V. Mosby Company, pp. 249–278, 1981.

Swanson, D.: Cancer of the bladder and prostate: the impact of therapy on sexual function. *In* von Eschenbach, A. and Rodriguez, D. (eds.): Sexual Rehabilitation of the Urologic Cancer Patient. Boston, G.K. Hall Medical Publishers, pp. 88–108, 1981.

17

Gynecologic Cancers

ANN MARIE DOZIER, RN, MSN

GYNECOLOGIC OR PELVIC MALIGNANCIES

A. Normal anatomy (Fig. 17–1).
   1. Note proximity of cervix to bladder and rectum.
   2. Note lymphatic drainage (Fig. 17–2).
B. Separate malignancies identified for each structure, including Fallopian tube and vagina.
   1. Primary are endometrial, ovarian, and cervical (Table 17–1).
   2. All but ovarian cancers have an in situ form or precursor identified.

CERVICAL CANCER (CANCER OF THE UTERINE CERVIX)

A. Increasing attention paid to preinvasive disease.
   1. Nomenclature changed recently from dysplasia (mild, severe) to cervical intraepithelial neoplasia (CIN) I, II, or III.
      a. The three different degrees of CIN are defined by the extent of full thickness changes in the epithelium:
         (1) CIN I: undifferentiated neoplastic cells occupy the lower ⅓ of the epithelium (mild dysplasia).
         (2) CIN II: undifferentiated neoplastic cells occupy up to the lower ⅔ of the epithelium (inodevate dysplasia).
         (3) CIN III: undifferentiated neoplastic cells occupy to the full thickness of the epithelium (severe dysplasia to cancer in situ).
   2. Approximately 45,000 new cases annually.
   3. Increasing incidence of these early, pre-invasive changes or conditions possibly due to easy access to cervix (for tissue visualization and sampling), advent and refinement of Papanicolaou (Pap) smear and changes in diagnostic criteria since the 1940s; concomitant decrease in invasive cervical cancer incidence occurring.
B. Incidence of invasive cervical cancer decreasing; 14,000 cases in 1986, less than endometrial or ovarian cancer.
   1. Reported as invasive cancer of the uterine cervix as different from the uterine corpus (endometrium).

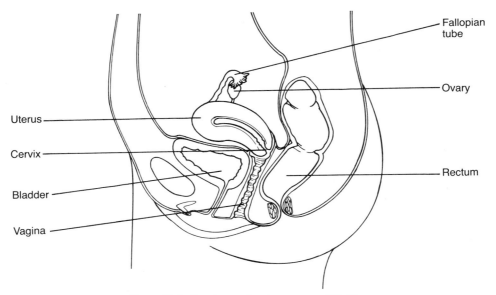

Figure 17–1. Female reproductive organs and bladder.

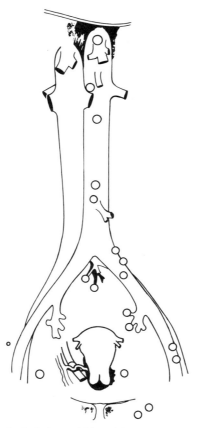

Figure 17–2. Gynecological lymphatic drainage. (Adapted from DiSaia, P., and Creasman, W. T.: Clinical Gynecologic Oncology, 2nd ed., St. Louis, C. V. Mosby Co., 1984.)

Table 17-1. DISTRIBUTION OF
INVASIVE GYNECOLOGIC
CANCERS

Site	Incidence (%)
Uterine corpus	38
Ovary	25
Uterine cervix	31
Vulva	3
Vagina	1
Fallopian tubes	<1
Trophoblastic tumors	<1

    2. Microinvasion has been defined, on spectrum between CIN and frank invasion.

C. Mortality decreasing since the 1950s; ranks second of the three pelvic malignancies.
    1. Annual deaths are over twice that of endometrial cancer.
    2. No change in survival; decreasing number of deaths because of decreasing incidence.

D. Risk factors (exogenous):
    1. Multiple sexual partners.
    2. Frequent coitus at early age (i.e., teenage years).
    3. Under investigation:
        a. Human papilloma viruses that cause genital warts or condylomata; potential for neoplastic transformation.
        b. Herpes simplex virus—full relationship not established.
        c. Role of male in transmission of infectious or oncogenic agents via intercourse.
    4. Not considered as risk factors:
        a. Socioeconomic status.
        b. Parity.
        c. Race. Studies show that mortality rates differ between whites and nonwhites, but this is not indicative of risk factor differences but of health care patterns (i.e., delay in diagnosis, less access to health care, and so forth).

E. Signs and symptoms.
    1. Pre-invasive and early stages typically evidence no symptoms, and a visible lesion on the cervix may or may not be present.
    2. May find post-coital bleeding, dyspareunia, watery discharge between periods.

F. Diagnosis (key is to rule out invasive cancer and define extent and location of disease).
    1. Pap smear with bimanual pelvic examination for initial screening.
        a. Routine screening recommended for all women.
        b. Screening recommended every 1-3 years, depending on authority cited.
        c. Cost effectiveness of *annual* screening in question.
        d. American Cancer Society (ACS) recommends, for women of childbearing age, a Pap smear every 3 years after two negative annual

smears; American College of Obstretics and Gynecology (ACOG) recommends annual Pap smear, citing importance of pelvic exam, not just Pap smear.

    e. Over ¾ of women do not undergo routine Pap smear screening.

2. If Pap smear indicates abnormal cells, do examination of the cervix under magnification.

    a. Directed biopsies provide diagnostic confirmation of CIN vs. invasive disease upon which to determine optimal treatment.

    b. Endocervical curettage is also recommended.

    c. 95% of cancers are squamous cell, and usually originate at squamocolumnar junction.

3. If frank lesion observed, directed biopsies are used to confirm the diagnosis of invasive disease.

4. Additional diagnostic procedures for invasive disease:

    a. Intravenous pyelogram (IVP) evaluates presence or absence of ureteral obstruction.

    b. Computerized tomography (CT) scan and/or lymphangiogram evaluate lymph node involvement.

    c. Examination under anesthesia, cystoscopy, or sigmoidoscopy is used to palpate or evaluate the extent of disease and to visualize involvement of the bladder or rectal mucosa.

5. Staging (Table 17–2).

6. Treatment of pre-invasive disease (Fig. 17–3) is 100% curative (several procedures may be required). Objective is to destroy or remove affected area. Follow-up continues indefinitely beginning with every 3-month intervals.

    a. Cryotherapy—freezes cervix.

        (1) Outpatient procedure that requires approximately 20 minutes.

        (2) Minimal discomfort.

        (3) Use for in situ disease not recommended, owing to delay in evaluation of treatment outcome.

Table 17–2. STAGING OF CARCINOMA OF THE UTERINE CERVIX: PATTERNS OF EXTENSION*

Stage 0	Confinement to surface epithelium.
Stage Ia	As in Stage 0 plus microinvasive histologic pattern.
Stage Ib	Invasive cancer confined to the cervix.
Stage Ib	Invasion confined to the cervix but also involving the fundus of the uterus.
Stage IIa	Cervical and upper vaginal involvement without parametrial extension.
Stage IIb	Cervical plus parametrial extension but not to the pelvic side wall.
Stage IIb	Cervical, parametrial and upper vaginal involvement.
Stage IIIa	Cervical plus involvement of the lower third of the vagina.
Stage IIIa	As above (Stage IIIa) plus parametrial involvement but not to the side wall.
Stage IIIb	Involvement of cervix, pelvic wall and lower third of the vagina.
Stage IIIb	Cervical, pelvic side wall and upper vaginal involvement.
Stage IIIb	Cervical, pelvic side wall and upper vaginal involvement.
Stage IVa	Bladder involvement.
Stage IVa	Rectal involvement.
Stage IVb	Extension beyond the pelvis.

*Adapted from DiSara, P. and Creasmen, W. T.: Clinical Gynecological Oncology, 2nd ed. St. Louis, C. V. Mosby Co., pp. 73–74, 1984.

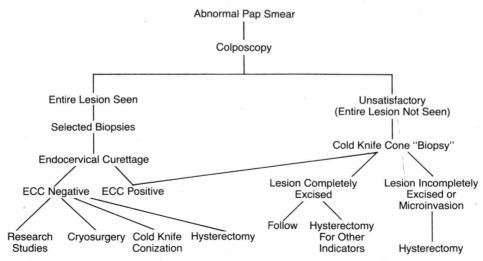

Cervical Intraepithelial Neoplasia

Abnormal Pap Smear

Colposcopy

Entire Lesion Seen

Selected Biopsies

Endocervical Curettage

ECC Negative   ECC Positive

Research   Cryosurgery   Cold Knife   Hysterectomy
Studies   Conization

Unsatisfactory
(Entire Lesion Not Seen)

Cold Knife Cone "Biopsy"

Lesion Completely   Lesion Incompletely
Excised   Excised or
                           Microinvasion

Follow   Hysterectomy
          For Other
          Indicators   Hysterectomy

Figure 17–3. *Schematic diagram of diagnosis and management of cervical intraepithelial neoplasia. (Redrawn from Wilbanks, G.: Cervical intraepithelial neoplasia. In Sciarra, J. J., ed.: Gynecology and Obstetrics, Vol. 4, Philadelphia, J. B. Lippincott, 1985.)*

    (4) Wastery discharge lasts 10–14 days.

    (5) Three-month interval after treatment required for healing before Pap smear can confirm success of treatment.

    (6) Nursing care includes:

        (a) Patient education regarding purpose, duration, and goal(s) of treatment; anticipated drainage from cell sloughing; perineal care; abstinence from sexual intercourse; return for follow-up (indefinitely, beginning 3 months after procedure).

        (b) Monitor for adverse reactions.

  b. CO_2 Laser treatment (Laser = light amplification by stimulated emission of radiation).

    (1) Tissue destruction via vaporization—less necrotic tissue created; healing more rapid.

    (2) Outpatient procedure that requires approximately 1 hour.

    (3) Moderate discomfort—warmth or heat sensed; more painful than cryosurgery.

    (4) Bleeding occasionally. Follow-up is possible within several weeks.

    (5) Nursing care includes:

        (a) Patient education (See Cervical Cancer).

        (b) Preparing environment for Laser hazards (e.g., placing signs in room, using appropriate eye wear, eliminating reflective surfaces).

        (c) Monitor for adverse reactions.

  c. Conization of cervix (cone biopsy) (Fig. 17–4).

    (1) Can be used effectively for in situ cervical cancer.

    (2) Successful outcome determined by pathologic assessment of free margins of specimen; follow-up Pap smears or colposcopy after 3 months.

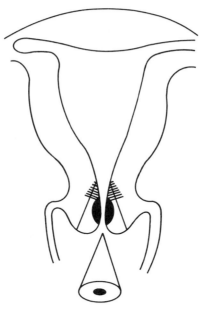

Figure 17–4. Cone biopsy. (Redrawn from DiSaia, P., and Creasman, W. T.: Clinical Gynecologic Oncology, 2nd ed., St. Louis, C. V. Mosby Co., 1984.)

      (3) Complications include:
         (a) Hemorrhage.
         (b) Uterine perforation.
         (c) Anesthetic risk.
         (d) In pregnancy, rupture of membranes and premature labor.
         (e) Cervical stenosis.
         (f) Infertility.
         (g) Incompetent cervix.
         (h) Increased risk of preterm delivery in the pregnant patient.
      (4) Nursing care:
         (a) Patient education regarding recuperative period (plus items noted under Cervical Cancer).
         (b) Routine postoperative care.
    d. Hysterectomy.
      (1) Increasingly uncommon unless other pelvic pathology or rationale indicates need.
      (2) Appropriate for in situ disease or recurrent or refractory disease or CIN.
      (3) See items under invasive cervical cancer for additional details and nursing care.
  7. Treatment for invasive disease.
    a. Surgery for early disease.
      (1) Stage Ia—total abdominal hysterectomy, with wide vaginal cuff but not pelvic lymphadenectomy.
      (2) Stage Ib—disease confined to cervix, but may encompass all of cervix (i.e., is a bulky tumor), requires radical surgery (radiation therapy may be used for bulky tumors).

       (a) Surgery includes radical hysterectomy, bilaterial pelvic lymphadenectomy. Choice of surgery influenced by age, desire for preservation of ovarian and sexual functioning, and history of pelvic infection or bowel disease.

  (3) Nursing care:

       (a) Preoperative preparation both physical and psychological; discussion of impact on fertility, sexuality, body image.

       (b) Supportive care during postoperative period, insuring frequent ambulation, adequate pulmonary toilet, and pain control.

       (c) Return of normal bladder function delayed until postoperative IVP indicates that bladder catheter can be removed. Maintain bladder decompression via catheters; normal bladder emptying-filling patterns reestablished via institutional policy. Discharge with catheter if no other need for hospitalization exists.

       (d) Carefully monitor all drainage because of the potential for fistula formation and fluid and electrolyte imbalance.

       (e) Monitor for signs and symptoms of infection.

       (f) Reestablish normal bowel evacuation pattern prior to discharge; use of natural laxative is preferred. Return of bowel function may be slowed owing to intraoperative retraction.

       (g) Discharge planning should include teaching about importance of ambulation, avoiding venous stasis, degree of fatigue anticipated (usually significant, but the patient rarely appreciates the level of exhaustion after surgery or hospitalization), information regarding medications, Foley catheter and leg bag care and use, and signs and symptoms necessitating physician notification. Initiate referral services; include family as appropriate.

       (h) Consistent follow-up necessary to evaluate vaginal apex, healing, long-term sequelae, nursing evaluation of problems identified above.

         i. Resumption of normal sexual activity.

           (i) Quell fears and dispel myths regarding hysterectomy or removal of ovaries and the long-term effects (e.g., weight gain, depression).

          (ii) Ovary removal often reduces normal vaginal secretions. A water-soluble lubricant should be recommended for sexual intercourse; oral estrogen used if vasomotor instability occurs (sometimes as early as 5 days after surgery). Current preference is a combination of estrogen and progesterone (to simulate normal hormonal pattern).

         (iii) Foreshortening of the vagina is rarely a problem if regular intercourse is resumed (usually 6 weeks after surgery).

 b. Radiation therapy for more extensive or regional disease.

  (1) Radiation therapy in Stage I disease is used primarily for bulky tumors and nonsurgical candidates. It involves 5 weeks of external beam treatment to the pelvis followed by two internal implants

(usually delivered by a Fletcher's applicator); for Stage I tumors a hysterectomy may be indicated following the radiation therapy.

(a) Lengthy, multiple modality treatment is used because of local recurrence pattern particularly prevalent in Stage I bulky tumors.

(b) Nursing care of patient undergoing radiation therapy (See Chapter 23):

    i. Assessment and intervention regarding potential home maintenance dysfunction, nutritional adequacy, family support, other medical conditions.

    ii. Patient education includes anticipated short-term side effects and actions and medications to ameliorate them. Also information about skin care, vaginal drainage, nutrition, fatigue, and gastrointestinal disturbances is given.

    iii. Involvement of family members for support, transportation, and assistance with activities of daily living is essential.

    iv. For internal implants (usually after-loaded) when the patient will be under general anesthesia:

        (i) Provide patient with information and reassurance. Clarify difference between internal and external implants, explain purpose of treatment, type of energy and source used.

        (ii) Provide or arrange for diversions because of activity restrictions and isolation.

        (iii) Provide staff protection and monitoring with respect to radiation hazards; the patient should be in a private room; employ principles of time, distance, and shielding (see Chapter 23).

        (iv) Cleanse bowel and decompress bladder before implant.

        (v) Cleanse vagina with antiseptic douche.

        (vi) Maintain bedrest, minimize bowel activity, decompress bladder, assist with personal hygiene as well, perineal care according to institutional policy.

        (vii) Minimize discomfort. Position change via logrolling, head of bed up 45°, according to institutional policy.

        (viii) Monitor for physiologic instability, especially temperature elevations and abdominal pain (may signal uterine perforation).

        (ix) Account for all radiation sources.

        (x) Post-implant, provide for bowel evacuation and resumption of recovery.

    v. Follow-up—assess patient fatigue level, GI irritation, nutritional status, monitor for signs of long-term sequelae, including ureteral structure, cystitis, fistulas, small bowel injury, and promote use of vaginal estrogens to increase lubrication and decrease atrophy.

(2) Stage II and III lesions undergo radiation therapy (internal and external) often with an extension along the para-aortic node chains.

(a) Work-up may also include surgical retroperitoneal node exploration to more specifically identify lymph node involvement.

(b) See Chapter 22 for surgical nursing care.

c. Progression and recurrence.

(1) Incidence of vaginal hemorrhage increased in patients with large friable lesions; vaginal packing and bedrest may suffice. Hemostasis can be established with transvaginal or external beam irradiation.

(2) Pain is not uncommon; it often occurs in conjunction with lymphedema. Need for comfort provided by a combination of analgesics (via narcotics, comfort measures, nerve stimulation or destruction).

(3) Fistula formation as disease progresses. Skin care is critical; odor may be significant (use of metronidazole orally or directly to necrotic area may eliminate odor).

(4) Support for adaptive coping and grieving mechanism/processes; maintain at home if appropriate and possible; provide supports and respite to family.

(5) For central recurrence in some patients, an extensive surgical procedure (pelvic exenteration) may be feasible.

(a) Goal of therapy is cure.

(b) Involves removal of bladder, rectum, vagina, uterus, Fallopian tubes, or ovaries (if still present), and all supportive structures.

(c) Urinary conduit *and* fecal stoma created.

(d) During or after recovery new vagina may be created.

(e) Nursing care:

i. Education and support throughout process, including self care issues, home care, re-entry into home environment, and roles as mother, wife, sexual partner, employee.

ii. Close physiologic monitoring, especially for hemodynamic and fluid instability.

iii. Long-term sequelae—monitor for:

(i) Recurrence.

(ii) Fistulae formation.

(iii) Stoma malfunction.

(iv) Ineffective coping.

(v) Sexual dysfunction.

OVARIAN CANCER

A. Overview.

1. Represents 26% of female genital cancer incidence (1986), but 52% of female deaths from genital cancer; despite treatment changes absolute and relative (%) death rate figures have remained stable for twenty years. Ovarian cancer is the *fourth highest* cause of cancer deaths in females.

2. Spreads intra-abdominally, growing locally, invading capsule of ovary then adjacent organs (contiguous spread implants onto peritoneal surfaces and spreads via lymphatics).

3. Survival determined by stage, grade, and residual tumor after surgery.
4. Diverse geographic and ethnic distribution.

B. Risk Factors:
1. Increasing incidence with peri- and postmenopausal women; possibility of hormonal influence.
2. Environmental carcinogen effect (by implication only). Highest incidence of ovarian cancer found in industrialized countries; talc also suspected.
3. Ovaries that have no opportunity to rest via pregnancy or use of birth control pills, or are hyperstimulated are likelier to develop abnormal changes and possibly cancer.
4. Higher incidence also occurs in:
   a. Nulliparous women.
   b. Women with other conditions in which the ovary is hyperstimulated.
   c. Women with dysmenorrhea and heavy menstrual flow.
   d. Single women.

C. Signs and symptoms:
1. Nonspecific complaints precede diagnosis by 2–6 months; vague abdominal discomfort, pelvic pressure, dyspepsia and other mild digestive disturbances, bowel or bladder complaints occur.
2. Irregular peri- or postmenopausal bleeding.
3. Postmenopausal enlarged ovary (found upon pelvic exam).
4. Absence of pain (except in advanced stages).
5. Early detection often serendipitous; frequent pelvic exams or culdocentesis have failed to impact earlier diagnosis.
6. Practical, cost-effective early diagnosis or screening mechanism is not currently available; future possibility of screening by use of tumor markers, such as a serum antigen screen, is currently under development.
7. Symptoms of advanced disease:
   a. Effusions (pleural or abdominal), shortness of breath, increasing abdominal girth.
   b. Intestinal obstruction.
   c. Anemia.
   d. Dehydration, malnutrition.

D. Diagnosis.
1. Preoperative radiologic tests may reveal little additional information and contribute to delay in diagnosis; possible tests include chest x-ray, barium enema, ultrasound (to identify tumor structure, omental involvement), or IVP; UGI and CT not routinely used because they yield limited information.
2. Work-up also includes thorough physical exam, laboratory studies, thoracentesis or paracentesis (if indicated, specimens sent to cytology).
3. Confirmed at surgical staging procedure, usually including a cytoreductive (de-bulking) effort. (This may improve quality, but not duration, of survival.) See Table 17–3.
   a. Diaphragmatic washings sent for cytologic evaluation.
   b. Carefully inspect and palpate diaphragm, liver, spleen, mesentery, pelvis, peritoneum.
      (1) Remove omentum.
      (2) Objective is to leave no lesions or nodules of > 2 cm.
      (3) Presence of adhesions or masses attached to bladder, rectum, or peritoneum changes the disease to a more advanced stage.

Table 17–3. INTERNATIONAL FEDERATION OF GYNECOLOGY AND
OBSTETRICS STAGING OF OVARIAN CARCINOMA*

Stage	Description
I	Growth limited to ovaries
IA	Growth limited to one ovary; no ascites
	(i) No tumor on the external surface; capsule intact
	(ii) Tumor present on the external surface or capsule ruptured (or both)
IB	Growth limited to both ovaries; no ascites
	(i) No tumor on external surface; capsule intact
	(ii) Tumor present on the external surface or capsule(s) rupture (or both)
IC	Tumor either stage IA or stage IB but with ascites present or positive peritoneal washings
II	Growth involving one or both ovaries with pelvic extension
IIA	Extension or metastases to the uterus or tubes
IIB	Extension to other pelvic tissues
IIC	Tumor either stage IIA or IIB but with ascites present or positive peritoneal washings
III	Growth involving one or both ovaries with intraperitoneal metastases outside the pelvis or positive retroperitoneal nodes; tumor limited to true pelvis, with histologically proved malignant extension to small bowel or omentum
IV	Growth involving one or both ovaries with distant metastases; if pleural effusion is present there must be positive cytology to allot a case to stage IV: parenchymal liver metastases equals stage IV
Special category	Unexplored cases thought to be ovarian carcinoma

*From Knapp, R., Berkowitz, R., and Leavitt, J.: *In* Sciarra, J. J. and Bushbaum, H. (eds.):
Gynecology and Obstetrics, Vol. 4. Philadelphia, J. B. Lippincott, 1985.

  E. Treatment.
     1. Borderline tumors (15% of all epithelial ovarian cancer) have a low malignant potential; surgery is usually adequate treatment. 95% have a 10-year survival rate.
     2. Postsurgical treatment for ovarian malignancies—adjuvant chemotherapy because of intra-abdominal and systemic nature of disease spread and the likelihood of recurrence outside the pelvic area.
       a. For Stage I or II disease.
         (1) If it is not residual disease and peritoneal washings are negative (the optimal situation), no further treatment is usually indicated.
         (2) If washings are positive, treat with radioactive isotopes (e.g., P^{32}), external beam (via strip field or field within field technique), or chemotherapy (use single oral alkylating agent).
         (3) For residual disease, treat with combination chemotherapy.
       b. For Stage III optimal and suboptimal and Stage IV disease.
         (1) Multiple agent chemotherapy.
         (2) Most common combination currently used involves cyclophosphamide, doxorubicin, and cisplatin for eight courses (approximately every 3-4 weeks).
         (3) Other combinations include hexamethylmelamine or melphalan with one or more of the other drugs mentioned.
     3. Post-treatment follow-up:
       a. "Second look" (only method to confirm absence of disease) via laparotomy and/or laparoscopy.
         (1) Evaluates disease status of inadequately staged patient.

(2) Evaluates effect of chemotherapy.

(3) Evaluates patients deemed free of clinical disease.

(4) Some institutions do serial examinations (e.g., every 6 months); usually laparotomy is required to rule out presence of disease.

    b. Following second look, if disease is present, second line chemotherapy is available, but results are disappointing.

F. Progression.

  1. Intestinal obstruction.

    a. Conservatively managed via decompression of bowel (e.g., via Cantor tube).

    b. Potential for surgical palliation if factors contributing to poorer outcomes are evaluated: age, nutritional status, prior treatment(s).

    c. Significant operative morbidity and mortality.

  2. Effusions (pleural or abdominal) may require frequent taps for fluid removal to provide patient comfort. Pleural effusions may require sclerosing of the pleura to minimize fluid accumulation.

G. Nursing care:

  1. During preoperative work-up:

    a. Establish baseline data, including nutritional intake pattern, usual weight, bowel evacuation pattern, existence of any chronic medical problems.

    b. Provide support, both physical and psychological.

      (1) Evaluation and correction of nutritional deficiencies.

      (2) Treatment of effusions (pleural or abdominal) to enhance comfort.

      (3) Provide information and education regarding disease process.

      (4) Assess family situation for potential ineffective coping or grieving.

      (5) Support and provide information regarding:

        (a) Coping and the grieving process.

        (b) Disease.

        (c) Delayed diagnosis due to nature of disease.

      (6) Preoperative preparation.

  2. After surgery:

    a. Routine postoperative care. Particular attention paid to resumption of normal intestinal and pulmonary function; monitor lung or abdominal fluid accumulation.

    b. Communication of findings and diagnosis.

    c. Encourage and provide information regarding maintenance of adequate nutritional intake; monitor parameters and use anthropometric measure.

    d. Preparation for subsequent treatments (e.g. chemotherapy)—information regarding purpose, anticipated side effects, duration and frequency of treatment.

    e. Assist with realistic goal setting.

    f. Assess, initiate, and mobilize family or community support resources.

    g. Assess adaptiveness of coping.

  3. During adjuvant treatment:

    a. See Chapters 23 and Chapter 24.

    b. Provide for patient and family education.

    c. Maintain adequate nutrition; this is often a key challenge due to weight loss prior to diagnosis. Stress the importance of family involvement.

        d. Maintain adequate hydration; determine requirements based on toxic effects of chemotherapy and effectiveness of antiemetics.
4. During disease progression:
     a. Provide for physical comfort and support.
        (1) Maintain nutrition and hydration, if possible; use dietary supplement.
        (2) Assess fluid build-up in lungs or abdomen.
        (3) Assess the patient's level of pain and provide for pain relief.
        (4) Assess GI status.
     b. Provide support for patient's and family's grieving process.
        (1) Involve family in care.
        (2) Maintain independence as long as possible.
        (3) Assist with realistic goal setting.
        (4) Assess and arrange for home maintenance needs.
        (5) Assess grieving process.
        (6) Listen.

CANCER OF ENDOMETRIUM (CORPUS OR FUNDUS OF UTERUS)

A. Overview.
1. Most common of the genital malignancies of females.
2. Anticipated incidence 36,000 cases (1986); anticipated mortality 2,900 (1986).
3. Increased incidence in 1970s may be due to:
     a. Earlier detection due to increased availability of medical care.
     b. Increase in number of women reaching age range for peak incidence; mean and median age at time of diagnosis is 61 years.
     c. Broadening criteria; improved reporting.
     d. Increased use of conjugated Estrogen Replacement Therapy (ERT).
     e. Incidence may be plateauing and decreasing in the 1980s.
4. Decrease in death rate simultaneous with the aforementioned increase may be due to earlier detection and, therefore, earlier treatment and higher likelihood of successful outcome.
5. Adenocarcinoma is most common.
B. Risk factors:
1. Obesity (> 15% over normal weight). Risk may be associated with estrogen deposit in fat.
2. Nulliparity.
3. Late menopause (i.e., after 52 years).
4. All three together increase risk five times.
5. Diabetes and high blood pressure are associated with this cancer but are also associated with obesity and age, so may be confounding variables.
6. Exogenous estrogen use is associated with increased risk; use of estrogen with progesterone reduces risk.
C. Signs and symptoms:
1. PMB (postmenopausal bleeding). Approximately 20% of women with PMB have a pelvic malignancy.
2. With increasing age, PMB is more likely to be cancer.
3. Presence of endometrial hyperplasia.

D. Diagnosis:
  1. Screening should be selective.
     a. A woman over 50 with an intact uterus.
     b. In high risk asymptomatic women regardless of age.
     c. Endometrial cavity sampling or endocervical curettage, using the vacuum aspiration technique, evaluates cervical involvement.
  2. Pelvic exam with thorough history and Pap smear is inadequate because less than 50% of the lesions show; Pap smear does not directly sample lesion.
  3. Fractional dilation and curettage. For a definitive diagnosis, specimens from the endocervix and exocervix should be obtained separately.
  4. Additional studies (e.g., cystoscopy or sigmoidscopy, IVP) are not cost effective because no additional information about disease spread is obtained.
  5. Surgical determination of extent of disease is based on degree of myometrial penetration and presence of lymph node metastases.
  6. Staging (Table 17–4).
E. Prognostic factors:
  1. Histologic type (pathology).
  2. Histologic differentiation.
  3. Uterine size.
  4. Stage of disease.
  5. Myometrial invasion.
  6. Peritoneal cytology.
  7. Lymph node metastasis.
  8. Adnexal metastasis.
F. Treatment:
  1. For Stage I (75% of patients present in this stage), exploratory laparotomy with total abdominal hysterectomy and bilateral salpingo-oophorectomy, nodal exploration, and selective periaortic or pelvic lymphadenectomy. Individualization of therapy not the use of a standard procedure is essential. Postoperative radiation therapy used only in patients with poor prognosis based on grade of tumor and percentage of invasion.

Table 17–4. INTERNATIONAL CLASSIFICATION OF CANCER OF THE UTERINE FUNDUS

Stage 0	Carcinoma in situ. Histologic findings suspicious of malignancy. Cases of Stage 0 should not be included in any therapeutic statistics.
Stage I	The carcinoma is confined to the corpus.
Stage Ia	The length of the uterine cavity is 8 cm or less.
Stage Ib	The length of the uterine cavity is more than 8 cm. The stage I cases should be sub-grouped with regard to the histologic type of adenocarcinoma as follows: G1—Highly differentiated adenomatous carcinomas. G2—Differentiated adenomatous carcinomas with partly solid areas. G3—Predominantly solid or entirely undifferentiated carcinomas.
Stage II	The carcinoma has involved the corpus and the cervix.
Stage III	The carcinoma has extended outside the uterus but not outside the true pelvis.
Stage IV	The carcinoma has extended outside the true pelvis or has obviously involved the mucosa of the bladder or rectum. A bullous edema as such does not permit allotment of a case of Stage IV.

2. For Stage II, external and intracavitary radiation followed by hysterectomy; order may be reversed.

3. Stage III or IV (rare for initial presentation) disease is treated with chemotherapy, surgery, radiation and/or hormonal manipulation. The goal is palliative not curative in most cases, individualization of treatment is essential.

4. Hormonal chemotherapy—progestational agents achieve responses in ⅓ of patients; appropriate for patients with extrapelvic metastases. Response more likely if tumor is well differentiated. Evaluation of estrogen and progesterone receptors on cells is under investigation as indicator of appropriateness of progestational agent use; use of adjuvant not supported.

5. Nonhormonal chemotherapy.
   a. Results have been disappointing. Agents that have been studied include:
      (1) Doxorubicin.
      (2) Malphalan, megestrol, 5-fluorouracil, and cyclophosphamide.
   b. Response rates are low. It is possible that patients with few estrogen and progesterone receptors respond better.

G. Nursing care:
   1. Provide patient education to resolve or address problems of lack of knowledge regarding normal anatomy and physiology, disease process, workup and treatment process.
   2. Provide support throughout diagnosis, treatment, and recovery to foster appropriate coping and grief reactions.
   3. Where indicated, provide pre- and postoperative care, monitor fluid and electrolyte concentration, maintain adequate pulmonary toilet, foster mobility and pain control, encourage resumption of self care activities.
   4. Prepare for recuperation after discharge; emphasize how to handle fatigue.
   5. During and after recovery provide regular assessments of return to normal activity level, sleep-rest pattern, sexual activity, nutritional intake, bowel and bladder function.
   6. For patients undergoing radiation therapy, see Chapter 23.
   7. For patients undergoing hormonal or nonhormonal therapy, see Chapter 24.

STUDY QUESTIONS

1. List risk factors for cervical cancer.
2. List risk factors for ovarian cancer.
3. List risk factors for endometrial cancer.
4. Develop a plan of care for a woman with a gynecologic malignancy.

Bibliography

Creasman, W. T.: Surgical treatment of endometrial carcinoma. *In* Sciarra, J. J. and Bushbaum, H. (eds.): Gynecology and Obstetrics, Vol. 4. Philadelphia, J. B. Lippincott, pp. 1–5, 1985.

Curry, S.: Surgical treatment of cervical cancer: Radical hysterectomy. *In* Sciarra, J. J. and Bushbaum, H. (eds.): Gynecology and Obstectrics, Vol. 4. Philadelphia, J. B. Lippincott, 1985.

DiSaia, P. and Creasman, W. T.: Clinical Gynecologic Oncology, 2nd ed. St. Louis, C. V. Mosby Co., 1984.

Ferenczy, A.: Methods for detecting endometrial carcinoma and its precursors. *In* Sciarra, J. J. and Bushbaum, H. (eds.): Gynecology and Obstetrics, Vol. 4. Philadelphia, J. B. Lippincott, 1985.

Gal, D. and Bushbaum, H.: The staging of cervical carcinoma. *In* Sciarra, J. J. and Bushbaum, H. (eds.): Gynecology and Obstetrics. Philadelphia, J. B. Lippincott, 1985.

Kessler, I.: Epidemiological aspects of uterine cervix cancer. *In* Sciarra, J. J. and Bushbaum, H. (eds.): Gynecology and Obstetrics, Vol. 4. Philadelphia, J. B. Lippincott, 1985.

Knapp, R. C., Berkowitz, R. S., and Leavitt, T.: Natural history and detection of ovarian cancer. *In* Sciarra, J. J. and Bushbaum, H. (eds.): Gynecology and Obstetrics, Vol. 4. Philadelphia, J. B. Lippincott, 1985.

Kohorn, E.: Hormonal and nonhormonal chemotherapy of endometrial carcinoma. *In* Sciarra, J. J. and Bushbaum, H. (eds.): Gynecology and Obstetrics. Philadelphia, J. B. Lippincott, 1985.

Rutledge, F.: Radical hysterectomy. *In* Ridley, J. H. (ed.): Gynecologic Surgery—Errors, Safeguards and Salvage. Baltimore, Williams & Wilkins, pp. 325–342, 1974.

Wharton, J. T., Smith, J. P., Delclos, L., and Fletcher, G. H.: Radiation therapy for cervical carcinoma. *In* Sciarra, J. J. and Bushbaum, H. (eds.): Gynecology and Obstetrics. Philadelphia, J. B. Lippincott, 1985.

Wilbanks, G. D.: Cervical intraepithelial neoplasia. *In* Sciarra, J. J. and Bushbaum, H. (eds.): Gynecology and Obstetrics. Philadelphia, J. B. Lippincott, 1985.

18

Head and Neck Cancer

CONNIE M. YUSKA, RN, MS

CHARACTERISTICS OF HEAD AND NECK CANCER

A. Accounts for 5% of all cancers in the U.S.
B. Early stage disease is curable with surgery and radiation.
C. Stage III or IV disease demonstrates local recurrence at a rate of 60% and distant metastases at a rate of 20–30%.
D. It is a locally aggressive disease that spreads quickly within the head and neck area.
E. Occurs most commonly in the fifth to seventh decade of life.
F. Male to female ratio is 3:1.
G. Histology—majority are squamous cell; in varying sites adenocarcinoma, sarcoma, and basal cell carcinoma are also seen.

ETIOLOGIC FACTORS

A. Aerodigestive tract has potential for contact with broad range of carcinogenic agents.
B. Tobacco in all forms, cigarettes, dipping snuff, and chewing tobacco.
C. Alcohol consumption—moderate to heavy drinking history is prevalent.
D. Evidence of synergistic effect between alcohol and tobacco.
E. Environmental factors:
   1. Wood dust (furniture industry).
   2. Nickel refining.
F. Viral etiology proposed as a factor in nasopharyngeal cancer. There is an association between the Epstein-Barr virus and the development of nasopharyngeal cancer.

SCREENING AND DETECTION

A. Assessment:
   1. Thorough head and neck exam should be done.
   2. Inspection and palpation of the oral cavity.

3. Many oral lesions are discovered on dental exam.
4. Bimanual palpation of the neck.
    a. Note size, number, and mobility of nodes in the neck.
    b. "Fixed" nodes carry poorer prognosis. They indicate invasion of tumor into underlying musculature of the neck.
    c. Characteristics of benign neck nodes: pain, fever, intermittent regression.
    d. Characteristics of malignant neck nodes: absence of pain, no regression, fast growth.
    e. 85% of masses in the neck in adults are metastatic from the head and neck area.
    f. Location of neck mass often suggests site of primary tumor.
        (1) A mass high in the cervical region often represents metastases from a nasopharyngeal tumor.
        (2) Subdigastric nodes often are the site of metastases from primary cancers of the oral cavity, oropharynx, or hypopharynx.
        (3) Submandibular triangle nodes may be site of metastases from the oral cavity.
        (4) Masses in the midcervical region are associated with tumors of the hypopharynx, base of the tongue, larynx, and the pyriform fossa.
        (5) Deep jugular chain nodes often suggest metastatic disease of the thyroid.
B. Physical examination.
    1. The patient should be in a sitting position with good light available.
    2. Lips and oral cavity:
        a. Vermilion border inspected for symmetry, ulcers, crusted lesions, and swelling.
        b. Examine the oral cavity with a penlight and tongue blade. Retract buccal mucosa bilaterally and gingival sulcus anteriorly.
        c. Note white patches or erythematous lesions on oral mucosa.
        d. Note status of dentition.
        e. Tongue examined at rest and with protrusion. Examine lateral and ventral surfaces.
        f. Taste sensation should be tested with salty, sour, sweet, and bitter reagents.
        g. Sublingual exam includes entire floor of mouth extending posteriorly to tonsillar pillars.
    3. Oropharynx examination includes tonsils, soft palate, lateral and posterior pharyngeal walls, and base of tongue.
        a. Base of tongue should be inspected and palpated. This is a common location for an occult primary tumor.
        b. Asymmetry of the tonsil may indicate a parapharyngeal tumor.
    4. Hypopharynx examination includes observation of the base of the tongue, epiglottis, and false and true vocal cords.
    5. A detailed larynx examination is not always possible to perform because of a hyperactive gag reflex. Thorough exam may be performed endoscopically by the physician.
    6. Nasopharynx examination of all areas for suspicious areas of ulceration or exophytic growth.
    7. Nose and paranasal sinus—nasal area examined with nasal speculum. Sinus examined with appropriate radiographic studies.

8. Ear is externally observed for ulceration, crusting, inflammation, masses. Presence of middle ear infusion noted, which may be suggestive of a nasopharyngeal tumor.

9. Psychosocial evaluation—large percentage of patients have a history of moderate to heavy alcohol intake. Important to assess motivation for cooperation with treatment plan.

10. Signs and symptoms of tumors in the head and neck area:
    a. Oral cavity—a swelling or ulcer that fails to heal, referred otalgia, local pain not always present.
    b. Oropharynx—"silent" area, symptoms delayed, dysphagia, local pain, odonophagia (painful swallowing), referred pain.
    c. Nose and sinuses—bloody nasal discharge, nasal obstruction, facial pain, swelling, diplopia.
    d. Hypopharynx—dysphagia, odonophagia, referred otalgia, neck mass.
    e. Nasopharynx—bloody discharge, nasal obstruction, conductive deafness.
    f. Larynx—hoarseness, pain, dysphagia, dyspnea and stridor, odonophagia, chronic cough, hemoptysis.

METHODS OF TREATMENT

A. Surgery.
   1. Principle of surgery is to remove all the cancer while preserving function and cosmesis.
   2. Surgical area often involves more than one area in the head and neck.
   3. Brief description of major surgical resections:
      a. *Composite resection* is used to indicate resection of more than one anatomic area through one incisional site. For example, a tumor that arises in the tongue and extends to the mandible and neck would be treated by surgical resection of these areas resulting in a glossectomy (partial, hemi, or subtotal), mandibulectomy (partial or hemi), in combination with a radical neck dissection.
      b. *Radical neck dissection* removes sternocleidomastoid muscle, spinal accessory nerve (may be spared in some cases), cervical lymphatics, and jugular vein.
      c. *Hemi-laryngectomy* preserves one set of vocal cords. Postoperatively patient experiences a hoarse but serviceable voice.
      d. *Supraglottic laryngectomy* involves removal of the epiglottis and superior portion of larynx. Postoperatively patient may experience aspiration.
      e. *Total laryngectomy.* Removal of entire larynx and two to three rings of the trachea, resulting in the remaining portion of the trachea being sutured to the skin to create a permanent tracheostoma.
   4. Preoperative teaching specific to head and neck surgical procedures:
      a. Care of the altered airway—review procedures of suctioning, cleaning inner cannula of tracheotomy tube, changing tracheotomy ties and dressing, care of the surgical site with hydrogen peroxide and normal saline.
      b. Alteration in communication—use of writing pads, communication board. Maintain sensitivity to patient's need to complete written

thought without interruption. Utilize system of marking nurse call light notifying that patient cannot speak.

   c. Nutritional management—enteral route used frequently since GI system remains intact in most cases. Delivered via nasogastric or gastrostomy tube. Method of administration may be continuous drip delivered via a feeding pump or bolus method per gavage bag.

   d. Wound care—will have wound drainage apparatus and exposed suture lines that will be cleansed with hydrogen peroxide and normal saline.

   e. Oral care—performed using solution delivered either per rinse, gavage bag, Water Pik, or power spray.

   f. Support systems—describe ancillary departments that provide therapeutic support (ie. social work, psychiatry, chaplain).

B. Chemotherapy.

  1. Goals of treatment:

   a. Adjuvant therapy is used in combination with other treatment modalities to increase chance of disease control.

   b. Palliative treatment may help to control the pain of recurrent disease by shrinking the tumor.

  2. Combination chemotherapy is used primarily in Stage III and IV disease. Cisplatin, methotrexate, bleomycin, and 5-fluorouracil have been used. Combinations of cisplatin and 5-fluorouracil have achieved responses of 30–50% after two or more cycles of treatment.

  3. Nursing management of patients receiving chemotherapy for head and neck cancer:

   a. Symptom management:

    (1) Nausea and vomiting—administer antiemetics as ordered. Note effectiveness and work with physician to determine an effective antiemetic regimen. Relaxation and guided imagery effective in reducing anticipatory nausea and vomiting.

    (2) Leukopenia—if white blood count falls below 4000 cu/mm, subsequent course of chemotherapy is altered. If white blood count falls below 1000 cu/mm, usual precautions against infection are intensified.

    (3) Oral care—incidence of oral infection decreases with frequent use of an oral care regimen. It is important for nursing staff to assess the oral cavity frequently using a tongue blade and light to examine thoroughly. If stomatitis develops, give the patient instructions on avoiding spicy foods, alcohol, and smoking. Frequency of oral hygiene should be increased. Local oral anesthetics will help to alleviate pain until lesions subside. If unable to swallow liquids, intravenous hydration will be necessary.

    (4) Nutrition—GI disturbances may contribute to alteration in nutritional status. Dietary assessment with appropriate supplements is indicated.

C. Radiotherapy.

  1. Used in combination with surgery and/or chemotherapy to control tumor bulk as well as microscopic disease.

  2. May be indicated as the definitive therapy in early lesions.

  3. Aim of postoperative radiotherapy is to control residual disease at the surgical resection margins.

4. Usually administered 3–4 weeks after surgery for a period of 5–6 weeks with a total dose of 5,500 rad.
5. Nursing management of patients receiving radiation therapy to the head and neck is discussed in Chapter 23.

POSTOPERATIVE NURSING MANAGEMENT

A. Symptom management.
 1. Care of the altered airway (tracheostomy or laryngectomy).
    a. Pulmonary stimulus performed every 1–2 hours for the first 24–48 hours following surgery. Pulmonary stimulus is defined as cough and deep breathing, deep tracheal suctioning, or instillation of normal saline. The method of pulmonary stimulus is determined by the nurse following assessment of the pulmonary status. Sterile technique is used for deep tracheal suctioning.
    b. Clean inner cannula of tracheotomy tube every 4 hours and PRN with hydrogen peroxide and saline or sterile water. Avoid using hydrogen peroxide on metal tracheotomy tubes; peroxide increases the oxidation rate leading to tarnishing of the metal.
    c. Clean around the tracheostomy site or laryngectomy stoma with cotton swabs moistened in hydrogen peroxide and then with swabs moistened in normal saline every shift. Observe site for erythema, crusting, and drainage.
    d. Change tracheostomy ties and dressing PRN when soiled.
    e. Normal humidifying mechanisms of the nose and mouth are bypassed with an altered airway; it becomes essential to provide some form of supplemental humidity.
       (1) Warm, humidified air may be provided in the immediate postoperative period delivered by a high humidity tracheotomy collar device.
       (2) Instillation of normal saline provides moisture to upper tracheobronchial tree.
          (a) Syringe method of instillation of normal saline—1½–2 cc of normal saline directly into tracheotomyy tube or laryngectomy stoma every 2–4 hours and PRN.
          (b) Atomizer method—fill bowl of nasal or other type of atomizer with normal saline and spray into tracheotomy tube or stoma every 2–4 hours and PRN.
          (c) Teach patient signs of inadequate humidity—thick, tenacious secretions, bloody secretions, secretions that are hard to cough out.
 2. Wound care.
    a. Assessment of skin flaps and grafts:
       (1) Temperature—should be warm to touch.
       (2) Color—should not be dusky in color; blanches well to indicate good capillary refill.
    b. Monitor and record drainage from wound suction apparatus every shift.

    c. Avoid pressure, kinking of flap, and use of constricting dressings or tracheotomy ties around neck area.

    d. Clean exposed suture lines with hydrogen peroxide and normal saline as ordered.

    e. Management of fistulas. Fistulas are most often a result of wound breakdown; a communication between the oral cavity and neck tissues occurs, resulting in a fistula. Small fistulas can be treated with frequent dressing changes utilizing packing to encourage the wound to granulate to closure. Large fistulas will need surgical closure with rotation of a skin flap to the area.

    f. Carotid blowout.

      (1) This is an oncologic emergency. Close assessment of the wound noting any changes in color, temperature, edema, size and shape of the lesion. Two warning signs: some patients complain of sternal or high epigastric pain several hours before a rupture. Small prodromal bleed may be noted 24–48 hours before a rupture.

      (2) Plan of preventive action should be developed. All nursing staff should be knowledgeable about nursing actions indicated in the event of a carotid blowout.

      (3) Emergency supplies to stabilize the patient for transport to the operating room should be placed at the bedside of any patient who is in danger of a carotid blowout (Table 18–1).

      (4) Goals of nursing intervention during carotid blowout—maintain airway and prevent aspiration, relieve discomfort and distress, provide psychological support to the patient and family.

3. Nutritional management.

    a. 40% of head and neck cancer patients present in good nutritional status; the remaining patients are in either fair (20%) or poor (40%) nutritional status.

    b. Nutritional assessment includes a diet history, anthropometrics, laboratory testing, history of weight loss.

    c. Large percentage of patients have functioning GI tract. Nutritional support is generally delivered orally with diet supplementation or with a nasogastric or gastrostomy tube.

Table 18–1. EMERGENCY SUPPLIES FOR CAROTID BLOWOUT*

Supplies include the following:
  Three bath towels
  Six packages of 4×4 gauze
  1 cuffed tracheostomy tube
  10cc syringe (used to inflate cuff on tracheostomy tube)
  Complete IV set-up with solutions and filter tubing for blood transfusions
  Cut-down or venesection tray
  Appropriate materials and requisitions to draw type and crossmatch
  Extra equipment for blood drawing (blood tubes, syringes, needles)
  Blood gas kit
  Alcohol wipes
Check that suction apparatus is available in the patient's room

* Place at bedside of any patient who is in danger of a carotid blowout.

    d. Continuous or intermittent feedings can be used.
      (1) Continuous—usually tolerated better than intermittent feedings in the immediate postoperative period. Started at ½ strength and advanced 25 cc per hour per day as tolerated.
      (2) Bolus—five to six feedings per day administered over a 20–30 minute period.
      (3) General nursing considerations in administration of tube feedings—elevate the head of the bed or place the patient in a sitting position to decrease the chance of aspiration. Note patient complaints of abdominal cramping, bloating, or diarrhea.
      (4) Feeding intolerance may be due to the method of administration or to the type of supplemental feeding used.
4. Oral care.
    a. Method of administration—assess ability to close lips and "swish" mouthwash. If unable to contain solution orally, will need to administer oral care via gavage bag or Water Pik used on the lowest setting.
    b. Solution—avoid commercially prepared mouthwash and lemon/glycerine swabs. May use ½ strength hydrogen peroxide or salt and soda mouthwash. Perform oral hygiene four times a day.
5. Speech rehabilitation.
    a. Options for the total laryngectomy patient:
      (1) Electrolarynx—mechanical, battery-operated device which when placed against the neck or cheek transmits sound into the oral cavity. The lips and tongue are used for articulation.
      (2) Esophageal speech—method of injecting air into the esophagus and forcing it back out creating a sound. The lips and tongue are used in articulation.
      (3) Tracheal-Esophageal puncture—a surgical procedure in which a small hole between the posterior wall of the trachea and the anterior wall of the esophagus is created. A one-way valve prosthesis is inserted which allows air to go into the esophagus but prevents back flow of food or fluid into the trachea. The lips and tongue are used for articulation.
    b. Options for the partial or hemiglossectomy patient:
      (1) Exercises to strengthen remaining musculature to improve the slurred speech that results postoperatively.
      (2) Prosthesis may be used to lower the palate for close approximation of the remaining tongue to increase the intelligibility of the speech.
6. Swallowing rehabilitation.
    a. Radiographic study as well as a bedside clinical exam of any patient suspected of aspiration should be done to identify presence of aspiration, define the etiology, design the appropriate therapy, and determine the best method of nutritional intake.
    b. Nursing should support and follow through on the individual teaching plan given by the speech pathologist.
    c. The cuff on the tracheostomy tube should be inflated for meals and for 30 minutes afterward if the patient is known to aspirate. When deflating the cuff, be prepared to suction the trachea.
7. Psychosocial concerns.
    a. Patient and family will need help coping with the alterations of surgery.

   b. There may be an alteration in speech, swallowing, and in the patient's body image.
   c. Provide an opportunity for the patient and family to express their concerns.
   d. The nurse's role becomes one of educator, listener, and supporter.
8. Methods of pain control.
   a. May be managed with narcotics, relaxation therapy, biofeedback. Common to have referred pain from the head and neck area to the ear.
   b. Refer to Chapter 29.

MULTIDISCIPLINARY APPROACH

A. Rehabilitation needs are diverse and complex.
B. One health care professional is not prepared to address all of the patient's needs.
C. Multidisciplinary approach with structured meetings between health care professionals from various disciplines smooths the transition from hospital to home.
D. The following disciplines may be represented: medicine, nursing, social work, dietary, speech pathology, physical therapy, pharmacy, and chaplaincy.
E. Use of the multidisciplinary format provides an opportunity for exchange of information regarding the rehabilitation treatment plan, including goals, progress, and expected date of discharge.

STUDY QUESTIONS

1. Identify the two most common risk factors in the development of head and neck cancer.
2. Describe the major components of preoperative teaching for the head and neck surgical patient.
3. Identify the rationale for a combined modality approach in the treatment of head and neck cancer.
4. Describe appropriate nursing interventions for the successful rehabilitation of the postoperative head and neck cancer patient.
5. Identify the oncologic emergency that is a possible complication of head and neck cancer. Identify essential nursing interventions when this emergency occurs.

Bibliography

Basset, M. R. and Dobie, R. A.: Patterns of nutritional deficiency in head and neck cancer. Otolaryngology Head and Neck Surgery, 91(2):119–125, 1983.
Beck, S.: Impact of a systemic oral care protocol on stomatitis after chemotherapy. Cancer Nursing, 2:185–199, 1979.
Kane, K.: Carotid artery rupture in advanced head and neck cancer patients. Oncology Nursing Forum, 10(1):14–18, 1983.
Keith, C. F.: Wound management following head and neck surgery. Nursing Clinics of North America, 14(4):761–778, 1979.

Kies, M. S., Levitan, N., and Hong, W.: Chemotherapy of head and neck cancer. Otolaryngologic Clinics of North America. *18*(3):533–541, 1985.

Logemann, J.: Evaluation and Treatment of Swallowing Disorders. San Diego, College Hill Press, 1983.

Morrow, G. and Morrell, C.: Behavioral treatment for the anticipatory nausea and vomiting induced by cancer chemotherapy. The New England Journal of Medicine, *307*:1476–1480, 1982.

Schwartz, S. L. and Barr, N. J.: Carotid catastrophe. American Journal of Nursing, *79*(9):1566–1567, 1979.

Suen, J. and Myers, E.: Cancer of the head and neck. New York, Churchill Livingstone, 1981.

19

Colorectal Cancer

JULENA LIND, RN, MS

RISK FACTORS

A. Geographic differences.
   1. High incidence in Western industrialized countries.
   2. Most common cancer among men and women in U.S.
   3. Second leading cause of cancer deaths in U.S.
   4. Low incidence of colon cancer in Japan, Finland, Africa.
   5. Japanese immigrants to U.S. have increased incidence compared to native Japanese.
   6. In recent years, has increased almost 50% in U.S. blacks; incidence now almost equal to that in whites.
B. Diet.
   1. High fiber intake associated with low incidence of colorectal cancer. Probably due to decreased transit time through colon.
   2. Influence of dietary fat under study. Not known how important a risk factor it is.
C. Medical history.
   1. Higher risk of developing colorectal cancer in patients with a history of ulcerative colitis (especially in those who have had it for over 10 years). Risk increases with younger age of onset and larger extent of bowel involvement.
   2. Crohn's disease increases risk, especially if onset occurs before 21 years of age.
   3. The risk associated with adenomatous polyps is controversial. Higher risk is associated with larger polyps.
D. Family history.
   1. Familial polyposis, a hereditary disease passed to offspring according to Mendelian laws, is a widespread proliferation of adenomatous polyps. Associated with a very high incidence of colon cancer.
   2. Patients with juvenile polyps are also at higher risk for colon cancer.
   3. There is a two to three time greater risk of colon cancer if immediate family member has cancer of the colon.

163

E. Site of presentation—approximate incidence:
 1. 16% in cecum and ascending colon.
 2. 8% in transverse colon.
 3. 20–35% in descending and sigmoid colon.
 4. 40–50% in the rectum.

SCREENING AND DETECTION

A. Screening.
 1. Digital rectal examination (measures occult blood in stool) screening.
 2. Fecal occult blood.
  a. Cost-effective method.
  b. Correct preparation important: meat-free diet for 3 days, no iron or Vitamin C; three sequential specimens should be sent.
 3. Proctosigmoidoscopy or colonoscopy.
  a. Should be used to screen high risk patients and all patients over 40 years old during routine physical examination.
  b. Almost 2/3 of colorectal cancers are detectable with flexible sigmoidoscopic exam.
B. Signs and symptoms (dependent on tumor location).
 1. Right colon:
  a. Unexplained anemia and GI bleeding.
  b. Abdominal pain (rare complaint).
  c. Occasionally a palpable mass.
  d. Weight loss.
 2. Left colon.
  a. Mucus in stools.
  b. Obstructive symptoms.
  c. Decreased caliber stools.
  d. Blood or blood mixed with stools.
 3. Sigmoid colon.
  a. Obstruction (from napkin ring growth).
  b. Blood per rectum (not common).
 4. Rectum:
  a. Mucus diarrhea.
  b. Rectal bleeding or pain.
  c. Tenesmus (straining on stool).
  d. Sensation of incomplete evacuation.
C. Diagnostic tests:
 1. Rectal examination.
 2. Sigmoidoscopy—to examine the distal 25–30 cm of the large bowel.
 3. Colonoscopy—flexible scope can visualize approximately 60 cm. of the colon.
 4. Barium enema—with air contrast to detect small lesions and visualize difficult areas.
 5. Chest x-ray and liver scan—detect metastases.
 6. Laboratory evaluations:
  a. CBC—to detect anemia.
  b. CEA (carcinoembryonic antigen)—a tumor marker used before and after surgery.

Table 19–1. STAGING SYSTEM FOR COLORECTAL CANCER (AS DESCRIBED BY INTERNATIONAL UNION AGAINST CANCER)

Colon

T	Primary tumor; no categories
NX	Regional lymph nodes (intra-abdominal and subdiaphragmatic), pathologic confirmation only, i.e., NX− = no metastases, NX+ = metastases present.
M	Distant metastases
M0	Absent
M1	Present
P	Histopathologic categories
P1	Confined to mucosa only
P2	Invasion to submucosa only
P3	Invasion of muscularis propria or to subserosa
P4	Invasion to serosa or beyond
G	Histopathologic grading
G1	Highly differentiated
G2	Moderately differentiated
G3	Anaplastic

Rectum

T	Primary tumor
T1	Primary occupies no more than one third of the length or circumference of the rectum; no invasion of muscle
T2	More than one third but no more than one half of rectal dimensions occupied, or invasion of muscle coat, no fixation of rectum
T3	More than one half of rectal dimensions occupied or fixation, but no extension to neighboring structures
T4	Tumor extends to neighboring structures

7. Laparotomy may be done to assess nodal involvement.
8. CT scan may detect local invasion of rectal cancer (to bladder, prostate, ureters, vagina, sacrum).

D. Staging:
1. Duke's Classification.
   a. Duke's A: Growth confined to mucosa; no nodal involvement.
   b. Duke's B: Growth spread to muscularis; no nodal involvement.
   c. Duke's C: Metastasis to regional lymph nodes.
   d. Duke's D: Distal metastasis.
2. TNM System (Table 19–1).

METHODS OF TREATMENT

A. Surgery is the treatment of choice for most patients.
   1. Types of surgical intervention for colon cancer:
      a. Resection with anastomosis.
      b. Resection with temporary or permanent colostomy.
      c. Abdominal-perineal resection.
   2. Extent of resection dependent on size of tumor and spread of disease.
      a. Lymph node spread especially important.
      b. Lymph nodes in the area of the colon follow the vascular supply to the area.

3. Right-sided colon tumors:
   a. Right hemicolectomy for smaller lesions.
   b. Right ascending colostomy or ileostomy for large, wide-spread lesion.
   c. Right-sided ostomies produce effluent liquid that is rich in enzymes and electrolytes.
4. Left-sided colon tumors:
   a. Left hemicolectomy for smaller lesions.
   b. Left descending colostomy for larger lesions.
   c. Left-sided ostomies produce effluence that is more formed and less liquid.
5. Sigmoid colon tumors:
   a. Sigmoid colectomy for smaller lesions.
   b. Sigmoid colostomy for larger lesions.
   c. Abdominal-perineal (A/P) resection for large, low sigmoid tumors.
      (1) A/P resection removes margin of sigmoid colon and rectum.
      (2) Levator muscles are left intact.
      (3) In women, uterus, ovaries, tubes, and posterior vaginal wall may also be removed.
      (4) Necessitates a colostomy.
6. Rectal cancer:
   a. Resection with anastomosis or pull-through procedure (which preserves the anal sphincter).
   b. Resection with permanent colostomy.
   c. Abdominal-perineal resection for large lesions.
7. Surgery may be used as palliative treatment:
   a. Pain relief.
   b. Prevent or relieve bowel obstruction.
B. Radiation Therapy.
   1. As a treatment for colon cancer:
      a. Has not played a major role.
      b. Sometimes used as palliative treatment.
   2. As a treatment for rectal cancer:
      a. May be used as curative treatment if patient is not a candidate for surgery.
      b. Occasionally used as an adjunct to surgery:
         (1) Preoperatively, it may make some unresectable lesions surgically resectable.
         (2) Postoperatively, it may decrease local recurrence.
      c. Localized symptomatic recurrence may be managed by radiation therapy.
      d. Used for palliation.
         (1) Pain relief in an unresectable primary tumor.
         (2) To treat metastases or malignant effusions.
C. Chemotherapy.
   1. Adjuvant chemotherapy for colon cancer:
      a. used to help prevent recurrence.
      b. Has had no major effect on survival.
      c. 5-Fluorouracil alone or 5-fluorouracil + methyl lomustine.
      d. Recently 5-fluorouracil + Cisplatin has demonstrated promising results.

2. For advanced colorectal cancer:
   a. Response rate of approximately 43% has been reported.
   b. Combination therapy:
      (1) Methyl lomustine–5-fluorouracil–vincristine.
      (2) Cisplatin-methotrexate-mitomycin C.
   c. Immunotherapy using BCG or MER has also been used.
3. Intrahepatic arterial chemotherapy:
   a. Used for colorectal patients with liver metastases.
      (1) Can give increased concentration of drug to the liver.
      (2) Decreases systemic toxicity.
      (3) Allows continuous exposure to the drug.
   b. FUDR (a 5-FU analogue) is the drug most commonly used.
   c. A silastic catheter is threaded into the hepatic artery.
   d. The catheter is attached to a device which delivers the drug:
      (1) External infusion pumps.
      (2) Implanted infusion pumps which are placed in a surgically con-
          structed subcutaneous pocket in the abdominal wall.

PROGNOSIS AND REHABILITATION

A. Prognosis. 5-year survival rates:
   1. Overall, considering all stages: 40%.
   2. Duke's A: 80%–90%.
   3. Duke's B: 60% with negative nodes.
   4. Duke's C: 25%–45%.
   5. Duke's D: less than 5%.
B. Rehabilitation.
   1. Discharge teaching.
      a. Include family.
      b. Give written instructions as needed.
   2. Referral to United Ostomy Association.
   3. Home Health Care follow-up; arrange referral.
   4. Odor control, e.g., charcoal, bismuth, ASA.
   5. Learning colostomy control:
      a. Problems: diarrhea, constipation, gas.
      b. Irrigation: timing.
      c. Diet: question of low residue; avoidance of foods that cause gas or
         odor.
   6. Sexuality concerns.

NURSING CARE

A. Potential psychosocial concerns:
   1. Body image changes.
   2. Social isolation.
   3. Threatened sexuality (related to surgical intervention).
   4. Fear of death.
B. Nursing assessment data related to psychosocial concerns:
   1. Patient's and family's reaction to prospect of an ostomy.
   2. Occupational and recreational activities.

    3. Available support systems.
    4. Degree of current anatomic knowledge.
    5. Level of general understanding.
    6. Importance of sexuality.
    7. Feelings regarding social acceptability of people with ostomies.
  C. Nursing interventions related to psychosocial concerns:
    1. Allow ventilation of feelings regarding ostomies.
    2. Refer to enterostomal therapist (ET) if available.
    3. Provide specific information on functional changes that will result from ostomy.
    4. Give permission for discussions regarding sexual concerns.
  D. Potential patient problems related to surgery:
    1. Fever.
    2. Anastomotic leak.
      a. Usually more common in lower resections.
      b. May result in abscesses and fistula formation.
      c. Usually self-limiting.
    3. Paralytic iteus.
    4. Urinary difficulties.
      a. Especially problematic in men.
      b. Aggravates previous nocturia problem.
    5. Impotency.
      a. Associated with abdominal-perineal resections.
      b. A result of damage to pelvic nerve fibers.
    6. Ostomy complications:
      a. Changes in peristomal skin integrity.
      b. Stoma prolapse.
      c. Stoma retraction.
  E. Nursing assessment data related to colorectal surgery:
    1. Nutritional status.
    2. Skin integrity.
    3. Laboratory tests (CEA, CBC, liver function tests).
    4. Location of tumor.
    5. Patient's knowledge of anatomy, functional changes, and stoma appearance.
    6. Signs of fever.
    7. Presence of bowel sounds, oral intake.
    8. Presence of normal effluence if ostomy is present.
    9. Changes in sexuality.
   10. Patient's or family's ability to incorporate stoma care into activities of daily living.
  F. Nursing interventions related to colorectal surgery:
    1. Preoperative instruction on:
      a. Usual coughing, deep breathing, and leg exercises.
      b. What a colostomy is and how it will affect the patient (including understanding of the GI tract).
      c. How the stoma will look immediately after surgery and how it will gradually reduce in size.
      d. The resumption of activities, normal dress, and so forth.
      e. The preoperative routine.

2. Physical preoperative preparation, which includes:
   a. Nutritional build-up.
   b. Sterilization of the bowel.
   c. Cleansing of the bowel.
   d. Preparation of the skin.
   e. Restriction of food and fluids.
3. Postoperative physical care:
   a. Provide peristomal skin care.
      (1) Clean skin gently with warm water. (Mild soap may be used, but should be thoroughly washed off.)
      (2) Allow skin to air dry. (Gauze may be used to retain liquid contents from stoma during skin care.)
      (3) Apply pouch with appropriate adhesive:
         (a) Ileostomy and cecostomy: skin barrier (e.g., Stomahesive [Squibb], Hollihesive, [Hollister]) or plasticized skin covering (e.g., Skin Prep [United], Skin Gel [Hollister]).
         (b) Transverse colostomy: same as for ileostomy.
         (c) Sigmoid/descending colostomy: possible to wear closed pouch or stoma covering if regulated with irrigation.
   b. Prevent or identify obstruction of output.
      (1) Assess frequency, color, and consistency of stools.
      (2) Auscultate bowel sounds.
      (3) Note signs and symptoms of obstruction.
      (4) If patient usually irrigates sigmoid or descending colostomy, may irrigate with 30 cc warm water. Teach colostomy patient to eat more fiber and drink more fluids.
      (5) If ileostomy stoma obstruction, consult physician. Do not irrigate.
   c. Provide adequate hydration.
4. Postoperative teaching of patient or family.
   a. When and how to irrigate colostomy.
   b. Appearance of a normal stoma:
      (1) Color (pink).
      (2) Texture (mucous membrane like inside of lips).
      (3) Absence of sensation in stoma.
   c. Provide printed information on stoma appliances.
   d. Provide information on community resources such as the United Ostomy Association.
   e. Instruct on diet:
      (1) Adequate milk and fluid intake.
      (2) Importance of small frequent meals.
      (3) Avoidance of gas and odor producing foods.
   f. Teach about signs and symptoms of bowel obstruction:
      (1) Cramping.
      (2) Diarrhea or absence of defecation.
      (3) Abdominal distension or pain.
      (4) Nausea and vomiting.
   g. Potential patient problems related to radiation therapy.
G. Potential patient problems related to radiation therapy:
   1. Skin changes (dry to wet desquamation).

    2. Fistula formation.

    3. Nutritional deficits as a result of nausea or indigestion.

    4. Diarrhea.

H. Nursing assessment data related to radiation therapy:

    1. Degree of skin changes and impact on activities of daily living.

    2. Changes in eating patterns.

    3. Changes in elimination patterns.

    4. Pattern of fatigue and its effect on lifestyle.

    5. Degree of physical dysfunction associated with fistula formation.

I. Nursing interventions related to radiation therapy:

    1. Explain physiologic effects of radiation therapy.

    2. Skin care (see Chapter 23).

    3. Fistula care.

    4. Provide eating hints to alleviate or diminish feelings of nausea or indigestion (see recommendations under Radiation therapy).

    5. Teach patient or family parameters for assessing severe diarrhea.

    6. Suggest dietary changes to control diarrhea (e.g., drink fluids in small amounts frequently and avoid high-bulk foods, fresh fruit and juices, milk products, highly spiced foods).

J. Potential patient problems related to chemotherapy:

    1. Diarrhea, stomatitis (5-FU).

    2. Delayed myelosuppression (methyl CCNU).

    3. GI symptoms (FUDR).

       a. Nausea.

       b. Epigastric burning.

       c. Abdominal pain, cramping.

       d. Lack of appetite.

    4. Peripheral neuropathies (vincristine).

    5. Nephrotoxicity, ototoxicity (Cisplatin).

K. Nursing assessment data related to chemotherapy:

    1. Platelet count (below 20,000).

    2. White blood cell count (below 1000).

    3. Signs of stomatitis.

    4. BUN, creatinine.

    5. Degree of diarrhea.

    6. Degree of GI discomfort.

L. Nursing assessment data related to hepatic artery infusion of chemotherapy:

    1. Ability to manage self care.

    2. Liver function tests.

    3. Signs of seroma at pump site.

    4. Signs of infection at pump site.

    5. Patient's and family's understanding of teaching plan.

    6. Coagulation studies (heparin usually given simultaneously).

M. Nursing interventions related to chemotherapy:

    1. Monitor platelet and white blood cell count.

    2. Good oral hygiene.

    3. Administer antiemetics.

    4. Hydrate well (if receiving Cisplatin).

    5. Provide foods high in protein and calories.

    6. Provide antacid for gastric distress.

    7. Suggest dietary changes to control diarrhea.

STUDY QUESTIONS

Mr. Keller is a 62-year-old married business executive who has just been diagnosed with a Duke's C lesion of the sigmoid colon. He has no evidence of liver involvement and is otherwise in good health.

1. Write a generic nursing care plan that could address Mr. Keller's potential problems during the diagnostic phase of his disease progression.
2. Write a generic nursing care plan that could address Mr. Keller's potential problems during the treatment phase of his illness.
3. Write a generic nursing care plan that could address Mr. Keller's potential problems during the rehabilitation phase of his illness.

Bibliography

Broadwell, D. and Jackson, B. (eds.): Principles of Ostomy Care. St. Louis, C. V. Mosby Co., 1982.

Cozzi, E., Hagle, M., McGregor, M., and Woodhouse, D.: Nursing management of patients receiving hepatic arterial chemotherapy through an implanted infusion pump. Cancer Nursing, 7(3): 229–234, 1984.

Crespi, M., Weissman, G. S., Gilbertsen, V. A., et al.: The role of proctosigmoidoscopy in screening for colorectal neoplasia. CA Cancer Journal for Clinicians, 34(3):158–166, 1984.

DeCosse, J. J.: Are we doing better with large-bowel cancer? New England Journal of Medicine, 310(12):782–783, 1984.

Moore, J. and LaMont, J. T.: Colorectal cancer—risk factors and screening strategies. Archives of Internal Medicine, 144:1819–1823, 1984.

Ramming, K., Haskell, C. M. and Tesler, A.: Gastrointestinal tract neoplasms. In Haskell, C. M. (ed.): Cancer Treatment. Philadelphia, W. B. Saunders Co., pp. 231–357, 1980.

Stearns, M. (ed.): Neoplasms of the Colon, Rectum and Anus. New York, John Wiley & Sons, 1980.

20

Leukemia

MARYELLEN MAGUIRE, RN, BSN

LEUKEMIA OVERVIEW

A. Definition:
  1. Leukemia is a malignant disorder of the blood and blood-forming organs (bone marrow, lymphatics, and spleen).
  2. Results in an accumulation of dysfunctional cells.
  3. Due to a loss of cell division regulation.
B. Perspectives:
  1. Leukemia represents 3% of the overall cancer incidence in the United States.
  2. Most commonly affects older people.
  3. Common form of cancer affecting children, representing 30% of all childhood malignancies.
  4. Some forms may be curable.
C. General classification is based on the predominant cell the and the rate of symptom onset. Incidence of leukemia:
  1. Acute leukemia = 60%.
    a. Acute lymphocytic leukemia (ALL) = 25%.
    b. Acute nonlymphocytic leukemia (ANLL) = 35%.
  2. Chronic leukemia = 40%.
    a. Chronic lymphocytic leukemia (CLL) = 25%.
    b. Chronic myelogenous leukemia (CML) = 15%.
  3. Detection and screening—Because of the biologic nature of the acute leukemias, symptom onset usually occurs over a brief period of time and reflects the replacement of normal bone marrow elements with abnormal cells. The chronic leukemias have a longer clinical course and are more commonly diagnosed during physical examination and blood work. Presently, there is no cost effective method for screening and early detection.
  4. Presenting symptoms—Involvement of the bone marrow may result in anemia, thrombocytopenia, and granulocytopenia, and infiltration of organs may result in splenomegaly, lymphadenopathy, and bone pain.

Table 20–1. CLINICAL SIGNS AND SYMPTOMS OF THE LEUKEMIAS*

Clinical Symptoms	Clinical Signs	Laboratory Findings	Cause
Malaise, fatigue, weakness	Pallor	Anemia	Marrow failure
Decreased weight	Weight loss	Hypoalbuminemia	Anorexia, increased metabolism
Easy bruising, gum bleeding, visual difficulties, tarry stools	Petechiae, ecchymosis, microscopic hematuria, hypertrophy or bleeding gums, retinal hemorrhage, guaiac positive stools	Thrombocytopenia Abnormal clotting	Marrow failure
Prolonged or recurrent viral or bacterial infection	Sinusitis, pneumonitis, urinary tract infection, decreased wound healing	Granulocytopenia	Marrow failure
Headache, nausea, vomiting	Meningismus Papilledema	Increased cerebrospinal fluid (CSF) protein, decreased CSF sugar, leukemic cells in CSF	Meningeal or central nervous system leukemic involvement
Bone pain	Bone tenderness	Abnormal roentgenogram	Leukemic infiltration
Swollen glands	Lymphadenopathy	Abnormal biopsy or scans	Leukemic infiltration
Abdominal fullness or pain	Splenomegaly or hepatomegaly	Abnormal liver function tests	Leukemic infiltration
Testicular swelling	Testicular mass	Abnormal biopsy	Leukemic infiltration

*Adapted from Williams, W. J., et al.: Hematology. New York, McGraw-Hill Book Co., 1977, pp. 992–1024.

These clinical signs and symptoms are commonly seen in the acute and chronic leukemias. See Table 20–1, which lists the clinical signs and symptoms with the specific laboratory findings and etiologic cause.

ACUTE LEUKEMIA

A. General overview:
   1. Risk factors in developing acute leukemia:
      a. Chromosome damage:
         (1) Radiation—therapeutic exposure for treatment of neoplastic and nonneoplastic diseases, exposure to atomic radiation such as in survivors of Nagasaki and Hiroshima.
         (2) Chemical—exposure to cytotoxic drugs (alkylating agents), benzene, chloramphenicol, and phenylbutazone.
         (3) Genetic abnormalities—Down's syndrome (Trisomy 21) increases the risk of developing leukemia eighteen times. Other abnormalities include Fanconi's anemia, Bloom's syndrome, Klinefelter's syndrome, and Turner's syndrome.

   b. Familial susceptibility—A greater incidence of leukemia occurs in certain families and in identical twins.
   c. Viral exposure—The human T cell lymphotrophic virus (HTLV-1) has been associated with T cell leukemia in males in both Japan and the Caribbean. At this time there is no proof that a virus plays a major role in the etiology of leukemia in the United States.
2. Age distribution of the acute leukemias:

	Acute Lymphocytic	Acute Nonlymphocytic
Children	85%	15%
Adults	13%	87%

3. Survival—There was a median survival of 5–6 months for untreated acute leukemia at a major cancer center between 1951 and 1966. See Figure 20–1.
4. Improved statistics—Over the past three decades the experience of treating acute leukemia has improved greatly, with complete remissions of 90% and 70% occuring in acute lymphocytic leukemia and acute nonlymphocytic leukemia, respectively. Factors influencing these statistics are:
   a. Introduction of combination and multimodality therapy.
   b. Improved support services; blood banking, more efficacious use of antibiotics.
   c. Coordinated and cooperative research efforts. See Figure 20–2 for an example of improved survival in children with acute lymphocytic leukemia treated on successive cooperative trials.
5. Theory of acute leukemia treatment:
   a. Remission induction—The initial treatment phase when multiple chemotherapeutic agents are administered in high doses to "empty" the bone marrow of all hematologic elements so that normal marrow constituents may repopulate. The goal of therapy is to achieve a complete remission. A complete remission requires:
   (1) The absence of all clinical signs and symptoms of leukemia.

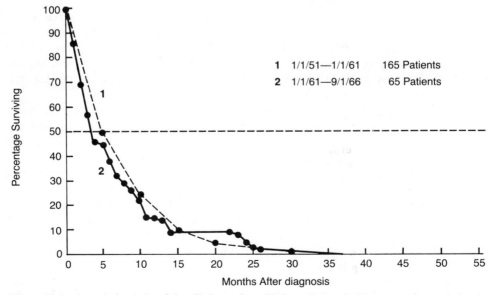

Figure 20–1. Acute leukemia in adults. (Redrawn from Clarkson, B., et al.: Treatment of acute leukemia. Cancer 37:775, 1975.)

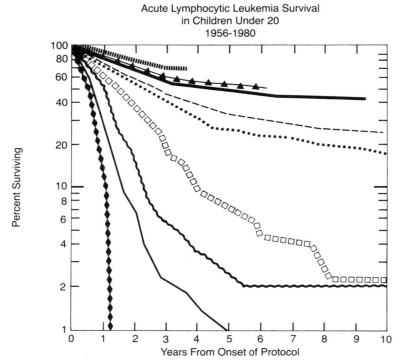

Figure 20–2. *Each line designates a different clinical trial. Successive controlled clinical trials in 3,072 children demonstrate the incremental steps to the cure of acute lymphocytic leukemia. (Redrawn from Holland, J.: Breaking the cure barrier. Journal of Clinical Oncology, 1:75, 1983.)*

    (2) Normal peripheral blood differential devoid of blasts.

    (3) Restoration of a normal bone marrow with less than 5% blasts; adequate numbers of maturing myeloid cells, megakaryocytes, and adequate numbers of erythroid and lymphoid precursors.

  b. Post remission therapy—Pharmacokinetic studies indicate that a successful induction regimen reduces the leukemic cell population, rendering it microscopically undetectable but undoubtedly present. Post remission therapy is initiated to further reduce or eliminate the remaining population of undetectable cells. Research to identify the most effective, least toxic treatment method continues.

  c. Intensification or consolidation therapy is the administration of intensive therapy given after remission to further reduce the leukemic cell population. The sequencing of this treatment is designed with consideration for optimal effect and tolerable toxicity.

  d. Maintenance is the administration of long-term therapy in moderate doses to "maintain" the disease-free state.

  e. Relapse is the reappearance of clinical and hematologic evidence of leukemia. This may occur in the bone marrow or in extramedullary sites (e.g., central nervous system, testes, skin).

B. Acute childhood lymphocytic leukemia (ALL).

  1. Overview:

    a. ALL is a disease of the blood resulting in an accumulation of immature lymphoid cells, lymphoblasts. This disease is believed to arise in the lymph system and invade the bone marrow.

b. ALL is a disease primarily of children, with 85% of cases occurring in that population.

c. It is the type of leukemia that has shown the most progress in treatment. Since Dr. Farber's initial treatment with aminopterin in the late 1940's, the rate of complete remission has increased from 20% to 85–95%.

d. Today more than 50% of patients will enjoy long-term remission and probably be cured of their disease.

2. Reasons for improved survival—Many of the treatment concepts that have resulted in improved survival have occurred because of a better understanding of the biology and behavior of this disease.

a. The introduction of combination chemotherapy in the 1960's increased complete remission rates from 45–50% to 80–90%.

b. The administration of prophylactic central nervous system radiation decreased the incidence of CNS relapse from 50% to less than 10%. See Figure 20–3. for an illustration of the effect of these factors on survival.

c. The identification of "high" risk factors resulted in the design of more intensive protocols for the high risk patients. High risk factors:

(1) Age <2 or >10 years.

(2) Male sex (risk of testicular relapse).

(3) White blood cell count >20,000 cu/mm.

(4) Presence of a mediastinal mass.

(5) Central nervous system disease.

d. A comparison of relapse rates of ALL patients having "standard" and "high" risk features is illustrated in Figure 20–4.

3. Treatment:

a. Induction of remission:

(1) The administration of vincristine, prednisone, and L-asparaginase results in an overall remission rate of approximately 95%. 85% of complete remissions are achieved in four weeks.

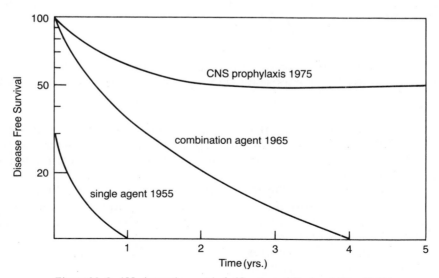

Figure 20–3. ALL: improving survival. (Courtesy of Stephen Sallan, M.D.)

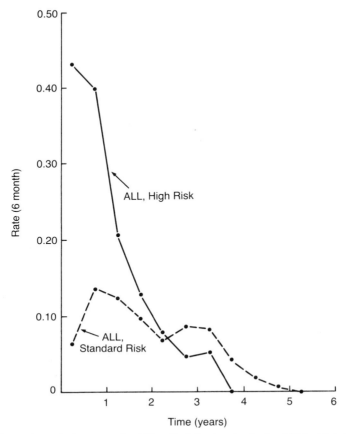

Figure 20–4. *Comparison of relapse rates for ALL patients having standard and high-risk features. A patient known to have at diagnosis at least one of the high-risk features (WBC 100,000/cu mm, mediastinal mass, CNS leukemia, or E^+ blasts) is considered as ALL, high risk. All other patients are considered in the ALL standard risk group. This data analysis has been prepared by Dr. Stephen George. (Redrawn from Mauer, A. M.: Therapy of acute lymphocytic leukemia in childhood. Blood 56:1, 1980.)*

      (2) The addition of an anthracycline does not appear to increase the induction response rate but some studies indicate that it may lead to an improvement in the long-term survival.

   b. Post remission therapy:

      (1) The administration of intensive post remission therapy along with central nervous system prophylaxis results in 50–65% of those whose disease remits initially remaining in complete remission at 5 years.

      (2) There is no standard post remission treatment. Much of the present research centers around defining the most effective, least toxic method of treatment during this phase. Therapy frequently consists of:

         (a) Repeated courses of combination chemotherapy administered over 2–3 years.

         (b) The consolidation of intensification phase may include high doses of combination therapy with vincristine, prednisone, cyclophosphamide, methotrexate, L-asparaginase, or 6-mercaptopurine.

  (c) Maintenance therapy frequently consists of a combination of methotrexate and 6-mercaptopurine. Vincristine and/or prednisone may also be added.

(3) The addition of an anthracycline as consolidation therapy in high risk patients has resulted in a 70% continuous complete remission rate at 2 years.

(4) Standard cranial nervous system prophylaxis consists of 1800–2400 rads to the cranium and four to six injections of intrathecal methotrexate. Alternate approaches include moderate dose intravenous methotrexate with intrathecal boluses of the same, or cytarabine and methotrexate intrathecally. High risk patients may receive higher doses of cranial irradiation.

c. Relapse and refractory treatment:

(1) 50% achieve a second complete remission.

(2) The original induction regimen may be reinitiated if the patient relapses after cessation of treatment.

(3) The testes and central nervous system are often the sites of extramedullary relapse. Radiation therapy should be administered locally and systemic therapy should be reinitiated as soon as possible.

(4) The combination of VM-26 and cytarabine has resulted in a substantial number of complete remissions in primary relapse and refractory disease. Other drugs used are high dose cytarabine with or without L-asparaginase, high dose methotrexate with citrovorum rescue, mAmsa, and mitoxantrone.

(5) The degree of success in attaining a subsequent remission is related to the number of previous treatments, with lower response rates seen in heavily pre-treated patients.

(6) Bone Marrow Transplantation is a treatment modality employed in second remission.

4. Controversies that persist in the treatment of childhood ALL are listed:

a. Role of cranial radiation and CNS prophylaxis.

b. Duration of maintenance therapy.

c. Prevention of testicular relapse.

5. Late effects of treatment: Long-term follow-up of childhood ALL studies indicate that children treated with combination chemotherapy and central nervous system prophylaxis are at risk for developing late physiologic and psychologic effects.

a. Characteristics of late effects:

(1) These effects may occur in any system and may develop after weeks or years of treatment.

(2) An increase in late effects is seen in children less than 5, and has been attributed to the toxic effect of treatment on developing tissue.

(3) The degree of impairment is related to the type and intensity of treatment.

b. Major areas of concern:

(1) Neuropsychiatric:

  (a) Reports of deficits in attention span, concentration, and short-term auditory memory.

(b) Decrease in overall level of intellectual functioning, as compared to siblings and peers.

(2) Alteration in growth and development:

(a) Majority of children are within normal parameters and any final loss is usually small.

(b) Impaired growth hormone response has been implicated as an etiologic factor.

(3) Development of secondary malignancies:

(a) Incidence of second malignances may be as high as 15%, which is 20 times greater than the normal population rate.

(b) Report of 2% incidence in brain tumors, gliomas and astrocytomas, following treatment in a Children's Cancer Study Group protocol.

(4) Psychosocial effects:

(a) Reports of anxiety, depression, and decreased self concept, varying from mild to severe.

(b) Reports of poor school performance.

(c) Fear of intimacy due to concerns about fertility.

C. ALL in adults

1. Overview:

a. ALL is far less common in adults, with only 15% of the new cases of acute leukemia occurring in this population per year.

b. Research in this disease is quite slow due to the limited number of cases. Many of the therapeutic conclusions have been drawn from pediatric studies.

c. With the realization that adult ALL most commonly resembled the "high risk" childhood type, more intensive induction regimens were introduced. The addition of an anthracycline to vincristine and prednisone increased the complete remission rate from 50% to 70–90%.

2. Treatment:

a. Induction of remission: See Table 20–2 for a list of induction regimens and response rates for previously untreated adults.

(1) Most induction regimens consist of combination therapy with vincristine, prednisone, and an anthracycline.

(2) The addition of other agents does not appear to significantly increase the remission rate.

Table 20–2. ADULT ALL: COMBINATION INDUCTION REGIMENS IN UNTREATED ADULT PATIENTS*

Chemotherapeutic Regimens	Response Rates
Vincristine, Prednisone, Daunomycin or Adriamycin	72–92%
Vincristine, Prednisone, Methotrexate	80%
Vincristine, Prednisone, Daunomycin, L-Asparaginase	71–72%
Vincristine, Prednisone, Methotrexate, L-Asparaginase	75%
Vincristine, Prednisone, L-Asparaginase, Cyclophosphamide	83%
Vincristine, Prednisone, Adriamycin, Cyclophosphamide	78–85%
Vincristine, Prednisone, Daunomycin, L-Asparaginase, Cyclophosphamide, Cytarabine, 6-Mercaptopurine	77%

*Adapted from Jacobs, A., and Gale, R.: Recent advances in the biology and treatment of acute lymphoblastic leukemia in adults. New England Journal of Medicine, *311*:(81) 1219–1231, 1984.

(3) It has been reported that 10% of patients have evidence of CNS involvement at the time of diagnosis and some studies incorporate therapy into this phase of treatment.
  b. Post remission therapy:
    (1) The administration of intensive post remission therapy results in a median duration of remission of 18–24 months.
    (2) Optimal therapy has not yet been determined, but many studies include reduced doses of drugs used during induction. Vincristine, prednisone, and an anthracycline are used in combination with 6-mercaptopurine and methotrexate over a 2–3 year period.
    (3) CNS prophylaxis is usually incorporated into this phase. This treatment has been found to decrease the incidence of CNS relapse but has not affected the duration of complete remission or survival.
  3. Remission duration: The overall long-term survival for adults in first remission in most recent studies is 25–35%. The duration of remission for adults, as compared to children treated on identical protocols, is shorter. See Figure 20–5 for an illustration of this point. Treatment of relapsed adult ALL is similar to that for relapsed childhood ALL.
D. Acute Non-Lymphocytic Leukemia (acute myelocytic, acute granulocytic) (ANLL)
  1. Overview: ANLL is a disease of the most primitive bone marrow cell and can arise in the myeloid, monocyte, erythroid, and megakaryocytic lines. Most commonly seen in adults, with 87% of cases occurring in this age

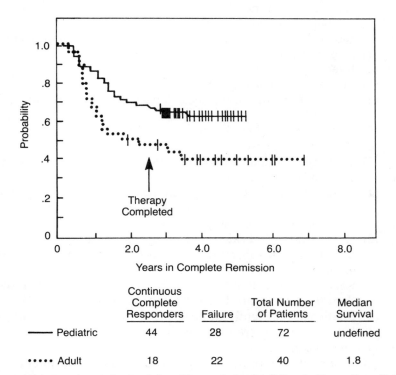

	Continuous Complete Responders	Failure	Total Number of Patients	Median Survival
—— Pediatric	44	28	72	undefined
••••• Adult	18	22	40	1.8

Figure 20–5. Duration of remission in adults with acute leukemia. (*Robert J. Mayer, Dana Farber Cancer Institute.*)

category. The median age of patients in most large studies is the sixth decade.

2. | Classification | Distribution |
|--|--------------|
| Acute myelocytic (AML) | 50% |
| Acute promyelocytic (APL) | 10% |
| Acute myelomonocytic (AMML) | 25% |
| Acute monocytic (AMOL) | 10% |
| Acute erythrocytic (AEL) | 5% |
| Acute megakaryocytic (AMeL) | <1% |

3. Treatment:
   a. Induction of remission:
      (1) Complete remissions have been reported in 50–85% of patients with the combination of daunorubicin and cytarabine with or without 6-thioguanine.
      (2) The remission induction rate is inversely correlated with age, and this is due to the inability of older patients to survive the rigors of intensive therapy rather than to a more resistant form of leukemia.
      (3) Standard induction therapy may include:
          (a) Daunorubicin, 30–60 mg/m^2, administered daily on each of the first 3 days of treatment. The drug is administered slowly, through the side arm of a well running IV line.
          (b) Cytarabine, 100–200 mg/m^2, administered as a continuous infusion, daily for 7 days, beginning on the first day of therapy.
          (c) 6-Thioguanine, 200 mg/m^2, administered orally for 5–7 days beginning on the first day of therapy.
   b. Prognostic factors that adversely influence induction outcome:
      (1) Age >60 years.
      (2) Infection at the time of diagnosis.
      (3) Multiple chromosome abnormalities.
      (4) Chronic bone marrow disease (aplastic anemia, myeloid metaplasia, etc.).
      (5) Leukemia occuring as a second malignancy.
      (6) Additional disease.
      (7) Leukocytosis (total leukocyte count greater than 100,000 cu/mm).
   c. Post remission therapy controversies:
      (1) Some studies indicate no additional benefit in the administration of post remission therapy; median durations of 10–14 months with or without post remission treatment.
      (2) Other studies indicate that it prolongs the duration of remission, but does not substantially increase the number of long-term survivors.
      (3) Reports indicate that the intensity of post remission therapy rather than the addition of therapy affects remission duration.
      (4) Studies are presently in progress to evaluate the efficacy and intensity of this therapy.
   d. Post remission therapy:
      (1) Post remission protocols may include single or combination therapy. Some chemotherapeutic agents commonly used in this phase of therapy are: cytarabine (in varying dose levels), daunorubicin, 6-thioguanine, and 5-azacytidine.

(2) Long-term survival rates of 10–25% are reported by most researchers.

(3) The duration of post remission therapy is highly variable and may range from 2–3 months of intensive therapy to 18–24 months of low dose maintenance.

4. Characteristics of ANLL in children:
   a. Predominance of monocytic subclassification.
   b. 5–15% of children present with CNS involvement at diagnosis; CNS prophylaxis is incorporated into the treatment regimen.
   c. Remission induction rates similar to those seen in adults are achieved.
   d. Report of a greater than 50% continuous complete remission rate with intensive non–cross resistant post remission therapy.

5. Bone marrow transplantation: Because of the poor overall survival rates some researchers recommend that patients in first remission who are under the age of 40 and have a matched sibling receive a bone marrow transplant.

6. Relapse: Approximately 65–90% of patients who previously achieved a complete remission will relapse before 2 years. Because second remissions are more difficult to attain and are often brief, the maintenance of initial remission is the major influencing factor on survival.
   a. Causes of relapse:
      (1) Ineffective elimination of the remaining leukemic cells.
      (2) Development of resistance by leukemic cells.
      (3) Presence of privileged sites or sanctuaries, i.e., CNS.
   b. Treatment of relapsed and refractory disease:
      (1) The original induction regimen may be utilized for re-induction in first relapse, especially if the patient relapses off therapy.
      (2) Second line treatments for relapsed or refractory disease usually consist of standard agents administered in novel dose schedules or new agents under investigation. Recent studies include high dose cytarabine with or without L-asparaginase, etoposide (VP-16), 5-azacytidine, 5-AZQ, mAmsa, and mitoxantrone.
      (3) Relapses occurring while on therapy as well as the number of previous treatment regimens have a negative influence on achieving a subsequent remission. Second remissions are achieved in approximately 50% of cases.

CHRONIC LEUKEMIA

A. General overview:
   1. Distinguishing characteristics:
      a. Chronic leukemia progresses over a period of years rather than weeks.
      b. Primarily affects older adults, and treatment is initiated to control the symptoms rather than to eradicate the disease.
      c. There are two major forms of chronic leukemia: myelocytic and lymphocytic.
      d. More common in men than women and rare in children.
   2. Risk factors:
      a. Research to determine the etiologic factors of chronic leukemia has been limited. Reasons for the lack of research include relative rarity of occurrence, difficulty in diagnosis, preponderance in the elderly, and lack of reliable statistics.

b. The present information implicates ionizing radiation as a risk factor for chronic myelogenous leukemia. Occasional associations with benzene exposure have also been reported.

c. Host and genetic factors appear to be important in the development of chronic lymphocytic leukemia.

3. General classification:
    a. Chronic myelocytic leukemia = CML (chronic granulocytic).
    b. Chronic lymphocytic leukemia = CLL.

4. Treatment: Because nonintensive treatment is available that can adequately and easily control these diseases for a number of years there has been limited research in developing more intensive methods that might prove to be more effective in the long term.

B. Chronic myelogenous leukemia.

1. Characteristics: Chronic myelogenous leukemia is a disease of the blood and blood-forming organs that results in an expanded myeloid cell population and organ infiltration. During the early stages the bone marrow functions adequately. However, in a period of months to years, 80% of patients develop a more aggressive picture with increasing immature forms. CML is the first human neoplasm to be associated with a nonrandom chromosome abnormality. The Philadelphia chromosome, a transfer of genetic material between chromosomes 9 and 22, is present in 95% of cases.

2. Disease phases: Three separate disease phases have been appreciated in terms of symptoms, clinical features, hematologic manifestations, treatment, and prognosis. See Table 20–3.

3. Chemotherapy:
    a. Single agent therapy is usually administered during the chronic phase to control the increasing number of myeloid cells and platelets. Agents most commonly used are hydroxyurea and busulfan.
        (1) Hydroxyurea is recommended because it provides rapid and tight control, rarely causes severe side effects, and lacks cross resistance with alkylating agents.
        (2) Busulfan is an inexpensive, effective chemotherapeutic agent. Side effects include hyperpigmentation, pulmonary fibrosis, xerostomia, and cataracts.
    b. With progression of disease, increasing doses of single agents may be administered, but combination treatment is often introduced.
    c. In the terminal or blast phase, the blast cells may be classified as either myeloid or lymphoid. A 60% complete remission rate may be achieved with the administration of vincristine and prednisone to patients with the lymphoid variant. Intensive therapy for the myeloid variant results in median survival of 2–4 months.

4. Alternative treatment:
    a. Radiation therapy:
        (1) Splenic radiation was the primary treatment, but has been replaced by chemotherapy, which results in longer survival.
        (2) Palliative treatment for splenic pain and extramedullary chloromas is effective but of short duration.
    b. Leukopheresis is a mechanical method of removing myeloid cells and can effectively reduce tumor mass. It has been used in cases of life-

Table 20–3. CHRONIC MYELOGENOUS LEUKEMIA

Phases	Chronic	Accelerated	Blastic
Duration	*30–40 months*	*3–9 months*	*2–3 months*
Hematologic picture	Total leukocyte count: 100,000–400,000/cu mm ↓ hemoglobin ↑ platelet count Bone marrow = 25% blasts	↑ number of peripheral blasts Less effective erythrocyte + platelet production Refractory leukostasis, progressive anemia + splenomegaly	↑ ↑ peripheral blasts = 30–50% Bone marrow >30% blasts Blasts may be classified as myeloid (75%) or lymphoid (25%)
Cytogenetics	95% pts, Philadelphia chromosome, translocation of genetic material between chromosomes 9 and 22	↑ no. of Philadelphia chromosomes noted + introduction of new abnormalities	Persistent ↑ in cytogenetic abnormalities 70–80% of patients have additional abnormalities— hyperdiploidy most common
Symptoms	Fever, night sweats, fatigue, anorexia, mild weight loss, pallor, abdominal mass 20% asymptomatic at diagnosis	Recrudescence of fever, fatigue, weight loss Spleen size	Massive hepatic splenomegaly in 80% of patients Infection Bleeding
Complications	Infection	Infection	Leukostasis Uric acid nephropathy Bone lesions
Treatment (chemical)	Hydroxyurea 1000 mg/m^2 every 8 hrs ↓ by 50% when WBC = 20,000/cu mm + again at 12,000/cu mm Maintenance: 500–2000 mg per day Busulfan: 4–6 mg/day, usually administered for 4–6 wks Restarted when WBC is greater than 20,000/cu mm	Increased doses of hydroxyurea 2–6 gm per day May be given in combination with 6-mercaptopurine, vincristine + prednisone	Myeloid High dose hydroxyurea High dose cytarabine Cyclophosphamide Cytarabine + 5-Azacytidine Lymphoid Vincristine, prednisone + doxorubicin/daunomycin

threatening leukostasis. The time involvement and economic expense of this treatment detract from its utility.

   c. Splenectomy is performed prophylactically to reduce the risk of late complications of splenic infarction and to alleviate platelet and red cell destruction.
   d. Bone marrow transplantation is available to only 15% of patients because of age restraints and the limited numbers of adequate donors; it is presently the only method of eliminating the Philadelphia chromosome cells.

C. Chronic lymphocytic leukemia.
   1. Characteristics: CLL is a neoplastic disease of the blood that results in a gradual accumulation of functionally abnormal, well differentiated lymphocytes. A disease of adults with a peak incidence in the fifth decade,

it occurs somewhat more commonly in men. Its onset may be insidious, and the course can be highly variable. The median survival is 71 months.

2. Presenting symptoms: The presenting symptoms are variable, with 25% of patients asymptomatic at diagnosis. Other symptoms noted are: fatigue, weight loss, anorexia, and night sweats. Hepatosplenomegaly is seen in 50% of patients, and lymphadenopathy in 60%. Laboratory examination may reveal a mild to moderate anemia, thrombocytopenia, granulocytopenia, and hypogammaglobulinemia.

3. Stages and prognosis: See Table 20–4.

4. Complications:
   a. Hypogammaglobulinemia and granulocytopenia result in an increased susceptibility to bacterial and fungal infections.
   b. Autoimmune hemolytic anemia occurs in about 20% of cases.
   c. Second malignancies are seen in 10% of cases.
   d. Transition to a resistant form of lymphoma occurs in 9% of cases (Richter's syndrome).

5. Treatment:
   a. Reasons for initiating therapy are:
      (1) Leukocyte count >200,000 cu/mm.
      (2) Autoimmune events result in hemolytic anemia.
      (3) Increased susceptibility to infection.
      (4) Progressive anemia and thrombocytopenia.
      (5) Increasing splenomegaly.
   b. Chemotherapeutic options:
      (1) Chlorambucil: 0.1–0.2 mg/kg/day initially and then 0.4 mg/kg/14 days. Responses of 70% are seen initially.
      (2) Prednisone: 15–60 mg/day for 6 weeks. May be used with or without chlorambucil. Safest way to treat patients in whom failure is already present.
      (3) Intensive chemotherapy is administered when chlorambucil and prednisone are no longer effective in controlling the disease. Cyclophosphamide, vincristine (Oncovin), and prednisone (COP) is the combination regimen most often initiated. The addition of doxorubicin to this program may also be effective.
   c. Radiation therapy:
      (1) The administration of radiation to the spleen and lymph nodes is

Table 20–4. STAGING OF CHRONIC LYMPHOCYTIC LEUKEMIA*

	Clinical Stage	Median Survival in Months
Stage 0	Absolute lymphocytosis >15,000/mm^3	>150
Stage 1	Absolute lymphocytosis plus lymphadenopathy	105
Stage 2	Absolute lymphocytosis and lymphadenopathy plus enlarged liver and/or spleen	71
Stage 3	Absolute lymphocytosis and lymphadenopathy plus anemia (hemoglobin <11 gm per 100 ml)	19
Stage 4	Absolute lymphocytosis and lymphadenopathy plus thrombocytopenia (platelet count <100,000 per cu mm)	19

*From Rai, K. R., Sawitsky, A., Jagathambal, K., Gartenhaus, W., and Phillips, E.: Chronic lymphocytic leukemia. Medical Clinics of North America, *68*:697–711, 1984.

a palliative measure to shrink the tumor mass and relieve symptoms.
   (2) Total body irradiation may be as effective as chemotherapy in the early stages of the disease.

BONE MARROW TRANSPLANTATION IN TREATMENT OF LEUKEMIA

A. Role of transplantation:
   1. Therapetic option in ALL (second remission), ANLL (first and second remission), CML (primarily chronic phase).
   2. It is the only potentially curative treatment for CML and ANLL in second remission. Best results are achieved in the chronic phase of CML.
   3. Allows for higher doses of cytotoxic drugs and radiation to be administered to eliminate the disease.
   4. Performed in patients less than 50 years of age, but less than 40 is preferable.
   5. Types:
      a. Allogeneic transplants are usually from a sibling.
      b. Autologous transplant is the re-infusion of the person's own marrow.
      c. Syngeneic transplantation is the transfusion of an identical twin's marrow.
   6. Marrow ablative doses of chemotherapy and/or total body irradiation are administered, followed by the intravenous re-infusion of the previously harvested marrow cells.
   7. Since only 25% of patients have an appropriately matched relative, autologous transplantation is being explored as an alternative. Techniques are presently being employed to "clean up" the marrow and eliminate the leukemic cells prior to its re-infusion.
B. Problems in transplantation:
   1. Graft versus host disease.
   2. Infection.
   3. Graft rejection.
C. Transplantation results are given in Table 20–5.

Table 20–5. CLINICAL OUTCOME OF BONE MARROW TRANSPLANTS: 1984*

Disease	Long-term Survival (%)	Relapse Rates (%)	Rejection Rates (%)
Acute lymphocytic leukemia			
1st or 2nd remission	25–50	30–40	<5
Relapse	10–20	50–70	<5
Acute myelogenous leukemia, 1st remission	40–45	10–35	<5
Chronic myelogenous leukemia			
Acute phase	5–15	–	<5
Accelerated phase	15–40	–	
Chronic phase	60–75	–	

*Adapted from Kamani, N., and August, C. S.: Bone marrow transplantation. Medical Clinics of North America, *68*:657–675, 1984.

TREATMENT COMPLICATIONS

A. Leukostasis (seen in AML and CML blast crisis)
  1. Characteristics: Absolute leukocyte counts greater than 100,000/cu mm comprised of primarily blast forms may result in capillary plugging, vessel rupture, bleeding, and organ dysfunction. The effects of this bleeding are most commonly seen in the central nervous system and the respiratory system.
  2. Clinical signs and symptoms: Symptoms of increased intracranial pressure and respiratory dysfunction may occur.
  3. Medical management: Immediate administration of fluids, allopurinol, and chemotherapy. The chemotherapy may be the specific leukemic regimen or hydroxyurea. Prophylactic radiation to the CNS and leukopheresis (mechanical removal of blast cells) may also be initiated.
  4. Nursing management:
    a. Continuous diligent assessment for subtle deterioration in clinical status.
    b. Education about the syndrome, its relationship to the disease, and rationale for immediate intervention.
    c. Emotional support.
B. Bleeding:
  1. Characteristics: Patients with leukemia are at risk for bleeding because of the pathophysiology of their disease as well as its treatment. Bleeding is usually a result of thrombocytopenia. The greatest risk of spontaneous hemorrhage occurs when the platelet count falls below 20,000/cu mm. Bleeding may also be a result of a bleeding syndrome, disseminated intravascular coagulation, which is commonly seen in acute promyelocytic leukemia and occasionally seen in blast crisis.
  2. Clinical signs and symptoms: Petechiae and ecchymosis may represent more serious bleeding such as gastrointestinal or intercranial. The patient with disseminated intravascular coagulation may exhibit gum bleeding, epistaxis, menorrhagia, hematuria, and gastrointestinal bleeding. Laboratory tests commonly show thrombocytopenia, hypofibrinogenemia, prolonged bleeding time, prolonged thrombin time, and an increase in fibrin degradation products.
  3. Medical management:
    a. Careful monitoring of coagulation parameters and signs and symptoms of increased bleeding.
    b. Replacement of clotting factors by the administration of fresh frozen plasma or coagulation factors.
    c. Although controversial, heparin is sometimes administered.
    d. Initiation of chemotherapy to control the underlying disease.
  4. Nursing management:
    a. Accurately assessing subtle changes and early intervention.
    b. Monitoring blood counts and coagulation studies.
    c. Minimizing blood loss.
    d. Accurately assessing blood loss.
    e. Educating patient and family about syndrome, symptoms, and rationale for treatment.
    f. Providing emotional support.
C. Infection:

1. Characteristics:
   a. Infection is still the major cause of morbidity and mortality.
   b. The disease and its treatment result in a prolonged period of marrow suppression and place the patient at risk for bacterial infection when the absolute granulocyte count is less than 500/cu mm.
   c. Septicemia is the most common infectious complication noted and results in a high mortality rate if effective antibiotic therapy is not initiated within 24 hours.
   d. The most common sites of infection are the pharynx and lungs; perirectal area infection is common in the monocytic type of ANLL.
   e. Infection with gram negative organisms is frequent and necessitates use of broad spectrum antibiotics.
2. Clinical signs and symptoms:
   a. The typical signs and symptoms of infection may be absent in the neutropenic patient. Temperature elevation is frequently the first or only sign.
   b. Any subtle sign or symptom should be noted.
3. Medical management:
   a. Initiate broad spectrum antibiotics when the temperature rises above 101 degrees Fahrenheit.
   b. Obtain cultures and x-rays.
   c. Antibiotics should be administered until marrow recovery, even if temperature returns to normal,
   d. Amphotericin may be added if the temperature is not controlled by antibiotics in 1 week.
4. Nursing management:
   a. Promote good hygiene and optimal health with frequent rest periods.
   b. Provide early identification of infection through systematic assessment and close observation.
   c. Reduce exposure to potential pathogens by placing the patient in a private room, allowing no visitors with viral or bacterial infections, minimizing invasive procedures.
   d. Institution of reverse isolation, when indicated.

REHABILITATION

A. Rehabilitation requires an understanding of the special needs and problems created by the disease and treatment. Goals of rehabilitation are maintenance of physical, personal, and social integrity.
B. Nursing rehabilitation interventions for patients with long-term effects of therapy:
   1. Educate patient and family about long-term or late effects.
   2. Assist in evaluation of intellectual functioning.
   3. Communicate to school and social agencies an assessment of strengths, weaknesses, and expectation of performance.
   4. Assist family in redefining goals in terms of degree of disability.
   5. Refer for remedial or tutorial assistance, when indicated.
   6. Offer opportunity to patient and family to verbalize concerns and frustrations.
   7. Provide for continued assessment after cessation of therapy to identify late effects.

NURSING CARE

A. Leukemia predisposes the individual and family to multiple stressors and problems. Continuous assessment to determine the effects of the diagnosis and treatment on functioning and performance is imperative. Nursing care should be designed to promote adaptation, with the goal of fostering hope, security, and cohesion.

B. Major areas of nursing intervention:

1. Coping.
    a. Factors that affect coping:
        (1) Fear of isolation and abandonment.
        (2) Fear of death or unknown.
        (3) Perception of meaning of disease.
    b. Goals of nursing intervention:
        (1) Relieve acute anxiety, confusion, and hopelessness.
        (2) Restore hope and sense of future.
        (3) Assist in exploring alternative solutions to problems.
        (4) Assist in developing a larger repertoire of coping behaviors.
    c. Nursing intervention:
        (1) Assess family structure and coping behavior.
        (2) Assess effects of illness on family functioning.
        (3) Develop a trusting relationship by being a good listener, offering honest answers, and being understanding of fears and concerns.
        (4) Create a warm, caring, therapeutic relationship for patient and family to ask questions.
        (5) Allow patient to regain control through education and participation in care.
        (6) Share insights into family and patient coping.
        (7) Instill realistic hope.
        (8) Assist in making contact with other patients, families, and professionals.

2. Information.
    a. Factors affecting learning ability:
        (1) Physical condition.
        (2) Stage of disease.
        (3) Emotional response to illness.
        (4) Social network.
        (5) Learning preference.
        (6) Desire to learn.
    b. Goals:
        (1) Provide accurate and adequate information so that patient can make informed decisions.
        (2) Lead patient to an understanding of disease process, treatment goals, side effects of treatment, self care responsibilities, and symptoms to report.
        (3) Assist patient in regaining a feeling of control.
    c. Nursing interventions:
        (1) Assess educational needs in terms of knowledge of disease, intellectual functioning, and ability to learn.
        (2) Develop goals and objectives in conjunction with family and in terms of patient and nursing evaluation.

(3) Provide formal and informal sessions as appropriate to physical and psychological endurance.
(4) Reinforce teaching with written materials.
(5) Evaluate learning in terms of behavioral objectives.

STUDY QUESTIONS

1. Distinguish between acute and chronic leukemia.
2. Describe induction, consolidation, and maintenance therapy.
3. Identify nursing measures to minimize infection in individuals with leukemia.

Bibliography

Adult Patient Education in Cancer: National Institute of Health Publication, No 83–2601, 1983.

Albo, V.: Proceedings of American Society of Clinical Oncology. 4:172, 1985.

Bennett, J. M.: The classification of the acute leukemias: Cytochemical and morphological considerations. *In* Wiernick, P. H. (ed.): Neoplastic Diseases of the Blood (Vol 1). New York, Churchill Livingstone, pp. 201–217, 1985.

Bennett, J. M., Catovsky, D., and Daniel, M. T.: Criteria for the diagnosis of acute leukemia of megakaryocyte lineage (M7). Annals of Internal Medicine, 103:460–462, 1985.

Cannelos, G. P.: Diagnosis and treatment of chronic granulocytic leukemia. *In* Wiernick, P. H. (ed.): Neoplastic Diseases of the Blood (Vol 1). New York, Churchill Livingstone, pp. 81–103, 1985.

Cassileth, P. A.: Adult acute nonlymphocytic leukemia. Medical Clinics of North America, 68:675–695, 1984.

Cassileth, P. A., Begg, C. B., Bennett, J. M., et al.: A randomized study of the efficacy of consolidation therapy in adult acute non lymphocytic leukemia. Blood, 63:843–847, 1984.

Clarkson, B. D., Dowling, M. D., Gee, T. S., et al.: Treatment of acute leukemia in adults. Cancer, 36:775–795, 1975.

Chessells, J. M.: Childhood acute lymphocytic leukaemia: The late effects of treatment. British Journal of Haematology, 54:369–378, 1983.

Davis, D. S.: Coping. *In* Johnson, B.L. (ed.): Handbook of Oncology Nursing. Bethany, Fleschner, pp. 129–144, 1985.

Ellerhorst-Ryan, J. M.: Complications of the myeloproliferative system: Infection and sepsis. Seminars in Oncology Nursing, 1:244–249, 1985.

Eyre, H. J., Ward, J. H., and Priebat, D. A.: Adult acute leukemia. Cancer, 51:2460–2468, 1983.

Foon, K. A., and Gale, R. P.: Controversies in the therapy of acute myelogenous leukemia. The American Journal of Medicine, 72:963–979, 1982.

Freeman, A. I., and Brecher, M. L.: Diagnosis and treatment of childhood acute lymphocytic leukemia. *In* Wiernick, P. H. (ed.): Neoplastic Diseases of the Blood (Vol 1). New York, Churchill Livingstone, pp. 267–293, 1985.

Gale, R. P., and Foon, K. A.: Chronic lymphocytic leukemia: Recent advances in biology and treatment. Annals of Internal Medicine, 103:101–120, 1985.

Gale, R. P., Champlin, R. E., and Jacobs, A.: Treatment of acute leukemia. Paper presented at the American Society of Hematology, New Orleans, 1985.

Giacquinta, B.: Helping families face the crisis of cancer. American Journal of Nursing, 77:1585–1588, 1977.

Glucksberg, H., Cheever, M. A., Farewell, V. T., et al.: Intensification therapy for acute nonlymphocytic leukemia in adults. Cancer, 52:198–205, 1983.

Griffin, J. D., Maguire, M. E., and Mayer, R. J.: Amsacrine in refractory acute leukemia. Cancer Treatment Reports, 69:787–789, 1985.

Heath, C. W.: Epidemiology and hereditary aspects of acute leukemia. *In* Wiernick, P. H. (ed.): Neoplastic Diseases of the Blood (Vol 1). New York, Churchill Livingstone, pp. 183–200, 1985.

Henderson, E. S.: Acute lymphocytic leukemia. *In* Gunz, F. W., and Henderson, E. S. (eds.): Leukemia. New York, Grune and Stratton, pp. 575–625, 1983.

Herbst, S. H.: Impairment as a result of cancer. *In* Martin, N. (ed.): Comprehensive Rehabilitation Nursing. New York, McGraw-Hill, pp. 552–578, 1981.

Hitchcock-Bryan, S., Gelber, R., Cassady, R. J., et al.: The impact of induction anthracycline in long term failure free survival in childhood acute lymphocytic leukemia. Unpublished Manuscript, Dana Farber Cancer Institute Department of Pediatric Oncology, 1986.

Holland, J. F.: Breaking the cure barrier. Journal of Clinical Oncology, 1:75–90, 1983.

Kamani, N., and August, C. S.: Bone marrow transplantation: Problems and prospects. Medical Clinics of North America, 68:657–674, 1984.

Li, F. P.: The chronic leukemias: Etiology and epidemiology. *In* Wiernick, P. H. (ed.): Neoplastic Diseases of the Blood (Vol 1). New York, Churchill Livingstone, pp. 7–71, 1985.

Liepman, M. K.: The chronic leukemias. Medical Clinics of North America, 64:705–727, 1980.

Martocchio, B. C.: Family coping: Helping families help themselves. Seminars in Oncology Nursing, 1:292–297, 1985.

Mauer, A. M.: Therapy of acute lymphocytic leukemia in childhood. Blood, 56:1–9, 1980.

Mayer, R. J.: Acute lymphocytic leukemia in adults. Annals of Internal Medicine, 101:552–554, 1984.

Mayer, R. J., Coral, F. S., Rosenthal, D. S., et al.: Treatment of non-T, non-B cell acute lymphoblastic leukemia (ALL) in adults. Proceedings of the Society of Clinical Oncology, 1:1–126, 1982.

Mayer, R. J., Schiffer, C. A., Peterson, B. A., et al.: Intensive postremission therapy in adults with Ara-C by continuous infusion or bolus administration: Preliminary results of a CALGB phase I study. Seminars in Oncology, 12:84–90, 1985.

Mayer, R. J., Weinstein, H. J., Coral, F. S., et al.: The role of intensive postinduction chemotherapy in the management of patients with acute myelogenous leukemia. Cancer Treatment Reports, 66:1455–1461, 1982.

Mayer, R. J., Weinstein, H. J., and Rosenthal, D. S.: VAPA: A treatment program for acute myelogenous leukemia. Haematology and Blood Transfusion, 26:45–52, 1981.

McCalla, J. L.: A multidisciplinary approach to identification and remedial intervention for adverse late effects of cancer therapy. Nursing Clinics of North America, 20:117–130, 1985.

Miller, D. R.: Acute lymphocytic leukemia. Pediatric Clinics of North America, 27:269–291, 1980.

Newman, K. A.: The leukemias. Nursing Clinics of North America, 20:227–234, 1985.

Rai, K. R., Sawitsky, A., Jagathambal, K., et al.: Chronic lymphocytic leukemia. Medical Clinics of North America, 68:697–711, 1984.

Sallan, S.: Personal Communication, January 15, 1986.

Siegrist, C. W. and Jones, J. J.: Disseminated intravascular coagulopathy and nursing implications. Seminars in Oncology Nursing, 1:237–243, 1985.

Spiers, A. S.: Chronic granulocytic leukemia. Medical Clinics of North America, 68:713–727, 1984.

Spiers, A. S.: Chronic lymphocytic leukemia. *In* Gunz, E. W., and Henderson, E. S. (eds.): Leukemia. New York, Grune and Stratton, pp. 663–708, 1983.

Spiers, A. S.: Chronic myelocytic leukemia. *In* Gunz, E. W., and Henderson, E. S. (eds.): Leukemia. New York, Grune and Stratton, pp. 709–740, 1983.

Stone, R. M., Maguire, M. E., Goldberg, M. A., et al.: Complete remission without bone marrow hypoplasia in acute promyelocytic leukemia. Unpublished Manuscript, Dana Farber Cancer Institute, Department of Medical Oncology, 1986.

Storb, R., Thomas, E. D., and Santos, G. W.: Marrow transplantation. Paper presented at the American Society of Hematologists, New Orleans, 1985.

Tamaroff, M., Salwen, R., Miller, D. R., et al.: Comparison of neuropsychologic performance in children treated for acute lymphoblastic leukemia (ALL) with 1800 rads cranial radiation plus intrathecal methotrexate or intrathecal methotrexate alone. Paper presented at the American Society of Clinical Oncologists, Toronto, 1984.

Waskerwitz, M. J., and Ruccione, K.: An overview of cancer in children in the 1980's. Nursing Clinics of North America, 20:5–29, 1985.

Weinstein, H. J.: Diagnosis and treatment of childhood acute nonlymphocytic leukemia. *In* Wiernick, P. H. (ed.): Neoplastic Diseases of the Blood (Vol. 5). New York, Churchill Livingstone, pp. 321–333, 1985.

Wessler, R. M.: Care of the hospitalized adult patient with leukemia. Nursing Clinics of North America, 17:649–663, 1982.

Wiernick, P. H.: Diagnosis and treatment of acute nonlymphocytic leukemia. *In* Wiernick, P. H. (ed.): Neoplastic Diseases of the Blood (Vol. 5). New York, Churchill Livingstone, pp. 335–355, 1985.

Woodruff, R.: Diagnosis and treatment of adult acute lymphocytic leukemia. *In* Wiernick, P. H. (ed.): Neoplastic Diseases of the Blood (Vol. 5). New York, Churchill Livingstone, pp. 295–319, 1985.

SECTION SIX

Treatment of Cancer

Section Editor
ROBERTA STROHL, RN, MN

21

Goals and Principles of Treatment

ROBERTA A. STROHL, RN, MN

GOALS AND GENERAL PRINCIPLES OF THERAPY

A. Cure.
   1. The goal of therapy is to eradicate the entire tumor. In viewing cancer within the conceptual framework of a chronic disease, the term "cure" may be inappropriate.
   2. Follow-up of patients considered cured is essential. Time at maximum risk for recurrence is determined by growth rate of the tumor and varies widely. Disease recurrence in patients with breast cancer may be as long as 20 years following initial diagnosis. Increased length of disease free survival decreases likelihood that tumor will recur, but follow-up is essential.
   3. People who have had one cancer may be at a greater risk for the development of other malignancies (e.g., breast and endometrium). The second malignancy may be one with similar etiologic factors (e.g., head and neck, lung, esophagus).
B. Control.
   1. "Control" is a more accurate term to use in discussing therapeutic goal of arresting tumor growth.
   2. Consider local control of primary lesion and identification and control of any distant metastatic disease.
C. Palliation.
   1. Therapeutic goal is to alleviate symptoms when disease is beyond control.
   2. May still involve radical treatment such as surgery, radiation therapy, or chemotherapy to control or prevent pain, obstruction, and bleeding without influencing survival.
   3. Important to consider the potential side effects of therapy in relation to ability to control more serious symptoms.

4. Patient and family need to understand goal of therapy. Important to maintain hope for comfort.
D. Prophylaxis.
   1. Treatment given when the host does not exhibit detectable tumor cells but is known to be at high risk for tumor spread based upon usual spread pattern for the tumor (cranial radiation in small cell lung cancer and in children with acute leukemia).
   2. Patient and family may have concerns about treating apparently disease free areas.
   3. Statistics are being compiled to determine risks of therapy and long-term effects of therapy vs. waiting to see if disease develops in at-risk areas and ability to control disease once it occurs.

SEQUENCE OF THERAPY

A. Primary.
   1. Any therapy can be used as a primary therapy, depending on tumor type and responsiveness of tumor to that modality.
   2. Need to consider tumor size and extent (metastases) as these factors will determine resectability and ability of radiotherapy alone to control disease.
   3. Host factors will determine the ability of the patient to tolerate the prescribed regimen. Debilitated patients will have difficulty tolerating any radical therapy.
B. Salvage.
   1. Therapy initiated to "cure" disease following recurrence.
   2. Any treatment modality may be considered salvage therapy if recurrent tumor is successfully eradicated.
C. Adjuvant.
   1. Therapy in addition to the primary therapy.
   2. Usually given to control metastatic disease in addition to primary local therapy.
   3. Goal is to eliminate microscopic disease.

THERAPEUTIC MODALITIES

A. Surgery.
   1. Surgery is a local treatment for cancer.
   2. May be used to resect primary or limited metastatic disease (solitary brain metastases).
   3. May be primary treatment or palliative treatment.
   4. Earliest modality for cancer control (reports of surgery for breast tumors in ancient Egypt).
   5. Surgery became more radical as supportive care measures became available. Lack of change in survival even with radical surgery (in tumors such as breast cancer) led to need for combined modality approaches.
B. Radiation therapy.
   1. Local or locoregional (including lymph node draining area) therapy.
   2. Cure, control, palliation, and prophylaxis are goals.
   3. First report of treatment for cancer with radiation was for basal cell carcinoma in 1899.

4. Larger field radiation (whole body prior to marrow transplant or half-body for control of widespread metastatic disease) may be used.

C. Chemotherapy.
   1. Systemic treatment for cancer.
   2. Cure, control, palliation, and prophylaxis are goals.
   3. Newest of major therapeutic modalities. Some reports in first century AD of colchicine used in tumors that had not spread. Arsenic, benzol, and urethane were used in early experiments. Majority of anticancer drugs tested following World War II.
   4. Need for systemic therapy documented by knowledge that even in early stages cancer may spread beyond primary site.

D. Combined approaches.
   1. Most patients will receive more than one modality of therapy.
   2. Combination often includes a local treatment (surgery and/or radiation) plus systemic chemotherapy.
   3. Philosophy of treatment varies from one center to another, but factors to consider include the tumor type, usual patterns of spread, extent of disease, and therapeutic goal.
   4. Order of therapy will vary with tumor site, treatment philosophy, and therapeutic goal.
   5. Therapies may be given concomitantly (chemotherapy plus radiation, especially with agents that enhance radiation effect).
   6. Combined therapy may lead to increased side effects. Monitor carefully for decreased blood counts, especially in patients receiving chemotherapy and radiation therapy to a bone marrow–producing area.
   7. In sequential therapy, be aware of nadir of counts and occurrence of late effects of therapy, which may occur when the second therapy is being given.
   8. Late effects of combined therapy may be greater than with either modality alone. Radiation and chemotherapy affect different types of cells within the same tissue. For example: in the heart, radiation alters fine vasculoconnective stroma of myocardium while chemotherapy (Adriamycin) results in cytotoxicity to cardiomyocytes. In the lung, radiation affects surfactant and chemotherapy (Bleomycin) affects alveolar type I cells. Patients currently receiving combined modalities will need to be followed carefully for the assessment and management of combined toxicities.
   9. Incidence of second malignancies in individuals receiving combined modalities is higher.
   10. Consider risks of toxicities vs. benefits of therapeutic effect.

STUDY QUESTIONS

1. Define the goals of therapy delivered for cure, control, and palliation.
2. Discuss the rationale for combined modality therapy.
3. Discuss the potential problems of combined modality therapy.

Bibliography

Beyers, M., Durburg, S., and Werner, J.: Complete Guide to Cancer Nursing. Oradell, New Jersey, Medical Economics Books, 1984.

Hill, G.: Historic Milestones in Cancer Surgery. Seminars in Oncology, 6:409–427, 1979.

Kaplan, H.: Historic Milestones in Radiobiology and Radiation Therapy. Seminars in Oncology, 6:479–485, 1979.

Marino, L.: Cancer Nursing. St. Louis, C. V. Mosby Co., 1981.

Rubin, P.: Clinical Oncology for Medical Students and Physicians, 6th ed. New York, American Cancer Society, 1983.

Rubin, P.: The Franz Buschke Lecture: Late Effects of Chemotherapy and Radiation Therapy: A New Hypothesis. International Journal of Radiation Oncology, Biology and Physics, 10:5–34, 1984.

Zubrod, C. G.: Historic Milestones in Curative Chemotherapy. Seminars in Oncology, 6:490–500, 1979.

22

Surgery

THOMAS J. SZOPA, RN, MSN

PRINCIPLES OF SURGERY

A. Surgery remains an important treatment modality for cancer, sometimes being the primary treatment, and in some instances the only chance for cure.
B. Surgical excision of a tumor generally includes removal of the tumor beyond its margins and a portion of normal tissue surrounding the tumor. This ensures more complete removal of the tumor.
C. Surgical excision of a tumor is performed in a manner that will result in satisfactory appearance and function. Multidisciplinary planning of treatment is necessary to promote the best cosmetic effect.
D. Cancers that have long cell cycles, thereby being classified as slow-growing cancers, lend themselves best to surgical treatment. Metastasis in these cancers can be more easily controlled.
E. Combination treatment, or use of multimodality treatment, may decrease the adverse effects of each treatment modality by the conservation of normal tissue and improve treatment results. It is increasingly more common to use surgery in combination with other treatment modalities owing to the micrometastasis concept of cancer.

ROLE OF SURGERY

A. Establish tissue diagnosis—To obtain a sample of tissue for pathologic examination.
  1. Incisional biopsy—The removal of a portion of tissue for examination.
    a. Bite biopsy—Small portions of tumor are removed with special forceps, e.g., endoscopy.
  2. Excisional biopsy—The removal of the complete tumor with little or no margin of surrounding normal tissue removed. Most common type of biopsy performed, and usually done under local anesthesia.
    a. A disadvantage of this type of biopsy is that cells may be implanted into the tissue at the biopsy site and cause local recurrence.

3. Needle biopsy—The aspiration of fluid or tissue via a needle. This method is simple to perform, reliable, inexpensive, done under local anesthesia, and usually does not require hospitalization. A disadvantage of this procedure is the risk of injury to adjacent structures and possible implantation of tumor cells along needle tract.
4. Trend for a two-step process—The biopsy procedure is separate in time from the surgical procedure versus the biopsy and surgical removal of the tumor at the same time. The allows for the patient and family to assimilate the impact of the cancer diagnosis and make a better decision in regard to treatment options.

B. Determine surgical stage of disease.
1. Diagnostic laparotomy—Performed when there is intra-abdominal tumor involvement that cannot be adequately evaluated by other diagnostic methods.
   a. Performed prior to radical surgery so that occult intraperitoneal, lumboaortic, or liver metastasis can be ruled out.
   b. Performed to obtain tissue samplings and determine sites of disease to base treatment planning on. For example, in Hodgkin's disease, procedure includes an exploratory laparotomy with splenectomy, biopsy of the liver, and biopsy of the retroperitoneal nodes to determine stage of disease. Metal clips are placed on organs to mark location for future treatment with radiation therapy.
2. Second-look procedure—A follow-up surgery after the original surgery to check for the absence or presence of disease.
   a. Usually done for those cancers that have a propensity to recur locally (such as ovarian cancer).
   b. May be done to assess response to other treatment modalities, e.g., chemotherapy or radiation therapy, or to assess for residual disease following chemotherapy or radiation therapy.
   c. Becoming more uncommon because of the availability of other diagnostic procedures, laboratory tests, and tumor markers to evaluate response to treatment.

C. Definitive treatment.
1. Local excision—Simple excision of tumor with small margin of normal tissue, e.g., cancer of the skin.
2. Block dissection.
   a. Wide excision or "en bloc" dissection—Removal of tumor, any tissues containing primary nodal drainage area, and any involved contiguous structures. Also known as a "debulking" procedure, e.g., radical mastectomy, abdominal perineal resection, radical neck dissection, total pancreatectomy, radical nephrectomy.
   b. Extended wide excision—Removes wide infiltration of tumor in a particular region, which does not tend to metastasize to distant sites.
3. Surgical treatment of cancer in situ.
   a. Electrosurgery—Eradication of cancer cells by application of electrical current.
   b. Cryosurgery—Deep freezing with liquid nitrogen to selectively destroy tumor tissue. The site thaws naturally and then becomes gelatinous, healing spontaneously, e.g., cancer of the skin.
   c. Chemosurgery—The combined use of topically applied chemotherapeutic agents and layer-by-layer surgical excision of tissue, e.g., cancer of the skin.

      d. Endoscopy—Local excision after visual examination.

      e. CO_2 Laser—Use of laser for local excision, e.g., cancer of the larynx. Advantages include discharge to home on first postoperative day, no eating restrictions, use of speech, no tracheostomy, and less costly.

  4. Palliation—Surgery performed to promote patient comfort and quality of life without cure of disease.

      a. Removal of solitary metastasis—As in organ obstructions, subtotal-gastrectomy, nonseminomatous testicular cancer, solitary lung metastasis for Wilm's tumor.

      b. Cytoreductive surgery—Reduction of the number of cells within tumor for improving the effects of treatment; usually followed by adjuvant therapy.

      c. Treatment of oncologic emergencies—Exsanguinating hemorrhage, perforation, drainage of abscesses, laminectomy, bowel bypass surgery and ostomy creation, relief of side effects of other treatment modalities, e.g., radiation proctitis.

      d. Ablative surgery—Removal of hormonal influence, e.g., oophorectomy, adrenalectomy, orchiectomy, hypophysectomy.

      e. Insertion of therapeutic hardware—Insertion of gastrostomy tube or hyperalimentation lines.

      f. Neurosurgical management of cancer pain—Procedures for pain relief; relief may be time-limited.

        (1) Nerve blocks—A short-acting anesthetic may be tried first to determine what specific disruption in pain and side effects are caused, e.g., numbness, rectal sphincter and bladder dysfunction, muscle weakness.

          (a) Stellate ganglion block—To relieve pain of metastatic breast cancer.

          (b) Alcohol celiac (splanchnic plexus) block—Used to relieve pain of cancer of pancreas, stomach, liver and bile ducts, and gallbladder.

          (c) Intrathecal phenol block—Used to relieve pain of cancer of cervix, rectum, colon, bladder, kidney, bone, lung, pleura, and mediastinum.

          (d) Subarachnoid and extradural block—Used to relieve pain of cancer of the rectum, cervix, bronchus, breast, and colon.

          (e) Cranial nerve block—Used to relieve pain in cancer of the head, face, and neck.

        (2) Cordotomy.

          (a) Open cordotomy—A laminectomy is performed and a complete unilateral transection is made of the anterolateral quadrant of the cord at the thoracic or cervical level. There is loss of pain and temperature sensation. Motor function usually remains intact, but patients may experience weakness of one body side and bladder dysfunction.

          (b) Percutaneous cordotomy—The anterolateral quadrant of the cord is affected by the insertion of a coagulation probe in the upper or lower cervical level with the use of radiographic control.

D. Insertion and monitoring of therapeutic hardware—The insertion of various therapeutic hardware during active treatment periods to facilitate the delivery of treatment and increase patient comfort.

1. Ventricular reservoir—A mushroom-shaped silicone dome approximately 3.4 cm in diameter that is attached to a silicone catheter.
   a. Advantages:
      (1) Provides a convenient and direct access to ventricular cerebrospinal fluid, which ensures a more predictable and consistent distribution of medication into the subarachnoid space. Medication may not ascend into the head when a lumbar puncture method is used.
      (2) Increased patient tolerance of medication.
      (3) Increased remission duration rates experienced.
      (4) Decreased patient discomfort and anxiety secondary to easy access.
      (5) May be used in the home setting.
   b. Usage:
      (1) To more efficiently deliver medication (chemotherapeutic agents, pain medication) directly into the cerebrospinal fluid.
      (2) For measuring the cerebrospinal fluid pressure.
      (3) To obtain cerebrospinal fluid for examination.
   c. Disadvantages:
      (1) Infection.
      (2) Blockage of the catheter.
      (3) Displacement of the catheter.
2. Intra-arterial and venous access lines—A silicone catheter is placed into an artery or vein and is then threaded subcutaneously to an exit site in the chest region, e.g., Hickman catheter.
   a. Advantages:
      (1) Provides easy access to arterial or venous system for drug delivery, parenteral fluid administration, blood product administration, and for obtaining blood specimens.
      (2) Increases patient comfort; avoids multiple venipunctures.
      (3) May be connected to various external or internal pump systems for more continuous delivery of medication.
      (4) May be used in home setting.
      (5) Multiple lumen catheters available for simultaneous delivery of different parenteral fluids, e.g., double lumen, quadruple lumen.
   b. Disadvantages:
      (1) Possible complications include infection, catheter occlusion, displacement of catheter, and severed catheter.
      (2) May restrict patient activity.
      (3) May create body image disturbance.
3. Implantable vascular access device—A system for administration of drugs and fluids. The system consists of a self-sealing silicone septum encased in a port made of metal or plastic attached to a silicone catheter. The port is placed subcutaneously generally in the chest region and the catheter is threaded subcutaneously and placed into a vein or artery. Drugs, fluids, and blood products can be administered via the port with the use of a needle puncture through the skin into the septum of the port. The port also can be placed in the abdominal region for intraperitoneal chemotherapy.
   a. Advantages:
      (1) Easy access into vascular system and increased comfort.

(2) Not visible and reduces body image disturbance.
(3) Minimal maintenance care required.
b. Disadvantages:
(1) Complications include catheter occlusion, infection, and separation of port from catheter (in some models).
(2) May be difficult to access because of placement.
4. Central venous catheter may be placed into the superior vena cava for administration of total parenteral nutrition.
5. Radioactive implants (brachytherapy)—The insertion of a sealed radioactive isotope temporarily or permanently into hollow cavities, within body tissues, or on the body's surface. The radioactive isotope delivers a specific radiation dose continuously over hours or days. A highly concentrated radiation dose is given in or near the tumor site. This technique is generally combined with a course of external radiation therapy to increase the dosage to a specific site with minimal side effects.
a. Intracavitary—Gynecologic cancer. Source placed in cavity such as the uterus.
b. Interstitial—Placement of needles, seeds, wires, catheters of isotope for breast, lung, prostate, and head and neck cancers.
c. Experimental—Being used for brain and liver cancer.
6. Arterial catheter—For the purpose of regional therapy; the delivery of large doses of selected chemotherapeutic agents to a localized tumor with minimal systemic toxicity.
a. Catheter inserted into the arterial system to perfuse the organ or limb to be treated with a chemotherapeutic agent and a catheter for exit of the agent, e.g., regional limb hyperthermic perfusion for melanoma.
b. Catheter inserted into the arterial system to perfuse the organ with a chemotherapeutic agent; exit catheter is not needed due to body metabolization of drug, e.g., use of internal/external pump for treating colon metastasis to the liver.
E. Reconstructive surgery—The reconstruction of anatomic defects created by cancer surgery to improve function and cosmetic appearance, e.g., ostomies, breast reconstruction, head and neck reconstruction, and prostheses.
F. Prophylactic surgery—Surgery performed on nonvital organs that have an extremely high incidence of subsequent cancer (Table 22–1). The decision to perform surgery is based on the presence or absence of symptoms, statistical risk of cancer based on medical history, difficulty in early diagnosis

Table 22–1. PROPHYLACTIC SURGERY*

Underlying Condition	Associated Cancer	Surgery
Cryptorchidism	Testicular	Orchiopexy
Polyposis coli	Colon	Colectomy
Familial colon cancer	Colon	Colectomy
Ulcerative colitis	Colon	Colectomy
Multiple endocrine neoplasia types II and III	Medullary cancer of the thyroid	Thyroidectomy
Familial breast cancer	Breast	Mastectomy
Familial ovarian cancer	Ovary	Oophorectomy

* From DeVita, V., Hellman, S., and Rosenberg, S. (eds.): Cancer: Principles and Practice of Oncology, 2nd ed. Philadelphia, J. B. Lippincott, 1985.

of cancer should it develop, and the postoperative changes in appearance and function.

NURSING MANAGEMENT

A. Preoperative care.
  1. Diagnostic testing or biopsy:
     a. Be aware of any specific care or preparation of the patient prior to the procedure, e.g., bowel preparation, skin preparation, medications, positioning, and so forth.
     b. Provide for necessary testing equipment if needed.
     c. Patient and family teaching—Assess learning needs and provide information and explanation.
        (1) Plan of care and rationale for procedure.
        (2) What the patient may experience.
        (3) Rationale for what the patient may experience.
        (4) What the patient and family can do to help themselves. Assist in maintaining a sense of control by involvement in the planning of care.
     d. Emotional support—The diagnostic process is very anxiety-producing because of the many unknowns and the extensive testing that takes place.
        (1) Allow for ventilation of fears and anxieties.
        (2) Provide information as needed. Due to the effect of anxiety on one's listening and retention abilities, repetition of information may be necessary.
        (3) Reassure patients and families that diagnostic testing assists in determining the absence, as well as the presence of cancer. Individualized therapy is based on these findings.
  2. Surgical intervention.
     a. Be aware of any specific care or preparation of the patient prior to the procedure, e.g., bowel preparation, medications, and so forth.
     b. Conduct a nursing assessment of important patient parameters, e.g., nutritional status, elimination patterns, cardiac status, respiratory status, laboratory results, potential for postoperative complications.
     c. Provide for physical comfort. Debilitation prior to surgery may be due to the type of symptoms and length of time symptoms have been experienced or to advanced disease.
     d. Patient and family teaching—Assess learning needs and provide information and explanation.
        (1) Plan of care.
        (2) What to expect.
        (3) Rationale for procedures.
        (4) Self-care. Assist in maintaining a sense of control by involvement in the planning of care.
     e. Emotional support.
        (1) Explore fears—Fears of diagnosis, advanced disease, pain, death, findings from staging laparotomy, or second-look procedures.
        (2) Explore reactions, concerns, perceptions of disease.
        (3) Involve in the planning of care and decision-making process.

(4) Provide information as needed.

(5) Provide needed support for patients facing prophylactic surgery.

B. Postoperative care.

1. Diagnostic testing or biopsy.

   a. Be aware of any specific care following the procedure, e.g., wound or dressing care, positioning, medication, and so forth.

   b. Nursing assessment of status and recovery; observe for complications.

   c. Emotional support:

      (1) Provide a supportive environment when test results are presented.

      (2) Encourage involvement in the treatment planning and decision-making process.

      (3) Provide or reinforce information as needed.

      (4) Refer to any appropriate resources, e.g., support programs, as needed.

   d. Discharge care—Any special care required at home and how long it is needed. Teach:

      (1) Where to obtain needed supplies.

      (2) What follow-up care is required.

      (3) Where to call with questions and concerns.

      (4) Special skills or procedures.

2. Surgical intervention.

   a. Conduct a nursing assessment of important parameters, e.g., nutritional status, elimination patterns, cardiac and respiratory status, laboratory test results, and potential for complications (shock, hemorrhage, infection, thrombophlebitis, elimination difficulties, wound dehiscence).

   b. Provide for physical comfort—Enteral or parenteral nutrition, wound care and healing, pain relief, positioning, activity and rest periods.

   c. Provide teaching regarding activity, nutrition, medications, wound management, follow-up care and appointments, and other activities involved in the patient regaining self-care. Encourage family involvement.

   d. Emotional support.

      (1) Loss of a body part and/or function will cause a change in the patient's body image and self-esteem. Provide support in reaction to this loss.

      (2) Allow ventilation of fears and concerns.

      (3) Provide information as needed.

   e. Rehabilitation.

      (1) Make referrals to appropriate resources, e.g., social service, community health agency, physical therapy, occupational therapy, speech therapy, support groups, American Cancer Society programs (Reach to Recovery, Re-Con Group, Ostomy and Laryngectomee Visitor Program); Ostomy Association and outpatient clinics; International Association of Laryngectomees, and so forth.

      (2) Encourage family involvement in discharge planning.

      (3) Discharge care—Any special care required at home and how long it is needed. Teach:

         (a) Where to obtain needed supplies.

         (b) What follow-up care is required.

    (c) Where to call with questions and concerns.
    (d) Special skills or procedures.

STUDY QUESTIONS

1. List and describe the six roles surgery has in the treatment of cancer.
2. Describe at least four nursing interventions for patients prior to surgical diagnostic and/or treatment procedures.
3. Describe at least four nursing interventions for the patient after surgical diagnostic or treatment procedures.

Bibliography

Anderson, M., Aker, S., and Hickman, R.: The double-lumen Hickman catheter. American Journal of Nursing, *82*(2):272–273, 1982.

Brunner, L. and Suddarth, D.: The Lippincott Manual of Nursing Practice, 3rd ed. Philadelphia, J. B. Lippincott, 1982.

Bubela, N.: Technical and psychological problems and concerns arising from the outpatient treatment of cancer with direct intraarterial infusion. Cancer Nursing, *4*(4):305–309, 1981.

Carter, S., Glatstein, E., and Livingston, R.: Principles of Cancer Treatment. New York, McGraw-Hill Book Co., 1982.

DeVita, V., Hellman, S., and Rosenberg, S. (eds.): Cancer: Principles and Practice of Oncology, 2nd ed. Philadelphia, J. B. Lippincott, 1985.

Esparaza, D. and Weyland, J.: Nursing care for the patient with an ommaya reservoir. Oncology Nursing Forum, *9*(4):17–20, 1982.

Gullotte, M. and Foltz, A.: Hepatic chemotherapy via implantable pump. American Journal of Nursing, *83*(12):1674–1676, 1983.

Hassey, K.: Demystifying care of patients with radioactive implants. American Journal of Nursing, *85*(7):789–792, 1985.

Johnston, S. and Yehuda, P.: Caring for the patient on intraarterial chemotherapy . . . are you ready? Nursing, *11*(11):108–112, 1981.

Leoscher, L. and Leigh, S.: Isolated regional limb hyperthermic perfusion as treatment for melanoma. Cancer Nursing *7*(6):461–467, 1984.

Marino, L.: Cancer Nursing. St. Louis, C. V. Mosby Co., 1981.

Schahenbach, L. and Dennis, M.: And now, a quad-lumen I.V. catheter. Nursing, *15*(11):50, 1985.

Schmidt, A. and Williams, D.: The Hickman catheter: Sending your patient home safely. RN *45*(2):57–61, 1982.

Wilkes, G., Vannicola, P., and Starch, P.: Long-term venous access. American Journal of Nursing, *85*(7):793–796, 1985.

Winters, V.: Implantable vascular access device. Oncology Nursing Forum, *11*(6):25–30, 1984.

23

Radiation Therapy

JENNIFER BUCHOLTZ, RN, MSN

INTRODUCTION TO RADIATION THERAPY

A. Radiation therapy is the use of high energy radiation to treat diseases.
B. Indications:
   1. Used primarily to treat various cancers, especially solid tumors.
   2. Used occasionally to treat some benign diseases (for example, hyperthyroidism, desmoid tumors, benign brain tumors).
C. Extent of use:
   1. One of the three most commonly used cancer treatment modalities.
   2. Estimated that 50% of all persons in U.S. who have cancer will receive radiation therapy at some point during course of their disease.
   3. Can be used alone or in combination with other therapies for cure, control, or palliation of diseases.
   4. Generally used as a localized treatment.
D. History—Eras of radiation therapy and major accomplishments.
   1. Beginning years (1890–1920).
      a. Discoveries of x-rays, radium, and radioactivity.
      b. First treatment of skin cancer.
   2. Kilovoltage era (1920–1940).
      a. Invention of vacuum x-ray tube.
      b. Definition of radiation dose measurements.
      c. Use of daily dose fractions to treat diseases.
   3. Megavoltage era (1940–1960).
      a. Development of man-made radioactive cobalt (^{60}Co).
      b. Development of the linear accelerator.
      c. Better understanding of radiobiology.
   4. Modern era (1960–present).
      a. Refinement of radiation machines (linear accelerators, betatrons, gammatrons).
      b. Increased understanding of cancer and radiobiology.
      c. Use of computers in planning for accurate radiation dose distributions.

d. Increased number of radiation therapy–controlled clinical trials.

e. Specific training programs for radiation oncologists, radiation technologists.

PRINCIPLES AND PROPERTIES OF RADIATION

A. Radiation is the movement of energy through a space or medium.

B. Types of radiation:
   1. Electromagnetic—radiation in the form of waves.
      a. Examples of electromagnetic radiation (Fig. 23–1).
      b. Electromagnetic radiation used in therapy:
         (1) X-rays—delivered by machines, i.e., linear accelerators.
         (2) Electrons—delivered by machines, i.e., some linear accelerators, betatrons.
         (3) Gamma rays—delivered by machines that contain certain radioactive sources, e.g., Cobalt-60, Cesium-137, or emitted from radioactive substances in the form of seeds, threads, liquids, and so forth.
   2. Particulate—radiation in the form of heavy particles.
      a. Examples of particulate radiation:
         (1) Alpha particles (α)—positively charged particles with poor penetrating ability.
         (2) Beta particles (β)—high speed electrons with greater penetrating ability than alpha particles.
         (3) Pions (pimesons)—unstable nuclear particles.
         (4) Neutrons—uncharged particles.
      b. Particulate radiation used in therapy.
         (1) Beta particles—emitted from radioactive substances found in either liquid (unsealed) or solid (sealed) forms. Phosphorus-32, Strontium-90, Yttrium-90 are examples of pure beta radioactive substances.
         (2) Neutrons—used in some experimental treatments.
         (3) Pions—used in some experimental treatments.

Radio waves	Microwaves	Infrared light	Visible light	Ultraviolet light	X-rays	Gamma rays
*	*	*	*	*	*	*

Ionizing Radiation

Low Energy → High Energy

Long Wavelengths   Short Wavelengths

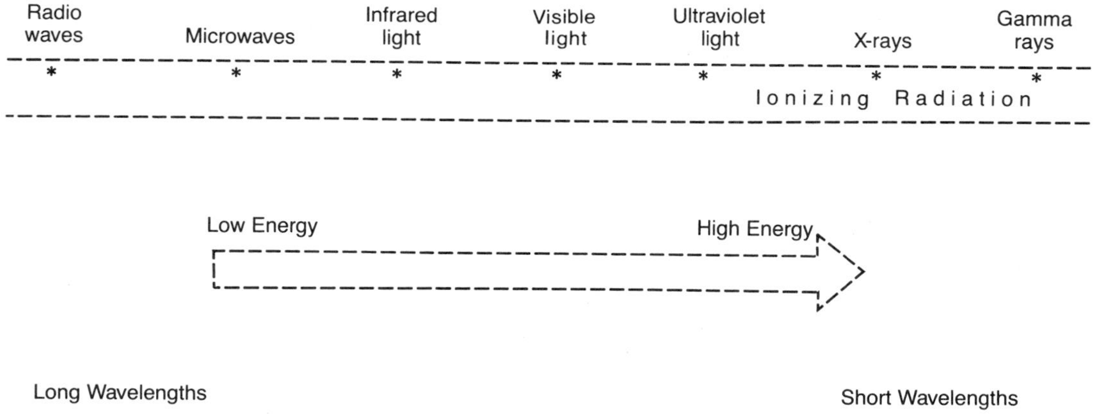

Figure 23–1. The electromagnetic spectrum.

EFFECTS OF IONIZING RADIATION ON CELLS

A. Ionizing radiation.
   1. Definition—high energy radiation that causes damage to cells or alters cells.
   2. Examples—x-rays, gamma rays, electrons, beta particles.
B. Cellular response to ionizing radiation—cells exposed to ionizing radiation undergo following stages of reaction (Fig. 23–2).
   1. Physical stage—cells' molecules become agitated and excited.
   2. Physiochemical stage—agitated molecules break into stable molecules and chemically active substances.
   3. Chemical stage—chemical reactions take place inside the cell, causing changes to DNA in nucleus.
   4. Biological stage—alterations to DNA take place and are expressed as a single chromosomal strand break or a double chromosomal strand break.
      a. Amount of DNA damage or cell radiosensitivity depends on:
         (1) Division rate of cell—rapidly dividing cells are more radiosensitive than slowly dividing cells.
         (2) Phase of cell life cycle—cells are more sensitive to radiation in phases of mitosis (M) and between G_1 and G_2 (see Fig. 24–2).
         (3) Cell oxygenation level—well oxygenated cells more radiosensitive than poorly oxygenated cells.
         (4) Degree of cell differentiation—poorly differentiated, immature cells are more radiosensitive than mature, well differentiated cells.
      b. Cell death due to DNA damage may occur.
         (1) Immediately—DNA in cell altered quickly and cannot be repaired.
         (2) At the time of cellular division—DNA damaged but cell continues to live and function until time of mitosis.
         (3) Due to cellular degeneration—cells become sterile, cannot divide, and die a natural death.

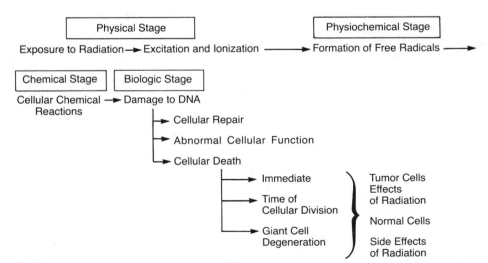

Figure 23–2. *Model of the stages of the cellular response to radiation. (Redrawn from Yasko, J.: Care of the Client Receiving External Radiation Therapy. Reston, VA, Reston Publishing Co., 1982.)*

C. Principles of ionizing radiation relevant to radiation therapy:
   1. Normal cell/tissue response vs. cancer cell/tissue response:
      a. Ionizing radiation damages both normal cells and cancer cells.
      b. Single chromosomal strand break in DNA of normal cells more easily repaired than single chromosomal strand breaks in cancer cells.
      c. Side effects of radiation therapy stem from radiation damage to normal cells treated.
   2. Principles of radiosensitivity related to treatment.
      a. Tumors containing cells that are rapidly dividing, well oxygenated, and poorly differentiated are the most radiosensitive. Table 23–1 lists various tumors by degree of radiosensitivity.
      b. Normal cells or tissues that are radiosensitive will exhibit more radiation side effects.
      c. Certain body tissues can tolerate only specified radiation doses before severe complications result (Table 23–2). Treatment is planned to avoid reaching these doses at specific organs.

GOALS OF RADIATION THERAPY

A. Cure—to eradicate the disease and have the individual live a normal life span. Examples of cancers often cured with radiation therapy:
   1. Hodgkin's disease (early stages with radiation alone; later stages with radiation and chemotherapy).
   2. Early stage breast cancer (following lumpectomy, preserving the breast).
   3. Seminoma of the testis.
   4. Cancer of the cervix (Stage II).
   5. Skin cancers (basal cell, squamous cell).
   6. Cancer of the larynx (disease confined to the vocal cords, sparing laryngectomy).
   7. Wilms' tumor (with chemotherapy).

Table 23–1. RELATIVE RADIOSENSITIVITY OF VARIOUS TUMORS AND TISSUES*

Tumors or Tissues	Relative Radiosensitivity
Lymphoma Leukemia Seminoma Dysgerminoma	High
Squamous cell cancer of the oropharyngeal, glottis, bladder, skin, and cervical epithelia; adenocarcinomas of the alimentary tract	Fairly high
Vascular and connective tissue elements of all tumors; secondary neurovascularization, astrocytomas	Medium
Salivary gland tumors, hepatoma, renal cancer, pancreatic cancer, chondrosarcoma, osteogenic sarcoma	Fairly low
Rhabdomyosarcoma, leiomyosarcoma, and ganglioneurofibrosarcoma	Low

* From Rubin, P.: Principles of radiation oncology and cancer radiotherapy. *In* Rubin, P. (ed.): Clinical Oncology for Medical Students and Physicians. New York, American Cancer Society, 1983, p. 60.

Table 23–2. MAXIMAL TOLERANCE* DOSE OF ORGANS
BY RADIATION†

Organ	Injury	Dose (rads)	Amount of Organ Treated (Field Size)
Bone marrow	aplasia	450	whole organ
	pancytopenia	4,000	segmental
Liver	acute, chronic	4,000	whole
	hepatitis	2,000	whole (strip)
Stomach	perforation, ulcer, hemorrhage	5,500	100 cm
Intestine	ulcer, perforation	5,500	400 cm
	hemorrhage	6,500	100 cm
Brain	infarction, necrosis	6,000	whole
Spinal cord	infarction, necrosis	5,500	10 cm
Heart	pericarditis	5,500	60%
	pancarditis	8,000	25%
Lung	acute, chronic	3,500	100 cm
	pneumonitis	2,500	whole
Kidney	acute, chronic	2,000	whole (strip)
	nephrosclerosis	2,500	whole
Fetus	death	400	whole

* Maximal tolerance dose is defined as the dose to which a given population of patients is exposed under a standard set of treatment conditions resulting in a 50% severe complication rate within 5 years of treatment.

† From Rubin, P.: Principles of radiation oncology and cancer radiotherapy. *In* Rubin, P. (ed.): Clinical Oncology for Medical Students and Physicians. New York, American Cancer Society, 1983, p. 68.

    8. Prostate cancer (early stages).

    9. Head and neck tumors (early stages) with or without surgery.

B. Control—to control the growth and spread of disease and have the individual live symptom-free for a period of time. Examples of cancers often controlled with radiation therapy:

    1. Cancer of the bladder (sometimes given preoperatively).

    2. Breast cancer (used in later stages, i.e., in chest wall recurrence).

    3. Head and neck cancers (tumors too large to cure).

    4. Brain tumors.

    5. Ovarian cancers.

    6. Lung cancers.

C. Prophylaxis—Radiation is sometimes used prophylactically to control disease that may be microscopic but not seen. For example, prophylactic cranial irradiation is used for certain lung cancers (oat cell, adenocarcinoma).

D. Palliation—to relieve or reduce distressing symptoms or impending complications. Examples of problems often palliated with radiation therapy:

    1. Pain from bony metastasis.

    2. Tumor obstructions in:

        a. Superior vena cava.

        b. G.I. tract.

        c. Kidney and ureters.

        d. Trachea.

    3. Spinal cord compression.

    4. Symptoms due to brain metastasis.

    5. Uncontrolled bleeding from tumor.

TYPES OF RADIATION THERAPY

A. External (external beam, teletherapy)—therapy in which source of ionizing radiation is outside of the body. Steps involved in external radiation therapy:
   1. Consultation.
      a. Individual meets radiation therapy physician (radiation oncologist, radiotherapist) and radiation therapy nurse.
      b. History and physical examination.
      c. Review of pre-treatment studies.
      d. Radiation therapy recommendations.
      e. Informed consent.
   2. Treatment planning—steps to outline treatment area and develop accurate treatment plan include:
      a. Simulation—planning session to tailor the external radiation beam to the individual's tumor volume area.
         (1) Individual lies on x-ray fluoroscope table that mimics treatment machine table.

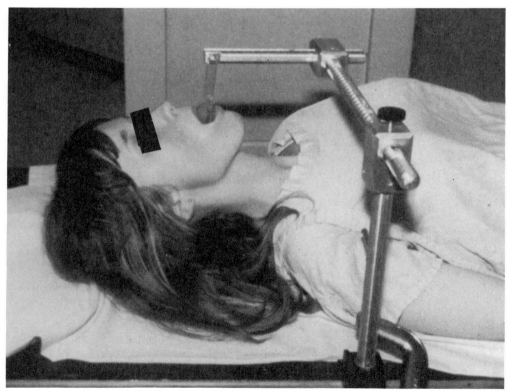

Figure 23–3. Immobilization bite block. (Courtesy of The Johns Hopkins Oncology Center, Department of Radiation Therapy, Baltimore, MD.)

(2) Immobilization devices may be used for exact body positioning (Fig. 23–3 and 23–4).

(3) Tumor volume area localized with fluoroscope (with help of pre-treatment studies, i.e., CT scans, MRI, x-rays, bone scans) and x-ray picture taken of area.

(4) Temporary marks placed on skin to outline tumor volume.

(5) Permanent tattoo mark (size of pen point) may be placed on skin in treatment area.

(6) Diagnostic studies may be done during simulation to locate vital structures (examples: I.V.P. dye given to locate kidneys, barium given to locate G.I. tract) if located in treatment field.

b. Construction of blocks.

(1) Simulation x-ray film ("sim film") marked by physician to show areas inside treatment field to be "blocked" or spared from the radiation beam (Fig. 23–5).

(2) From "sim film," technician outlines and constructs lead-like blocks to be placed in beam pathway during treatments. Blocks are mounted on plastic tray and inserted into machine before individual's treatment (Fig. 23–6).

c. Computerized treatment plans—Tumor volume and individual's body dimensions used to generate a computer plan showing dose distribution of radiation with particular machine set-ups (Fig. 23–7).

d. Not all treatment set-ups require simulation. Some set-ups are done

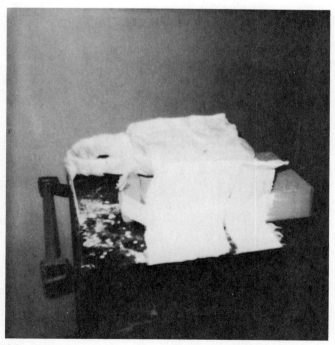

Figure 23–4. *Immobilization plaster of Paris cast. (Courtesy of The Johns Hopkins Oncology Center, Department of Radiation Therapy, Baltimore, MD.)*

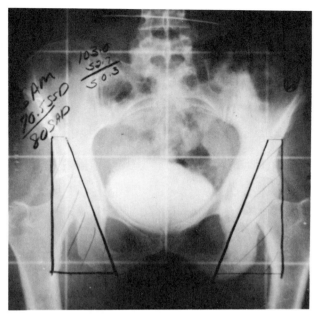

Figure 23–5. Simulation film. (Courtesy of The Johns Hopkins Oncology Center, Department of Radiation Therapy, Baltimore, MD.)

directly on treatment machine, "clinical set-up" (e.g., whole brain radiation, skin lesions).
e. Simulation may be done again during course of treatment if a smaller or a different tumor volume area is to be treated further.

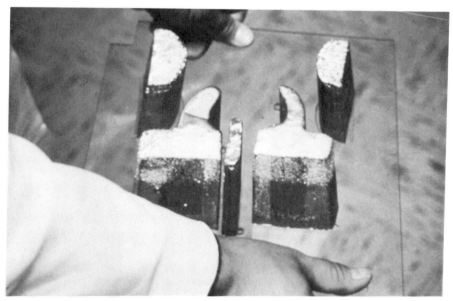

Figure 23–6. Treatment blocks. (Courtesy of The Johns Hopkins Oncology Center, Department of Radiation Therapy, Baltimore, MD.)

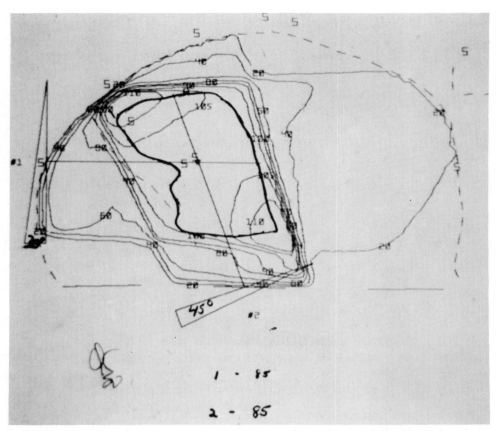

Figure 23–7. *Isodose curve. Radiation computerized treatment plan. (Courtesy of The Johns Hopkins Oncology Center, Department of Radiation Therapy, Baltimore, MD.)*

3. Radiation treatments:
   a. Treatment delivery—high energy x-rays, electrons, or gamma rays delivered by machines:
   (1) Linear accelerators (Fig. 23–8).
      (a) Deliver x-rays, electrons in energies from 4–35 MEV (million electron volts).
         Note: The deeper the tumor inside the body, the higher the energy needed to penetrate the tumor.
      (b) Deliver beam of radiation in exact paths with very little radiation scatter.
      (c) Are skin-sparing, i.e., the maximum dose is deposited where it is needed, not on skin surface (except electrons, which are meant to be given to superficial tumors).
   (2) Machines with radioactive sources:
      (a) Deliver gamma rays from radioactive cobalt (^{60}Co) or radioactive cesium (^{137}Cs).
      (b) Require periodic replacement of radioactive source owing to its decay.

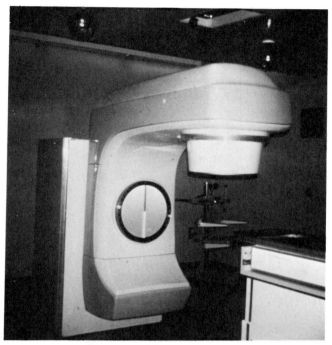

Figure 23–8. *The linear accelerator. (Courtesy of The Johns Hopkins Oncology Center, Department of Radiation Therapy, Baltimore, MD.)*

4. Treatment prescription:
   a. Radiation dose to be given and schedule are written by radiation oncologist or radiotherapist. Examples:
      (1) 200 rads to R breast 5 fractions per week to 5000 rads total.
      (2) 300 rads to lumbar spine 4 fractions per week to total dose of 3000 rads.
   b. Dose prescribed and treatment schedule depend on many factors including:
      (1) Radiosensitivity of tumor or normal cells to be treated.
      (2) Tumor location and extent.
      (3) Volume of tissues/normal cells to be treated.
      (4) Radiation dose/time relationship.
      (5) Goal of treatment: cure, control, palliation.
5. Treatment experience.
   a. Consists of lying on hard x-ray table.
   b. Feels like regular diagnostic x-ray procedure, i.e., nothing touches person, no pain, no sensations, no injections.
      Note: For some individuals, lying on hard table may be uncomfortable.
   c. Amount of time for each treatment varies, depending on dose and treatment delivery. (Most treatments last only a few minutes. Positioning for each treatment may take 10–15 minutes.)
   d. Machine rotates around individual, depending on how radiation beam is aimed.
   e. Individual is only one in room when radiation beam is in "on" position.

     f. Individual is constantly monitored in room via a window or TV screen and can talk with technologists via an intercom.

     g. Machines may make clicking or humming noises.

     h. Some individuals (mostly small children) may require daily sedation for each treatment.

     i. Individuals are never radioactive with external beam treatments.

  6. Treatment course monitoring:

     a. Weekly check-up with radiation oncologist.

     b. Weekly "port film" (an x-ray film taken directly on machine to double-check that treatment set-up is accurately done).

     c. Periodic blood counts.

     d. Ongoing nursing assessment of how individual and family are coping with treatment: nutritional status, side effects, and so forth.

     e. Treatment breaks may be given if untoward effects present: low blood counts, skin reactions, diarrhea.

     f. At completion of treatment follow-up schedules are established.

B. Internal radiation therapy (brachytherapy).

  1. Definition—the use of high energy radioactive sources placed into or directly on the body to treat disease.

  2. Uses:

     a. Delivers high, concentrated dose of radiation to specific body areas, minimizing radiation to normal tissues.

     b. Used to treat tumors or diseases that can be practically reached for therapy.

     c. Generally used for curative or control purposes.

  3. Types of internal radiation (Table 23–3).

     a. Mechanically positioned—positioning a radioactive source in a specific body site.

       (1) Uses sealed radioactive sources (radioactive seeds, threads, ribbons).

       (2) Radioactive sources implanted may be permanent or temporary.

Table 23–3. EXAMPLES OF INTERNAL RADIATION PROCEDURES

Type of Treatment	Disease	Radioisotope Used	Permanent/ Temporary
Mechanically positioned radiation			
Intrauterine implant	Ca cervix Ca uterus	Radium-226	Temporary
Intra-ocular implant	Melanoma of choroid	Iodine-125	Temporary
Interstitial implant of prostate	Ca prostate	Iodine-125	Permanent
Eye surface application	Pterygium	Strontium-90	Temporary
Oral ribbons/needles	Ca head, neck	Iridium-192	Temporary
Interstitial implants of breast	Ca breast	Iridium-192	Temporary
Metabolized or absorbed radiation			
Oral ingestion	Hyperthyroidism	Iodine-131	
Intrapleural	Pleural metastasis	Phosphorus-32	
Intraperitoneal	Peritoneal metastasis	Phosphorus-32	

(3) Methods of mechanically positioned radiation:
   (a) Intracavitary—inserting a radioactive source into a body cavity (example: gynecologic implant for cancer of the cervix using Cesium-137).
   (b) Interstitial—sewing or inserting a radioactive source directly into a body tissue (example: an interstitial breast implant using Iridium-192).
   (c) Surface—placing a radioactive source onto a surface tumor (example: a surface application of Strontium-90 to a superficial eye tumor [pterygium]).
   b. Metabolized or absorbed radiation.
   (1) Uses nonsealed sources of radiation.
   (2) Methods of metabolized or absorbed radiation:
      (a) Oral—administering an oral radioactive substance (example: an oral capsule of Iodine-131 to treat hyperthyroidism).
      (b) Intravenous—administering a liquid radioactive substance into a vein (example: administering intravenous Phosphorus-32 for bony metastatic lesions).
      (c) Intrapleural—instilling a radioactive colloidal substance into the pleural space via thoracentesis (example: instilling Phosphorus-32 intrapleurally for mesothelioma).
      (d) Intraperitoneal—instilling a radioactive colloidal substance into the peritoneal sac (example: instilling Phosphorus-32 intraperitoneally for metastasis to the peritoneum from breast cancer).
4. Internal radiation treatment planning.
   a. Selection of radioactive substance (radioisotope) dependent on many factors including: size, location, type of tumor, half-life of substance, method of internal radiation.
   b. Simulation film may be taken with some mechanically positioned radiation and computerized dosimetry done.

RADIATION SAFETY MEASURES AND PRACTICES

A. Purpose of radiation protection measures: low level ionizing radiation believed to cause following unwanted side effects:
   1. Somatic effects (nonstochastic): actual body tissue alterations in individual exposed. Examples:
      a. Solid tumors. Higher incidence of breast cancer than normal found in women in Nova Scotia who had frequent fluoroscopic treatments to the chest for T.B. follow-up care.
      b. Leukemias: Higher incidence of leukemia than normal found in Japanese atomic bomb survivors and in individuals in Great Britain whose spines were frequently x-rayed for ankylosing spondylitis.
   2. Genetic effects (stochastic): potential damage to offspring or future generations of individuals exposed to ionizing radiation.
      a. Genetic mutations shown in offspring of animals (fruit flies, mice) exposed to ionizing radiation and in some offspring of survivors of the atomic bomb.

     b. Most human studies of genetic effects of ionizing radiation based on high doses of ionizing radiation. Low level exposure risks not conclusive.

B. Measurements of radiation exposure:
1. Roentgen: unit of radiation exposure in air. Measures x-rays and gamma rays only.
2. Rad: unit of amount of absorbed radiation (*radiation absorbed dose*). 1 Gray = 100 rads.
3. Rem: unit of dose equivalent or how the body tissues handle the type of radiation absorbed. 1 Sievert = 100 rems.
   Note: For x-rays, gamma rays, and beta rays 1 rad = 1 rem = 1 Roentgen.
4. Curie: unit of amount of radioactivity in a radioactive substance. Based on the disintegrations/time of radium, which has 3.7×10^{10} disintegrations/second. 1 Becquerel = 1 transformation/second.
5. Specific activity: the number of Curies per gram of material.

C. Sources of radiation exposure:
1. Nonoccupational—background radiation that includes:
   a. Cosmic: from atmosphere. The higher the altitude, the more radiation exposure.
   b. Terrestrial: in building materials, ground water, soil, tobacco.
   c. Man: radioactive potassium ^{40}K found naturally in humans.
   d. 210 mrem/year is average American radiation exposure from nonoccupational sources.
2. Occupational:
   a. Nonmedical: includes nuclear power plants and use of ionizing radiation for scientific studies.
   b. Medical:
      (1) Diagnostic: x-rays, nuclear medicine. Generally employs low doses. Chest x-ray = 10 mrem.
      (2) Therapeutic: external and internal radiation therapy generally employ high doses, since the intent is to damage cells.

D. Maximum permissible dose limits of radiation exposure.
1. Established guidelines by the National Council on Radiation Protection (NCRP) for dose *limits* of radiation exposure.
2. Based on postulated amount of radiation exposure that would cause damage to ovaries and testes.
3. Guidelines are not intended to be used as threshold dose. Intent is to keep radiation exposure as low as reasonably achievable (ALARA).
4. Present recommended maximum permissible dose (Table 23–4).
5. Nurses may fall into either occupationally exposed or general public category, depending on their institution.
6. Few nurses exceed NCRP guidelines.

E. Radiation safety measures and practices:
1. Factors that determine type and amount of radiation safety measures.
   a. Type of radiation used.
      (a) Alpha, beta, and gamma radiation differ in penetrating abilities and in type of material needed to shield one from exposure (Fig. 23–9).
   b. Half-life of isotope used.
      (1) Half-life refers to amount of time for the radioisotope to be reduced to half of its amount of radioactivity.

Table 23–4. MAXIMUM PERMISSIBLE DOSES AND DOSE
LIMITS*

Exposure Site	Maximum Permissible Dose Equivalent
Occupational exposure	
Whole body	5 rem in any one year after age 18
Skin	15 rem in any one year
Hands	75 rem in any one year
Forearms	30 rem in any one year
Other organs	15 rem in any one year
Pregnant women (with respect to the fetus)	0.5 rem during gestation period
General public or occasionally exposed persons	**Dose Limit**
Whole body	0.5 rem in any one year

* From Radiation protection for medical and allied personnel. NCRP Report No. 48, Washington, D.C., U.S. Government Printing Office, 1976.

    (2) Isotopes with very long half-lives never used in permanent implants.

    (3) Table 23–5 lists half-lives of commonly used radioisotopes.

  c. Amount of the radioisotope used (specific activity).

    (1) The higher the amount, generally, the more radiation protection measures are needed, especially for gamma radiation.

    (2) Example: 8 mCi (8 millicuries) of ^{131}I given orally for hyperthyroidism can be done on outpatient basis, but 100 mCi would require the individual to be in isolation in the hospital.

  d. Method of isotope delivery:

    (1) When radioisotopes are mechanically positioned, implant itself is radioactive, not individual.

    (2) When radioisotope given orally or systemically, patient and his or her body secretions may be radioactive.

2. Radiation protection measures and practices:

  a. Assess factors discussed above.

  b. If radiation protection measures needed, utilize principles of time, distance, shielding.

    (1) Minimize *time* in contact with radioactive source or radioactive individual.

    (2) Maximize *distance* in contact with radioactive source or radioactive individual.

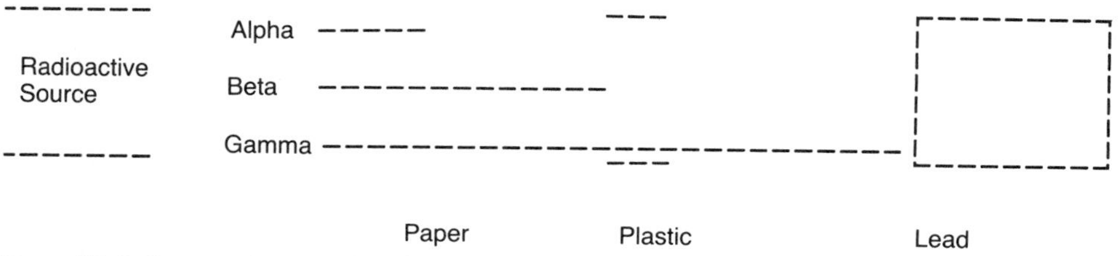

Figure 23–9. Range and penetration of alpha, beta and gamma radiation. (Redrawn from Yasko, J.: Care of the Client Receiving External Radiation Therapy. Reston, VA, Reston Publishing Co., 1982.)

Table 23–5. HALF-LIVES
OF COMMONLY USED
RADIOISOTOPES

Radioisotope	Half-life
Cesium-137	30.0 years
Cobalt-60	5.26 years
Gold-198	2.7 days
Iodine-125	60.2 days
Iodine-131	8.05 days
Iridium-192	74.2 days
Radium-226	1,602.0 years
Yttrium-90	64.0 hours
Phosphorus-32	14.28 days

(3) Utilize required *shielding* needed to decrease exposure based on source activity and penetration.

c. Examples of general guidelines for minimizing radiation exposure from high gamma radiation.

  (1) Mechanically positioned high energy gamma radiation:

    (a) Assess the patient's self-care status.

    (b) Assign patient to private room.

    (c) Limit the amount of contact time with the patient's implant as possible.

    (d) Keep the shield between you and the implanted source.

    (e) Check linens, clothing, and bedpans for any signs of a dislodged source.

    (f) Monitor your radiation exposure by use of a film badge or other monitoring device.

    (g) Avoid caring for these patients if you are pregnant or *might* be pregnant.

    (h) Patient's excretions do not need to be handled as radioactive.

    (i) Never touch a dislodged sealed source. Contact the radiation safety or radiation therapy department if the source is dislodged.

    (j) Make sure the patient's room and chart are marked with radiation precaution directions.

    (k) Do not allow pregnant visitors or children under 18 into patient's room.

    (l) Limit visitors to a specified amount of time per day based on the amount of radiation present.

  (2) Metabolized or absorbed gamma radiation:

    (a) Assess the patient's self-care status.

    (b) Assign patient to private room.

    (c) Limit the amount of time spent with the patient and keep your distance when inside the patient's room.

    (d) Wear waterproof gloves when handling any body secretions or items in contact with the patient's body secretions.

    (e) Provide disposable eating trays and utensils.

    (f) Keep all linens and trash in patient's room and have these scanned before their release.

(g) Do not take care of patient if you are or might be pregnant.

(h) Make sure the patient's room and chart are marked with radioactive caution directions.

(i) Have the patient scanned before he or she is discharged.

SIDE EFFECTS OF RADIATION THERAPY

A. Occur when normal cells inside radiated area are temporarily or permanently damaged (Table 23–6).

B. Types of side effects:
    1. Acute—those that occur during or shortly after the course of radiation therapy.

Table 23–6. EXAMPLES OF NURSING INTERVENTIONS FOR SIDE EFFECTS FROM SPECIFIC SITES OF RADIATION THERAPY

Body Site	Side Effect	Nursing Interventions
Scalp (whole brain)	Alopecia	Instruct in actions to minimize scalp irritation: avoid excessive shampooing, hair dryers, rollers, hair pins, hair spray, sun, cold exposure to head. Advise use of wigs, scarf, turban before hair loss.
Head and neck	Mouth dryness	Instruct in keeping oral mucous membranes moist with fluids, atomizer mist, mouth sprays, artificial saliva.
	Mucositis	Instruct in good mouth care; write down specific mouth care protocol. Advise measures to avoid trauma to mucous membranes: avoid alcohol, tobacco, irritating foods.
Chest	Esophagitis	Instruct in diet that contains foods that are comfortable to esophagus: creamy foods. Instruct in use of medication for esophagitis, e.g., Maalox, benadryl, lidocaine mixture. Reassure that esophagitis is temporary.
Abdomen	Nausea/vomiting	Instruct in dietary alterations helpful to individual: particular foods well tolerated per individual; remove non-tolerated food sights and smells, etc. Instruct in use of antiemetics, relaxation, distraction. Monitor fluid and electrolyte status.
Pelvis	Diarrhea	Instruct in use of low-residue diet to begin day one of treatment. Instruct in use and side effects of antidiarrheal medications.
	Cystitis	Instruct in good fluid intake (3,000 cc/day unless contraindicated). Instruct in avoidance of foods irritating to bladder epithelium: spicy foods, alcoholic beverages, coffee, tea.
Skin	Erythema Dry desquamation	Instruct in skin care: wash with water only; avoid soaps, lotions, perfumes, heating pads, sun exposure, irritating fabrics, chlorinated pools, straight razors to skin in treatment field.
	Wet desquamation	Instruct in skin care: cleanse with half strength peroxide, saline—rinse with saline. Dress as prescribed.

2. Chronic—those that occur months to years after the course of radiation therapy.
C. Factors that influence the occurrence and degree of side effects:
1. Body site irradiated—only body tissues inside radiation field are affected (i.e., if the scalp is not treated, individual will not lose hair on head).
2. Dose of radiation given (daily dose and/or total dose)—the more radiation given, the higher the potential for side effects. Most side effects occur after a certain dose to specific tissues.
3. Extent of body area treated—the larger the field of radiation, the more potential for side effects.
4. Method of radiation delivery—machines that deliver less penetrating radiation (i.e., electrons) will cause more skin reactions than machines that deliver higher penetrating radiation of same dose.
D. Examples of some side effects of radiation to specific body sites.
1. Scalp:
   a. Alopecia.
   b. Erythema.
   c. Edema.
2. Head and neck:
   a. Dry mouth (xerostomia).
   b. Mucositis.
   c. Taste alterations.
   d. Cataracts (if lens of eye treated).
   e. Pharyngitis/esophagitis.
   f. Skin erythema.
3. Chest:
   a. Esophagitis.
   b. Nausea.
   c. Pneumonitis.
4. Abdomen:
   a. Nausea.
   b. Vomiting.
5. Pelvis:
   a. Diarrhea.
   b. Cystitis.
   c. Decreased sexual function (if ovaries or testes treated).
6. Skin:
   a. Erythema.
   b. Dry desquamation.
   c. Moist desquamation.
7. Bone marrow:
   a. Leukopenia.
   b. Thrombocytopenia.
   c. Anemia.

NURSING MANAGEMENT OF PERSONS RECEIVING RADIATION THERAPY

A. Roles and actions of the nurse:
1. Teacher.
   a. Assesses the individual's and significant others' understanding of the diagnosis, disease process, present status, and treatment.

   b. Assesses the individual's and significant others' readiness to learn.
   c. Assesses the individual's and significant others' past experience, or
      fears associated with radiation therapy.
   d. Instructs the individual, significant others, and other health care pro-
      viders in information related to radiation therapy.
   e. Evaluates the individual's and significant others' learning.
  2. Direct care provider.
   a. Provides direct care to individuals undergoing radiation therapy.
   b. Promotes comfort to individuals undergoing radiation therapy.
   c. Continually evaluates individuals for side effects and response to
      treatment.
  3. Counselor.
   a. Assesses individual's and significant others' coping abilities.
   b. Supports and encourages positive coping strategies.

STUDY QUESTIONS

1. How is ionizing radiation effective in treating cancers?
2. Why is ionizing radiation used in treating some cancers and not others?
3. A patient tells you that she knows nothing about radiation treatments. How
   would you describe the actual treatments and the steps involved in treatment
   planning?
4. A patient is scheduled to have a radioactive implant. What questions would
   you ask in order to plan your radiation safety measures?
5. What factors influence the side effects of radiation treatments?

Bibliography

Dietz, K. A.: Radiation therapy—external radiation, part I. Cancer Nursing, 2:129–138, 1979.
Dietz, K. A.: Radiation therapy—external radiation, part II. Cancer Nursing, 2:233–244, 1979.
Gillick, K. M.: Radiation therapy—internal radiation, part I. Cancer Nursing, 2:313–325, 1979.
Gillick, K. M.: Radiation therapy—internal radiation, part II. Cancer Nursing, 2:393–402, 1979.
Godwin, C., Bucholtz, J., and Wall, S.: Hidden hazards on the job: radiation. Nursing Life, No-
    vember/December: pp. 43–47, 1985.
Hassey, K.: Demystifying care of patients with radioactive implants. American Journal of Nursing,
    85:788–792, 1985.
Hassey, K. M.: Altered skin integrity in patients receiving radiation therapy. Oncology Nursing
    Forum, 9(4): 44–50, 1982.
Hilderley, L. J.: Skin care in radiation therapy—a review of the literature. Oncology Nursing Forum,
    10(1):51–56, 1983.
Hilderley, L. J.: The role of the nurse in radiation oncology. Seminars in Oncology, 7(1):39–47, 1980.
Kelly, P. P. and Tinsley, C.: Planning care for the patient receiving external radiation. American
    Journal of Nursing, 81:338–342, 1981.
Leahy, I. M., St. Germain, J. M., and Varricchio, C. G.: The Nurse and Radiotherapy. St. Louis,
    C.V. Mosby Co., 1979.
Radiation protection for medical and allied personnel. NCRP Report No. 48, Washington, D.C.,
    U.S. Government Printing Office, 1976.
Rubin, P. (ed.): Clinical Oncology for Medical Students and Physicians: A Multidisciplinary Ap-
    proach, 6th ed. New York, The American Cancer Society, 1983.
Strohl, R. A. and Salazar, O. M.: Management of the patient receiving hemibody irradiation. On-
    cology Nursing Forum, 9(4):13–16, 1982.
Thompson, L.: Radiotherapy: Gynecologic malignancies. Nursing Mirror, 152(12):13–16, 1981.
Varricchio, C. G.: The patient on radiation therapy. American Journal of Nursing, 81:334–337, 1981.
Wilson, C. A. and Strohl, R. A.: Radiation therapy as primary treatment for breast cancer. Oncology
    Nursing Forum, 9(1):12–15, 1982.
Yasko, J. M.: Care of the Client Receiving External Radiation Therapy. Reston, VA, Reston Publishing
    Co., 1982.

24

Chemotherapy

CATHERINE M. BENDER, RN, MN

PRETREATMENT CONSIDERATIONS

A. Assessment of the patient receiving chemotherapy.
B. Initial treatment.
   1. Physical and emotional status of patient and family.
   2. Knowledge of chemotherapy, treatment plan, adverse effects, self-care strategies aimed at prevention or control of adverse effects.
   3. Resources available to ensure compliance with treatment plan.
   4. Goal of treatment.
   5. Allergies.
   6. Pertinent laboratory data.
   7. Chemotherapy agents to be administered.
   8. Method of administration.
   9. Dose, frequency, and nadir of chemotherapy agents.
   10. Mechanism of action of chemotherapy agents.
C. Subsequent treatments (in addition to the data collected prior to initial treatment):
   1. Date of first chemotherapy treatment.
   2. Date of last chemotherapy treatment.
   3. Compliance with treatment schedule.
   4. Problems experienced during administration.
   5. Side effects experienced, current status.
   6. Measures that relieved side effects.
   7. Last site of administration (if not orally).
   8. Potential side effects of chemotherapy agents.
D. Education of patient and family. Provide information related to:
   1. Rationale for chemotherapy.
   2. General mechanism of action of chemotherapeutic agents.
   3. Potential therapeutic outcome of treatment.
   4. Rationale for the occurrence of side effects.
   5. Treatment plan:
      a. Chemotherapy agents to be used.

    b. Rationale and schedule of laboratory studies to be performed prior to treatment.
    c. Method of administration.
    d. Schedule of administration.
    e. Potential side effects.
    f. Signs and symptoms that must be reported to health care professionals.
  6. Methods of self-care aimed at the prevention and control of side effects.
  7. Dietary and medication restrictions.
  8. Written materials available as an adjunct to individualized education.

MECHANISMS OF ACTION

A. Normal cell function and division.
  1. Deoxyribonucleic acid (DNA):
    a. Controls all cellular activity and function in the body.
    b. Consists of four types of nucleotides, which differ in structure according to the type of nitrogenous base present. The four bases are adenine, cytosine, guanine, and thymine.
    c. Nucleotides are connected in a single chain. DNA consists of a double chain of two single-chain nitrogenous bases connected by hydrogen bonding. The double chain of DNA is found in the form of a helix as shown in Figure 24–1.
    d. Bonding that occurs between nitrogenous bases may only occur as follows:
      ○ Adenine-Thymine
      ○ Cytosine-Guanine
    e. Separating the double strands of DNA exposes the nitrogenous bases, which can only reconnect with a base as described above.
      Therefore, as each single strand couples with a new single chain, the result will be two identical new double-stranded chains of DNA.
  2. Ribonucleic acid (RNA) is a chemical substance that transfers DNA from the nucleus of the cell to the cytoplasm of the cell, where protein synthesis takes place.
  3. Cell Cycle—process of reproduction that occurs in normal and malignant cells (Fig. 24–2).
    a. G_0 (Resting phase)—cells are temporarily out of cycle and not in the process of division (length of time is highly variable).
    b. G_1—cells activated into the cell cycle enter the G_1 phase. Many enzymes needed for DNA synthesis are produced (approximately 18 hours).
    c. S (Synthesis)—cellular DNA component is duplicated in preparation for division (approximately 20 hours).
    d. G_2—protein and RNA synthesis takes place, production of the mitotic spindle apparatus.
    e. Mitosis—actual cell division, four phases, very brief (about one hour).
      (1) Prophase—nuclear membrane breaks down, chromosomes clump.
      (2) Metaphase—chromosomes line up in middle of cell.
      (3) Anaphase—chromosomes segregate to centrioles.
      (4) Telophase—cell division, production of two new cells.

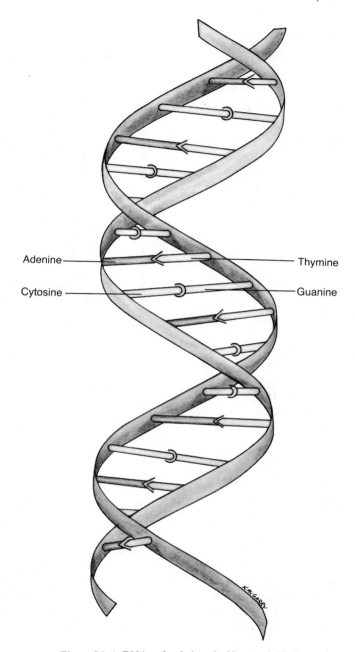

Adenine

Thymine

Cytosine

Guanine

Figure 24–1. DNA molecule in a double-stranded helix.

    f. The amount of time needed for the completion of this cycle varies with the cell type. The G_0 phase, the most variable in time, is the major determinant of the length of time of the cell cycle.

    g. Following mitosis, cells differentiate into mature cells.

  4. Cancer cell cycle and function.

    a. May divide into several new cells instead of the usual two.

    b. Cellular proliferation continues without the normal mechanisms for inhibition of cell division.

Phases of Cell Cycle   Stages of Mitosis

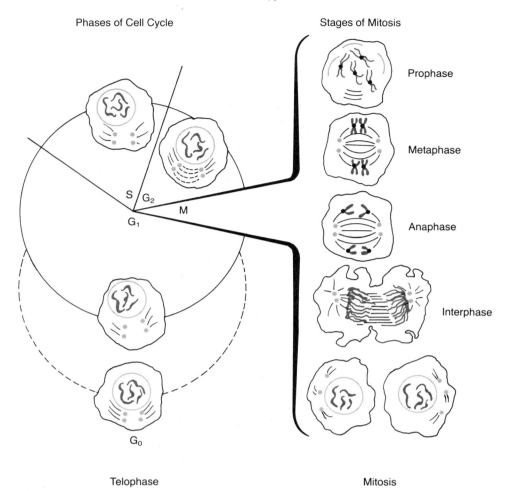

Figure 24–2. The cell cycle. (Redrawn from Marino, L.: Cancer Nursing. St. Louis, C. V. Mosby Co., 1981.)

B. Cancer chemotherapy, general mechanism of action.
   1. Chemotherapy functions at a cellular level by interrupting the cell life cycle. It modifies the proliferation kinetics of normal and malignant cells.
      a. Most agents function by modifying or interfering with DNA synthesis.
      b. Due to the nature of their function, most agents are effective in eradicating cells that are preparing for or are in the process of cell reproduction.
      c. Therefore, malignant as well as normal cells that are most rapidly dividing are most affected by chemotherapeutic agents.
C. Cell cycle–specific versus nonspecific agents.
   1. Cell cycle–specific agents:
      a. Major cytotoxic effects of the agent are sustained during a particular phase of the cell cycle.
      b. Greater cytotoxic effect can be achieved if these agents are given in divided doses.
      c. These agents are most effective in tumors in which a large number of cells are dividing.

2. Cell cycle nonspecific agents:
   a. Effective against resting and dividing cells.
   b. Cytotoxic effects of these agents take place at some point during the cell cycle and are then expressed when the cell attempts to divide or repair itself.
   c. The number of cells that are affected is proportional to the amount of drug given.

GOALS OF CHEMOTHERAPY TREATMENT

A. Cure.
   1. Cure of some malignancies may be achieved with the use of chemotherapy as the primary mode of treatment. Examples of these malignancies may include acute lymphocytic leukemia (in children), Hodgkin's disease, lymphosarcomas, Burkitt's lymphoma, testicular tumors, Wilms' tumor, and neuroblastoma.
   2. Cure may also be achieved with the use of chemotherapy in conjunction with other primary modes of therapy as radiation or surgery. This use of chemotherapy is known as adjuvant chemotherapy. Chemotherapy is used in this instance in an attempt to eradicate any micrometastases remaining after surgery or radiation.
B. Control.
   1. Control may be the goal of therapy when the hope of cure is not realistic. The aim of control of the disease with chemotherapy is to extend the length and improve the quality of life.
   2. Malignancies that may be controlled with the use of chemotherapy include breast cancer, Ewing's sarcoma, prostatic cancer, multiple myeloma, lung cancer (small cell).
C. Palliation.
   1. In the event that neither cure nor control of the malignancy is possible, palliation may be the goal of chemotherapy. Palliative therapy is aimed at the comfort of the patient.
   2. Comfort may be achieved through the use of chemotherapy by relieving pressure on nerves, lymphatics, and vasculature, and by easing organ obstruction.

ROUTE OF ADMINISTRATION

A. The administration of chemotherapeutic agents, regardless of the route, is an important responsibility for the nurse. Though the nurse may not be directly responsible for the administration of the agent, the nurse must be knowledgeable about the agent's dose, mechanism of action, potential toxicities, and methods and potential problems of administration. The nurse must also impart information to patients that will address their concerns about chemotherapy treatment and provide them with self-care strategies aimed at the prevention and control of side effects.
B. Oral route—commonly used for chemotherapy administration. Though the oral route seems innocuous in comparison with the other routes of administration, the nature of chemotherapy agents compels the nurse to administer these agents with equal regard to safety.

C. Intramuscular, subcutaneous route.
　　1. Infrequently used, agents are not vesicants.
　　2. The nurse will:
　　　　a. Use a small gauge needle.
　　　　b. Cleanse the area of administration with an antiseptic solution.
　　　　c. Be assured of adequate muscle or subcutaneous tissue at the site of administration.
　　　　d. Assess thrombocytopenic patients for bleeding at the site of administration.
D. Intravenous route.
　　1. Most common route of administration:
　　　　a. Provides for better absorption of the agent.
　　　　b. Vesicants are administered via this route.
　　2. Complications: Infection and phlebitis. To prevent these complications:
　　　　a. Wash hands.
　　　　b. Prepare skin as indicated by institution policy.
　　　　c. Employ smallest gauge needle possible with regard to vein size and objective of therapy.
　　　　d. Change intravenous fluid every 24 hours and change tubing according to institutional policy.
　　　　e. Maintain aseptic technique in managing the intravenous system.
　　　　f. Assess intravenous insertion site and along venous route for signs of infection, redness, edema, warmth, pain, discharge, and odor.
E. Central venous catheter infusion route.
　　1. Silicone catheters are inserted under general or local anesthesia through the superior vena cava into the right atrium of the heart.
　　2. May be used for continuous or intermittent infusions.
　　3. Potential complications include:
　　　　a. Malposition—verify placement with x-ray prior to use.
　　　　b. Infection at insertion site.
　　　　　　(1) Care for insertion site according to institutional guidelines using aseptic technique.
　　　　　　(2) Assess site for redness, edema, pain, discharge, warmth, or odor.
　　　　　　(3) Culture site if infection is suspected.
　　　　c. Clotting—catheters being used intermittently should be flushed daily and/or between each use with a heparin solution according to institutional policy.
　　　　d. Sepsis:
　　　　　　(1) Maintain aseptic technique in the care and removal of the catheter.
　　　　　　(2) Assess patient for early signs of sepsis.
F. Venous access via an implantable access device.
　　1. Designed for patients requiring prolonged venous access.
　　2. Venous approach (subclavian vein) used for systemic drug therapy. Arterial approach used for specific regional drug therapy.
　　3. Heparinization is required once a month or after each injection to maintain patency.
　　4. Complications:
　　　　a. Infection.
　　　　　　(1) Assess for redness, tenderness, drainage at port or tract site.
　　　　　　(2) Assess for signs of systemic infection, fever, malaise.

       b. Infiltration secondary to malposition.

       c. Occlusion.

G. Intraarterial route.

  1. Delivers high concentrations of chemotherapeutic agents directly to the tumor while decreasing the agents' toxic effects systemically.

  2. Placement of catheter determined by tumor location. Two methods:

    a. Percutaneous—catheter placed through small incision in skin.

    b. Surgically placed.

  3. Catheter may be connected to an infusion pump externally or to an implantable access port as described previously.

  4. Complications:

    a. Infection at catheter site.

      (1) Assess for local and systemic signs of infection.

      (2) Change dressing at site daily with aseptic technique.

    b. Bleeding at catheter site.

      (1) Apply pressure dressing.

      (2) Notify physician.

    c. Clotting of catheter.

      (1) Irrigate with heparin solution according to institutional policy.

      (2) Avoid kinks in tubing.

      (3) Check all tubing connections.

    d. Pump malfunction.

      (1) Check all pump attachments.

      (2) Change battery.

      (3) Patient should have backup battery available at all times.

    e. Catheter misplacement—check radiologically.

H. Intraperitoneal chemotherapy.

  1. Adapted from the technique used in peritoneal dialysis. Used for ovarian and colon cancer.

  2. High concentrations of chemotherapy are delivered to the peritoneal cavity via a catheter that is inserted through a small incision below the umbilicus, threaded through a subcutaneous tunnel, and out a small incision 5 to 10 cm from the insertion site.

  3. Dialysis with chemotherapy begins 7 to 10 days after catheter placement.

  4. Chemotherapeutic agents are instilled via a bottle or bag of dialysis solution and flow into the peritoneal cavity by gravity.

  5. The solution is then drained from the peritoneal cavity following a prescribed "dwell time."

  6. The number of exchanges, the dwell time, and treatment schedules vary.

  7. Complications.

    a. Abdominal pain due to:

      (1) Peritoneal irritation.

      (2) Incomplete drainage of solution.

      (3) Dialysate solution at a temperature below normal body temperature.

      (4) Chemical peritonitis.

      (5) Bacterial peritonitis.

    b. Potential side effects of chemotherapeutic agents used (methotrexate, 5-fluorouracil, Adriamycin):

      (1) Myelosuppression.

      (2) Nausea/Vomiting.

(3) Mucositis.

(4) Skin rash.

(5) Diarrhea.

(6) Alopecia.

I. Intrapleural chemotherapy.

1. Introduction of certain medications into the pleural cavity via a thoracotomy tube.

2. Produces sclerosing of the pleural lining aimed at prevention of reinvasion of the pleural cavity with fluid.

3. Agents that produce this sclerosing effect include nitrogen mustard, 5-FU, bleomycin, tetracycline.

4. Following instillation of the sclerosing agent, the patient is repositioned in bed every 10 to 15 minutes to allow for circulation of the sclerosing agent through the pleural cavity.

J. Intrathecal chemotherapy.

1. Utilized in the instance of potential or diagnosed central nervous system involvement with tumor cells due to the inability of most chemotherapeutic agents to pass the blood-brain barrier.

2. Chemotherapy is delivered to the central nervous system via the spinal fluid by means of a lumbar puncture.

3. May be used in the following malignancies in which meningeal involvement can occur: acute leukemia, breast cancer, non-Hodgkin's lymphoma, lung cancer, prostatic cancer, stomach and pancreatic cancers.

4. Agents that may be used: methotrexate, arabinoside-C, thiotepa.

5. Adverse effects:

   a. Side effects that may occur with specific agents.

   b. Headaches, stiff neck, lethargy, nausea/vomiting, confusion, seizures.

K. Ventricular reservoir.

1. Alternative method of delivering chemotherapy to the central nervous system to achieve more consistent cerebrospinal fluid levels and reach higher cavities of the brain due to its direct contact with the subarachnoid space.

2. Device is surgically implanted subcutaneously in the right frontal region over the coronal suture and through a burr hole into the lateral ventricle in the area of the foramen of Monro.

3. Chemotherapy is injected through the reservoir.

4. Complications:

   a. Infection.

      (1) Observe site for tenderness, redness, and drainage.

      (2) Fever, neck stiffness, headache with or without vomiting.

   b. Reservoir malfunction secondary to blockage.

   c. Displacement of the catheter.

      (1) Check for placement by "pumping" the reservoir (push down gently with finger on top of reservoir and release several times).

   d. Side effects of chemotherapeutic agent used.

DRUG CLASSIFICATIONS (Table 24–1)

A. Alkylating agents.

1. Products of the development of chemical warfare.

Table 24–1. CHEMOTHERAPEUTIC AGENTS ACCORDING
TO CLASSIFICATION

Alkylating Agents
  AMSA (Methanesulfon-M-Anisidide)
  Busulfan (Myleran)
  Chlorambucil (Leukeran)
  Cyclophosphamide (Cytoxan)
  Dacarbazine (DTIC)
  Mechlorethamine (Nitrogen Mustard)
  Melphalan (Alkeran)
  Triethylenethiophosphoramide (Thiotepa)
Antitumor Antibiotics
  Actinomycin-D (Dactinomycin)
  Bleomycin Sulfate (Blenoxane)
  Daunorubicin Hydrochloride (Rubidomycin
    HCl)
  Doxorubicin Hydrochloride (Adriamycin)
  Mitomycin-C (Mitomycin)
  Plicamycin (Mithramycin)
  Streptozotocin (Zanosar)
Vinca Alkaloids
  Teniposide (VM-26)
  Vinblastine Sulfate (Velban)
  Vincristine Sulfate (Oncovin)
  Vindesine (Eldisine)
  VP-16-213 (Vepesid)

Nitrosoureas
  BCNU (Carmustine BiCNU)
  CCNU (Lomustine)
  DCNU (Chlorozotocin)
  Methyl-CCNU (Semustine)
Antimetabolites
  5-Azacytidine (Ladakamycin)
  Cytarabine (Cytosar-U)
  Floxuridine (FUDR)
  5-Fluorouracil (5-FU)
  6 Mercaptopurine (6 MP)
  Methotrexate Sodium (Mexate)
  Tegafur (Ftorafur)
  6-Thioguanine (6-TG)
  Triazinate (BAF)
Miscellaneous
  Aminoglutethimide (Elipten)
  Cis-Diamine Dichloroplatinum (Platinol)
  L-Asparaginase (Elspar)
  Procarbazine Hydrochloride (Matulone)

2. Cause cross-linking and abnormal base pairing of proteins and interfere with the replication of DNA.
3. Most are cell cycle nonspecific.
4. Major toxicities are to the hematopoietic system, gastrointestinal system, and gonads.

B. Nitrosoureas.
1. Effects are similar to the alkylating agents.
2. Also inhibit DNA repair.
3. Nitrosoureas are cell cycle nonspecific and cross the blood-brain barrier.
4. Major toxicities are to the hematopoietic system and gastrointestinal system.

C. Antimetabolites.
1. Major activity exerted during S phase of cell cycle.
2. May inhibit protein synthesis or deceive the cell by introducing an erroneous metabolite along the metabolic pathway for DNA synthesis.
3. Antimetabolites are usually structural analogues of naturally occurring metabolites that are falsely substituted along metabolic pathways.
4. Cell cycle specific agents.
5. Major toxicities are to the hematopoietic system and gastrointestinal system.

D. Antitumor Antibiotics.
1. Most have some anti-infective qualities, but major effect is cytotoxic.
2. Interfere with nucleic acid synthesis, inhibit RNA synthesis, and react with or bind with DNA, therefore inhibiting DNA synthesis.
3. Cell cycle nonspecific agents.

    4. Major toxicities are similar to those of alkylating agents; also toxic to the cardiac system with cumulative doses.
- E. Vinca Alkaloids.
  1. Derived from the periwinkle plant.
  2. Bind with microtubular proteins that crystallize the mitotic spindle, resulting in metaphase arrest.
  3. Inhibit RNA and protein synthesis.
  4. Cell cycle specific agents.
  5. Major toxicities are to the hematopoietic system, neurotoxicity.
- F. Miscellaneous Agents.
  1. Agents whose mechanisms of action differ from those of the major classifications.
- G. Hormones.
  1. Steroidal hormones interfere with the synthesis of protein and alter cell metabolism by altering the hormonal environment of the cell.
  2. Palliative effects may include reduction of edema with the use of adrenocorticosteroids and improved appetite with steroidal hormones.
- H. Combination chemotherapy.
  1. Cancer chemotherapy is most often administered in combinations, which can potentially triple or quadruple the response rates of single agent use.
  2. Agents of differing classes may be used to afford the use of their various modes of action.
  3. Agents are used for synergistic activity.
  4. Agents with differing toxicities are used.

NURSING MANAGEMENT OF PERSONS RECEIVING CHEMOTHERAPY

- A. Obtain a baseline assessment to provide data regarding:
  1. Diagnosis.
  2. Treatment plan.
  3. Current physical status.
  4. History.
  5. Psychosocial resources and deficits.
  6. Knowledge base regarding these data.
- B. Understand the chemotherapy agent's mechanism of action, dose, method of administration, potential side effects, and nursing management of those side effects.
  1. Most of the side effects occur as a result of the action of chemotherapy on normal cells. The normal cells that are most predisposed to the effects of chemotherapy include:
     - a. Bone marrow stem cells.
     - b. Epithelial cells of the gastrointestinal tract.
     - c. Epithelial cells of hair follicles.
     - d. Cells of the gonads.
  2. Therefore, potential side effects include:
     - a. Bone marrow suppression.
     - b. Stomatitis or mucositis.
     - c. Esophagitis.
     - d. Nausea and vomiting.
     - e. Anorexia.
     - f. Taste changes.

g. Constipation or diarrhea.
h. Alopecia.
i. Extravasation.
j. Cutaneous reactions.
k. Sexual dysfunction.
3. Plan care to prevent and/or control these side effects.

STUDY QUESTIONS

1. Distinguish between cell cycle specific and nonspecific chemotherapy.
2. Identify the major toxicities of chemotherapy.
3. Develop a nursing care plan for the individual receiving chemotherapy.

Bibliography

Anderson, M., Aker, S., and Hickman, R.: The double-lumen Hickman catheter. American Journal of Nursing, *82*(2):272–277, 1982.

Becker, T.: Cancer Chemotherapy Manual for Nurses. Boston, Little, Brown and Company, 1981.

Bender, C., Bast, J., Drapac, D., and Kray, C.: Patient teaching in hepatic artery infusions. Oncology Nursing Forum, *11*(2):61–65, 1984.

Bjeletich, J. and Hickman, R.: The Hickman indwelling catheter. American Journal of Nursing, *80*(1):62–65, 1980.

Brager, B. L. and Yasko, J. M.: Care of the Client Receiving Chemotherapy. Reston, VA, Reston Publishing Company, Inc., 1984.

Bubela, N.: Technical and psychological problems and concerns arising from the outpatient treatment of cancer with direct intraarterial infusion. Cancer Nursing, *4*(4):305–309, 1981.

Crowley, M. and Baker, M.: Preparing nurses for Hickman catheter care: A self learning module. Oncology Nursing Forum, *7*(4):17–19, 1980.

Dodd, M. J.: Cancer patients knowledge of chemotherapy: Assessment and informational interventions. Oncology Nursing Forum, *9*(3):39–44, 1982.

Dodd, M. J. and Mood, D. W.: Chemotherapy: Helping patients to know the drugs they are receiving and their possible side effects. Cancer Nursing, *4*(4):311–318, 1981.

Dorr, T. T. and Fritz, W. L.: Cancer Chemotherapy Handbook. New York, Elsevier, 1980.

Esparza, D. M. and Weyland, J. B.: Nursing care for the patient with an Ommaya reservoir. Oncology Nursing Forum, *9*(4):17–20, 1982.

Garvey, E. C. and Manganaro, M.: Nursing implications of hepatic artery infusion. Cancer Nursing, *5*(1):51–55, 1982.

Jenkins, J. F., Hubbard, S. M., and Howser, D. M.: Managing intraperitoneal chemotherapy. Nursing 82, *12*(5):76–83, 1982.

Knobf, T.: Intravenous therapy guidelines for oncology practice. Oncology Nursing Forum, *9*(2):30–34, 1982.

Knobf, T., Fischer, D. S., and Welsh-McCaffrey, D.: Cancer Chemotherapy Treatment and Care, 2nd ed. Boston, G.K. Hall Medical Publishers, 1984.

Krakoff, I. H.: Cancer chemotherapeutic agents. Ca—A Cancer Journal for Clinicians, *31*(3):4–14, 1981.

Marino, L. B.: Cancer Nursing. St. Louis, C. V. Mosby Co., 1981.

McNally, J. C., Stair, J. C., and Somerville, E. T. (eds.): Guidelines for Cancer Nursing Practice. New York, Grune & Stratton, 1985.

Oncology Nursing Society and American Nurses' Association: Outcome standards for cancer nursing practice. Kansas City, American Nurses' Association, 1979.

Oncology Nursing Society and American Nurses' Association: Outcome standards for public cancer education. Kansas City, American Nurses' Association, 1983.

Trester, A. K.: Nursing management of patients receiving cancer chemotherapy. Cancer Nursing, *5*(3):201–210, 1982.

Walter, J.: Care of the patient receiving antineoplastic drugs. Nursing Clinics of North America, *17*(4):607–629, 1982.

Winters, V.: Implantable vascular access devices. Oncology Nursing Forum, *11*(6):25–30, 1984.

Yasko, J. M.: Guidelines for Cancer Care: Symptom Management. Reston, VA, Reston Publishing Company, 1983.

25

Investigational Cancer Treatment Modalities

DEBORAH K. MAYER, RN, MSN, CRNP, OCN
ROBERTA STROHL, RN, MN

IMMUNOTHERAPY

A. Based on association of immune system and the development of cancers (see Chapter 3). Crude immunotherapeutic agents used as stimulants capable of augmenting a variety of immune functions. Often referred to as the fourth cancer treatment modality.
B. Immunotherapy began in the late 1960's after positive results in improving survival in childhood leukemia were reported when bacille Calmette-Guérin (BCG) was administered.
C. A variety of agents were used in clinical trials in the 1970's with mixed results. Problems were related to study design, and to a lack of relatively pure and consistent immunotherapeutic agents. Interrelationships and control mechanisms of agents on immune system are not clear.
D. Major classifications of immunotherapeutic agents included:
1. Active specific—administration of tumor-related (antigens) vaccines, which were modified in vitro to stimulate the immune system.
2. Active nonspecific—administration of bacterial vaccine to boost overall immune system (e.g., BCG, MER [methanol extraction residue], C. parvum [Corynebacterium parvum], levamisole).
3. Passive—serotherapy when immune serum or antitumor lymphocytes are infused; effects are usually transient in nature.
4. Adoptive—transfer of extracts from sensitized lymphocytes; effects are more lasting in nature.
E. Administration may be oral, intralesional, intradermal, intravenous, or intravesical.
F. Side effects may be local, systemic, or allergic.

237

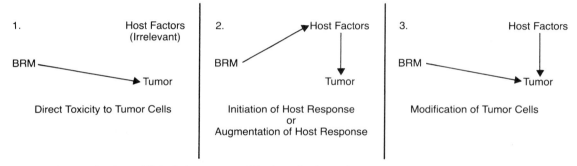

Figure 25–1. *Mechanisms of biological response modifications. (Redrawn from Scogna, D., and Schoenberger, C.: Biological response modifiers: an overview and nursing implications. Oncology Nursing Forum, 9(1):47, 1982.)*

BIOLOGIC RESPONSE MODIFIERS (BRM)

A. BRM are agents or approaches that modify the relationship between tumor and host (with resultant therapeutic benefit intended). Overall mechanisms of action are outlined in Figure 25–1.

B. Refinement and evolution of immunotherapy to BRM is related to scientific advances in genetic engineering and hybridoma technology. This has made production of large amounts of relatively pure and well defined biologic agents possible for clinical trials in the 1980's. Interferons are the prototype BRM.

C. Major classifications include:
   1. Immunomodulating agents.
   2. Interferons and interferon inducers.
   3. Thymosins.
   4. Lymphokines and cytokines.
   5. Antigens.
   6. Effector cells.
   7. Monoclonal antibodies.
   8. Miscellaneous approaches.
      See Table 25–1 for a more complete listing of specific BRM agents.

D. Administration may be oral, intralesional, intradermal, intravenous, or intravesical.

E. Side effects may be local, systemic, or allergic.

HYPERTHERMIA

A. Hyperthermia is the use of artificially induced high temperatures to treat cancer. Historically, it is based on clinical observation of tumor regression in febrile patients.

B. Rationale for use:
   1. Heat kills tumor cells; it inhibits production of DNA, RNA, and protein. Tumor cells lack ability to repair DNA damaged by heat. Difference in blood supply and vascular dynamics of tumor causes tumor to lack capacity for heat dissipation. Tumors may be necrotic and outgrow blood supply, which leads to heat trapping in tumor and sparing of normal tissue.
   2. Cells in relatively radioresistant S phase are killed and radiosensitized by heat.

Table 25–1. BIOLOGICALS AND BIOLOGICAL
RESPONSE MODIFIERS*

Immunomodulating Agents	Chalones
Alkyl lysophospholipids (ALP)	Colony-stimulating factor (CSF)
Azimexon	Growth factors (transforming growth
BCG	factor-TGF)
Bestatin	Lymphocyte activation factor
Brucella abortus	[LAF-interleukin 1 (IL-1)]
Corynebacterium parvum	Lymphotoxin
Cimetidine	Macrophage activation factor (MAF)
Sodium diethyldithiocarbamate (DTC)	Macrophage chemotactic factor
Endotoxin	Macrophage cytotoxic factor (MCF)
Glucan	Macrophage growth factor (MGF)
"Immune" RNAs	Migration inhibitory factor (MIF)
Krestin	Maturation factors
Lentinan	T-cell growth factor [TCGF-interleukin 2
Levamisole	(IL-2)]
Muramyldipeptide (MDP)	Interleukin 3 (IL-3)
Maleic anhydride-divinyl ether (MVE-2)	T-cell replacing factor (TRF)
Mixed bacterial vaccines	Thymocyte mitogenic factor (TMF)
N-137	Transfer factor
Nocardia rubra cell wall skeleton (CWS)	B-cell growth factor (BCGF)
Picibanil (OK432)	Tumor necrosis factor (TNF)
Prostaglandin inhibitors (aspirin,	**Antigens**
indomethacin)	Tumor-associated antigens
Thiabendazole	Vaccines
Tuftsin	**Effector Cells**
Interferons and Interferon Inducers	Macrophages
Interferons (alpha, beta, and gamma)	NK cells
Poly IC–LC	Cytotoxic T-cell clones
Poly A:U	T-helper cells
Tilorone	**Miscellaneous Approaches**
Brucella abortus	Allogeneic immunization
Viruses	Liposome-encapsulated biologicals
Pyrimidines	Bone marrow transplantation and
Thymosins	reconstitution
Thymosin alpha-1	Plasmapheresis and ex vivo treatments
Other thymic factors	(activation columns and
Thymosin fraction V	immunoabsorbents)
Lymphokines and Cytokines	Virus infection of cells (oncolysates)
Antigrowth factors	

* From Oldham, R. and Smalley, R.: Biologicals and biological response modifiers. *In* DeVita,
V., Hellman, S. and Rosenberg, S. (eds.): Cancer Principles and Practices of Oncology. Philadelphia,
J. B. Lippincott, p. 2224, 1985.

3. Hypoxic tumor cells may be more sensitive to heat. Altered metabolism
   (anaerobic) in tumor may exist because of hypoxic state. Heat increases
   cells' need for O_2 by increasing metabolic rate, which blood supply cannot
   meet.
4. Heat inhibits repair of radiation damage thereby increasing radiation effect. Heat prevents repair of single-stranded DNA breaks and chromosomal alterations.
5. Addition of hyperthermia to chemotherapy may enhance cell killing potential. Local heat can increase effect of chemotherapy in area of tumor
   by increasing blood supply. May increase permeability of cell membrane
   to allow greater drug penetration. Heat inhibits repair of damage.

6. Heat is not mutagenic.
7. Heat may stimulate immune system.
8. Heating chemicals that are not cytotoxic at 37°C may create cytotoxic agents at higher temperatures. Amphotericin B and lidocaine have been used in animal studies.

C. Historical background.
1. Reports as early as 1891 noting regression of inoperable tumors in febrile patients. Trials began in artificially raising temperature to induce tumor regression.
2. Fever therapy used in benign diseases such as syphilis and gonorrhea.
3. Whole body hyperthermia used in 1935 by Warren for patients with advanced disease.
4. Problem was in the development of technology to deliver heat to tumor in a consistent and regulated manner while sparing the surrounding normal tissue. Problems also exist in recording dosimetry of heat effect.

D. Therapeutic range.
1. Temperatures in range of 41–45°C used in most clinical trials.
2. Controversies exist relating to timing of heat (before, during, after) other treatments such as radiation, length of heating, number of times heat should be administered.

E. Delivery systems.
1. Local, regional, or whole body hyperthermia may be delivered.
2. Local, regional heating may be produced by radiofrequency, microwaves, or ultrasound. Heat is produced by molecular motion in tissue. Probes may be inserted into the tumor or the patient may sit in a cylindrical machine. Ultrasound uses a transducer. Penetration depends on frequency and tissue composition; ultrasound waves will not penetrate bone. Regional heating has been tried using heated blood for treatment of extremities. Limb may be isolated with a tourniquet. Perfusing organs with heated solution has been used (hot bladder irrigation).
3. Problems include need for invasive probes to measure temperature and possible development of thermal tolerance.
4. Whole body hyperthermia is used to treat widespread disease. Temperature does not go above 42°C (may cause heat necrosis). Patient may be immersed in heated water, hot paraffin wax, or in a heated suit. May require sedation and fluid replacement.

F. Patient care issues (See Nursing Management of Persons Receiving Investigational Cancer Treatment Modalities). Patient problems in whole body treatment may include:
1. Fatigue.
2. Hypotension.
3. Peripheral neuropathy.
4. Nausea.
5. Vomiting.
6. Diarrhea.
7. Hypomagnesemia and hypophosphatemia.

G. General patient care guidelines (local or regional and whole body hyperthermia):
1. Patient should demonstrate understanding of rationale for treatment and method of heating. (Specific information will depend on what type of heating is done.)

2. If probe is used and is kept in place, a dry dressing is applied. Patient should not shower and should inspect site for infection.
3. Void before treatment if bladder is to be heated. (Heating of urine may lead to neurogenic bladder.) Prevent constipation, as heat may be retained in stool.
4. Observe patient during treatment. If patient is isolated (some microwave units require patient to be in an enclosure as waves are not in FCC frequency), assure patient that he or she is being carefully monitored.
5. Encourage fluid intake after treatment.
6. Encourage rest if fatigue is present.

NURSING MANAGEMENT OF PERSONS RECEIVING INVESTIGATIONAL CANCER TREATMENT MODALITIES

A. Provide information.
   1. Understand purpose of research protocol.
   2. Assess individual's and family's understanding of treatment and anticipated side effects to ensure adequacy of informed consent (this should be done initially and periodically throughout treatment course); provide a copy of consent form.
   3. Provide information to individual and family about management of treatment-related effects to promote self-care.
   4. Instruct patient and family in documenting and reporting treatment-related effects.
   5. Instruct patient, family member, or other health care professional in treatment administration if off-site administration is planned.
B. Administer investigational therapy.
   1. Verify that informed consent has been obtained.
   2. Assess parameters (e.g., laboratory studies, clinical) prior to administration.
   3. Ensure availability of emergency support equipment and medications.
   4. Verify treatment orders.
   5. Premedicate if required.
   6. Administer treatment.
   7. Coordinate off-site treatment administration when necessary.
C. Monitor and manage treatment-related effects.
   1. Check investigational protocol for monitoring requirements (e.g., vital signs, lab studies).
   2. Monitor vital signs (particularly blood pressure), treatment site(s), systemic symptoms, allergic responses (particularly anaphylactic or anaphylactoid reactions).
   3. Monitor tumor response if appropriate (e.g., change in tumor size, tumor-associated symptoms).
   4. Management of local reactions to BRM (erythema, induration, pruritus, drainage)—instruct patient to keep site clean and dry for 24 hours after administration, wear loose fitting clothing, avoid scratching, and avoid use of creams or lotions unless prescribed.
   5. Management of systemic reactions to BRM (flu-like syndrome including fever, chills, myalgia, headache, fatigue, anorexia)—increase fluid intake to 2–3 L/d, administer acetaminophen for fever reduction and analgesia,

Table 25–2. CARE PLAN FOR PATIENT RECEIVING IFN*†

Nursing Diagnosis	Expected Patient Outcome	Nursing Intervention
Knowledge deficit related to new cancer therapy with IFN	Patient will have adequate information to be able to participate in decision making and self care	Make sure patient has a copy of consent form Explain plans for treatment Encourage and answer questions Review expected side effects and self-care measures to deal with them Have family member present, if possible Give written material to reinforce verbal information
Altered protective mechanisms with fever and chills related to IFN therapy	Patient will manage measures to prevent or treat fever and chills	Acetaminophen q.4° or p.r.n. (No ASA or NSAID products allowed) while chilled: Have patient wear socks, hats Have extra blankets available Have hypothermia blanket available for T > 105°F Use cool sponging for prolonged elevated temperatures Monitor for cardiovascular changes: Observe changes in v.s., obtain EKG for chest pain, irregular pulses Monitor for CNS change: somnolence, confusion, seizures Maintain intake > 3 L/day to prevent dehydration during febrile episodes Monitor intake and output on treatment days Monitor vital signs regularly
Potential alteration in comfort related to myalgias and headaches secondary to IFN therapy	Patient will identify and manage factors to influence comfort	Acetaminophen q.4° or p.r.n. Tylox or Percoset if more severe Place cool compresses on forehead Avoid use of aspirin-containing products Use of heat and/or massage to relieve symptoms Darken room if photophobia develops
Potential alteration in nutrition related to anorexia, occasional nausea and vomiting secondary to IFN therapy	Patient will identify and manage factors to maintain adequate nutritional status without weight loss	Monitor weight regularly (3 times per week) Instruct patient in ways to increase caloric and protein intake, and stress importance to eat despite anorexia Offer small, frequent meals Try to maintain fluid intake ≥ 3 L/day (p.o. or i.v.) Use antiemetics as needed Reassure patient that symptoms are not necessarily related to tumor progression Dietary consult p.r.n.
Potential alteration in protective mechanisms related to leukopenia and/or thrombocytopenia secondary to IFN therapy	Patient will identify and manage factors to prevent infection or bleeding and/or report early signs	Instruct patient about bleeding precautions if platelet count ≤ 50,000 Instruct patient to report signs or symptoms of infection, bleeding Have patient monitor temperature, report if > 101°F on nontreatment days Pressure at injection sites if platelet count < 50,000 Assess respiratory, urinary, integumentary systems for possible infection, bleeding Strict handwashing

Table 25–2. CARE PLAN FOR PATIENT RECEIVING IFN*†
(*continued*)

Nursing Diagnosis	Expected Patient Outcome	Nursing Intervention
Potential alteration in mobility related to fatigue secondary to IFN therapy	Patient will maintain activities of daily living and prevent sequelae from prolonged bedrest	Instruct patient to arrange most important activities in morning Allow for frequent rest periods Encourage patient to maintain mobility with frequent change in positions, sitting out of bed, ambulation TCDB q.2° if bedridden Range of motion if mobility is compromised Reassure patient that fatigue is not necessarily related to tumor progression
Potential alteration in coping related to changes in disease status and new therapy	Patient will manage stress to facilitate his/her own coping strategies	Encourage verbalization Encourage use of available resources, i.e., support groups, chaplain, social worker Instruct in use of relaxation techniques Social work or psychology consult p.r.n.

* Based on the ONS/ANA *Outcome Standards for Cancer Nursing Practice*, 1979.
† From Mayer, D. and Smalley, R.: Interferon: Current status. Oncology Nursing Forum, *10*(4):18–19, 1983.

provide adequate rest periods, provide adequate nutrition to maintain weight (may need dietary adjustments for anorexia).

6. Management of allergic reactions to BRM (urticaria, pruritus, dyspnea, hypotension, tachycardia)—premedicate if indicated, have emergency medications available, monitor closely during administration and for the first hour after treatment administration, notify physician at first signs of systemic allergic response.

D. Document treatment and treatment effects.
   1. Document questions, concerns, or comments individual and family member express.
   2. Document treatment administration (dose, route, site, time, other associated medications).
   3. Document short- and long-term side effects (description of type, quantity, quality, duration, aggravating or alleviating factors). Have individual keep own records if outpatient to assist in monitoring and documenting.
   4. Document tumor response if appropriate.

   See Table 25–2 for sample care plan of an individual receiving an interferon.

STUDY QUESTIONS

1. Describe the major nursing responsibilities when administering investigational cancer treatments.
2. Explain the rationale for the use of hyperthermia in the treatment of cancer.
3. Explain the rationale for the use of biologic response modifiers in the treatment of cancer.
4. Identify the commonly anticipated toxicities of hyperthermia.
5. Identify the commonly anticipated toxicities of biologic response modifiers.
6. Develop a nursing care plan for an individual receiving hyperthermia.
7. Develop a nursing care plan for an individual receiving a biologic response modifier.

Bibliography

Bull, J.: An update on the anticancer effects of a combination of chemotherapy and hyperthermia. Cancer Research (suppl), 44:4853–4856, 1984.

Cox, K. and Ern, M.: Immunology immunotherapy II. Cancer Nursing, 3:307–321, 1980.

DiJulio, J. and Bedigan, J.: Hybridoma monoclonal antibody treatment of T-cell lymphomas: Clinical experience and nursing management. Oncology Nursing Forum, 10(2):22–27, 1983.

Ern, M.: Immunology immunotherapy I. Cancer Nursing, 3:229–238, 1980.

Hall, E. and Towle-Roizin, L.: Biological effects of heat. Cancer Research (Suppl), 44:4708–4713, 1984.

Jeffs, C. and Laszlo, J.: A coordinating role for the nurse clinician in a phase I interferon study. Cancer Nursing, 6:379–386, 1983.

Hahn, G.: Hyperthermia and Cancer. New York, Plenum Press, 1982.

Hersh, E.: New cancer immunobiology—an overview. The Cancer Bulletin, 33(5):187–191, 1981.

Hubbard, S.: Principles of clinical research. In Johnson, B. and Gross, J. (eds.): Handbook of Oncology Nursing. New York, John Wiley and Sons, pp. 67–91, 1985.

Kirkwood, J. and Ernstoff, M.: Interferons in the treatment of cancer. Journal of Clinical Oncology, 2:336–352, 1984.

Klimaszewski, A.: Knowledge deficit related to immunotherapy. In McNally, J., Stair, J., and Somerville, E. (eds.): Guidelines for Clinical Practice of Oncology Nursing. New York, Grune & Stratton, pp. 50–53, 1985.

Mayer, D., Hetrick, K., Riggs, C., and Sherwin, S.: Weight loss in patients receiving recombinant leukocyte A interferon: A brief report. Cancer Nursing, 7:53–56, 1984.

Mayer, D. and Smalley, R.: Interferon: Current status. Oncology Nursing Forum, 10(4):14–19, 1983.

Miller, R., Conner, W., Heusinkveld, R., and Boone, M.: Prospects for hyperthermia in human cancer therapy. Radiology, 123:489–495, 1977.

Moldawer, N. and Murray, J.: The clinical uses of monoclonal antibodies in cancer research. Cancer Nursing, 8:207–213, 1985.

Moore, C.: Hyperthermia: A modern experiment in cancer treatment. Oncology Nursing Forum, 11:31–37, 1984.

Moore, C.: Nursing management of the patient receiving local or regional hyperthermia. Oncology Nursing Forum, 11:40–45, 1984.

Oldham, R.: Monoclonal antibodies in cancer therapy. Journal of Clinical Oncology, 1:582–590, 1983.

Oldham, R. and Smalley, R.: Biologicals and biological response modifiers. In DeVita, V., Hellman, S., and Rosenberg, S. (eds.): Cancer Principles and Practices of Oncology. Philadelphia, J. B. Lippincott, pp. 2223–2245, 1985.

Pestka, S.: The purification and manufacture of human interferons. Scientific American, 249(2):36–43, 1983.

Scogna, D. and Schoenberger, C.: Biological response modifiers: An overview and nursing implications. Oncology Nursing Forum, 9(1):45–49, 1982.

Suppers, V. and McClamrock, E.: Biologicals in cancer treatment: Future effects on nursing practice. Oncology Nursing Forum, 12(3):27–32, 1985.

26

Nutrition

ARLENE GORDON, RN, MSN

EFFECTS OF CANCER ON THE NUTRITIONAL STATUS

A. Overt malnutrition is seen in approximately 40% of patients hospitalized for cancer treatment. The exact mechanism of metabolic demands made on the body by the tumor is unknown. There is, however, a competition for essential nutrients that exists between the tumor and host. The tumor utilizes specific nutrients that may contribute to cachexia. The constant nutritional and metabolic demands result in:
   1. Increase in basal metabolic rate, thereby leading to increase in energy expenditure.
   2. Increased utilization of protein stores.
   3. Increased utilization of fat stores.
B. Alteration of CHO metabolism.
   1. Purpose is to produce energy.
   2. Energy production is achieved by two metabolic processes.
      a. Process of glycolysis:
         (1) Glycolysis = glucose converts to lactic acid and pyruvic acid; lactic acid released into blood stream → production of energy.
         (2) Not the most efficient means of energy production.
      b. Process of oxidation of hydrogen atoms:
         (1) Glucose molecule oxidized to acetic acid. Acetic acid is broken down to carbon dioxide and hydrogen. Hydrogen ion is oxidized to release energy in the form of ATP.
         (2) This is the most efficient process for energy production.
      c. Patient with cancer will utilize the least efficient process for energy production; therefore, metabolic demand for CHO production is decreased.
      d. To compensate for inefficiency, gluconeogenesis provides additional glucose for CHO metabolism.
         (1) Gluconeogenesis = synthesis of glucose in liver and renal cortex from lactic acid and amino acids.

        (2) Glucose is then released to cells and tumor.

        (3) Gluconeogenesis process is accelerated beyond the norm, thereby contributing to protein-calorie malnutrition.

C. Alteration in protein metabolism.

  1. Protein normally present in muscle tissue is broken down to be utilized as glucose (energy source) → wasting of skeletal muscle.

  2. Patient with cancer also has decrease in protein synthesis due to alteration in regulatory mechanism of insulin.

    a. Normally insulin facilitates the synthesis of protein from amino acids.

    b. Patient with cancer has an abnormal glucose tolerance and cannot appropriately utilize insulin to control blood sugar levels or facilitate protein synthesis.

  3. Protein loss is clinically described in terms of nitrogen.

  4. Effects of negative nitrogen balance can lead to:

    a. Anemia.

    b. Muscle wasting.

    c. Weakness.

    d. Increased susceptibility to infection.

    e. Impaired wound healing.

    f. Decubiti.

    g. Edema of gastrointestinal tract.

D. Alteration in fat metabolism.

  1. Fat is normally stored in adipose tissue in the form of triglycerides; it is composed of fatty acids.

  2. Patient with cancer undergoes lipolysis, a process of mobilization of fatty acids → blood stream to be used for energy.

    a. Normally insulin inhibits this occurrence.

    b. Patient with cancer with an alteration in insulin utilization aggravates lipolysis, causing a depletion of body fat.

E. Cachexia.

  1. Symptoms:

    a. Anorexia.

    b. Wasting of tissues (usually muscle and fat).

    c. Excess metabolism of nutrients.

    d. Weight loss.

  2. Characterized by nutritional depletion despite normal or increased food intake.

  3. If cancer treated successfully, cachexia will disappear.

F. Anorexia due to disease process.

  1. Anorexia is a loss of appetite.

  2. Physiologic factors of anorexia:

    a. Delayed digestion due to atrophic changes of the gastrointestinal tract.

    b. Metabolites (peptides and oligonucleotides), end products of the cancer cells, are destroyed by treatment modalities.

    c. General side effects of treatment: nausea and vomiting, diarrhea, oral irritations, and irritation after surgery of the gastrointestinal tract.

    d. Alterations in taste.

  3. Psychosocial factors that contribute to anorexia:

    a. Depression.

    b. Pain.

    c. Anxiety.

      d. Fatigue.
      e. Fear.
      f. Anger.
      g. Insomnia.
      h. Hospital environment.
      i. Variance of ethnic and cultural food preferences.

G. Mechanical interference due to tumor.
  1. Head and neck tumors:
      a. May have difficulty chewing and swallowing.
      b. Pain associated with tumor.
  2. Esophageal tumors: dysphagia with solid foods.
  3. Stomach and small bowel tumors:
      a. Persistent vomiting → decreased fluid and electrolytes.
      b. Ascites.
      c. Protein losing enteropathy → direct loss of serum protein.
         (1) Small bowel lymphoma.
         (2) Intestinal mucosal atrophy → diarrhea.
  4. Biliary and pancreatic obstruction:
      a. Malabsorption of fat.
      b. Steatorrhea.
      c. Deficiencies of calcium uptake from fat-soluble vitamins and electrolytes.
  5. Hepatocellular cancer:
      a. Anorexia.
      b. Protein depletion.
  6. Paraendocrine syndromes:
      a. Production of parathyroid substances.
           Hypercalcemia → anorexia, nausea and vomiting.
      b. Gastrointestinal and lung tumors.
           Increased production of gastrin → peptic ulcer.
      c. Diarrhea and pellagra.
      d. Thyroid tumors.
           Secrete calcitonin → diarrhea.

EFFECTS OF CANCER THERAPY ON NUTRITIONAL STATUS

A. Complications or side effects of cancer therapy can adversely affect the nutritional status. It is essential that patients are adequately supported nutritionally before, during, and after therapy. Nutritional requirements of the surgical patient:
  1. Increased need for CHO due to increased energy expenditure.
  2. Increased need for protein to assist with tissue repair and wound healing.
      a. Decrease in visceral protein stores.
      b. Increased risk of infection.
      c. Increase in gluconeogenesis → nitrogen loss.
  3. Specific surgical interventions.
      a. Radical head and neck resection:
         (1) Loss of normal mastication and deglutition.
         (2) Management: soft → liquid diets, tube feeding (TF).

Table 26–1. NUTRITIONAL COMPLICATIONS
OF RADIATION

Anatomic Site	Adverse Effect	Nursing Management
Head and Neck	Anorexia	Small frequent meals high in protein and calories
		Pleasant atmosphere
		Wine or beer (with physician's approval) may stimulate appetite
		Serve meals attractively
		Exercise before meals
		Eat with family or friends
		Avoid fluids at mealtime
	Taste alteration	Experiment with herbs and spices
		Experiment with high protein and calorie foods; add fruits and sauces to desserts
		If food aversions develop, try bland high calorie and protein foods: cheese, peanut butter, ice cream, gelatin salads
	Dry mouth	Eat moist, cool, bland foods and liquids
		Moisten foods with gravies, broth, sauces
		Hard (sugar-free) candy or gum
		Popsicles
		Artificial saliva
		Avoid hot, spicy foods
	Mucositis/ gingivitis	Soft, bland, cool foods
		Small, frequent meals
		Avoid acidic, spicy foods and beverages
		Force fluids
		Frequent mouth rinses with warm normal saline
		Brush teeth with soft toothbrush
		Keep lips moist
		Analgesics per physician order for relief of pain
		Solution of 40 ml 2% viscous Xylocaine, 40 ml Benadryl (12.5 mg/5 ml), 40 ml Maalox, to relieve pain
	Dysphagia	Depending on extent, food should be soft and cooked well
		Sauces, gravies to moisten food
		Liquids high in calories and protein
		Pureed foods may be necessary
		Avoid hard, dry foods
	Dental caries	Dental consultation
		Frequent fluoride treatment (daily)
		Avoid high sugar intake
		Good oral hygiene after each meal and at bedtime
Thorax	Esophagitis	Analgesics to relieve discomfort
		Use mixture of 40 ml viscous Xylocaine, 40 ml Benadryl, 40 ml Maalox, before meals
		Bland, soft, cool foods and liquids
		Foods high in protein and calories
	Indigestion	Avoid overeating
		Avoid spicy foods
		Bland diet
		Small, frequent meals
	Fatigue	Rest when fatigue is experienced
		Avoid doing too much at one time
		Seek help with household duties
		Maintain optimal nutrition

Table 26–1. NUTRITIONAL COMPLICATIONS
OF RADIATION (*continued*)

Anatomic Site	Adverse Effect	Nursing Management
Abdomen and Pelvis	Nausea and vomiting	Small, frequent feedings, eaten slowly
		Carbonated beverages
		Clear liquids
		Bland, cool foods
		Sour foods sometimes desirable
		Rest after meals
		Avoid sweet, spicy, salty, or fatty foods
		Avoid foods with strong odors
		Keep environment pleasant
		Antiemetics per physician's order
	Diarrhea	Eat smaller portions of food
		Avoid extremely hot or cold beverages, which tend to increase intestinal motility
		Decrease roughage
		Encourage fluid intake, avoiding acidic beverages
		Encourage potassium-rich foods
		Low residue diet high in protein and calories
		Avoid milk products
		Avoid caffeine
		Antidiarrheal agents per physician's order
	Acute enteritis	Low residue, low fat, gluten and milk-free liquid diet
		Elemental diets
		Antidiarrheal agents, corticosteroids per physician's order
	Fistulas	Bowel rest with TPN
		Elemental diet
		Surgery

b. Esophagectomy with reconstruction:
   (1) Gastric stasis, malabsorption of fat.
   (2) Management: long term TF.
c. Gastrectomy:
   (1) Fat and protein malabsorption.
   (2) Vitamin and iron deficiencies.
   (3) Dumping syndrome.
   (4) Hypoglycemia.
   (5) Management: small frequent feedings, parenteral vitamin B_{12}, increased protein and fat, low CHO diet.
d. Pancreatectomy:
   (1) Protein and fat malabsorption.
   (2) Vitamin and mineral deficiencies.
   (3) Diabetes mellitus.
   (4) Fistulas.
   (5) Management: pancreatic extract, vitamin and mineral supplements, insulin.
e. Proximal small bowel resection:
   (1) Protein and fat malabsorption.
   (2) Vitamin and mineral deficiencies.

        (3) Management: high protein diet, pancreatic extracts may be indicated, vitamin supplements.

    f. Distal small bowel/colon resection:

        (1) Diarrhea due to bile salt malabsorption.

        (2) Vitamin B_{12} malabsorption.

        (3) Fluid and electrolyte loss.

        (4) Management: parenteral vitamin B_{12}, high protein diet.

    g. Urinary diversion:

        (1) Acid-base imbalances due to renal deterioration.

        (2) Electrolyte abnormalities (decreased potassium).

        (3) Management: no specific nutritional intervention is necessary.

B. Nutritional requirements of the patient receiving radiation therapy.

  1. Increased need for protein/calorie intake to aid in repair of normal cells within the treatment field.

  2. Side effects of radiation as it relates to altering nutritional status are directly associated with the specific anatomic treatment site (Table 26–1).

  3. Head and neck irradiation:

    a. Anorexia.

    b. Taste alterations (mouth blindness).

    c. Dry mouth.

    d. Mucositis.

    e. Gingivitis.

    f. Dysphagia.

    g. Trismus.

    h. Dental caries.

  4. Thoracic irradiation:

    a. Esophagitis.

    b. Dysphagia.

    c. Indigestion or nausea.

    d. Fatigue.

  5. Abdominal and pelvic irradiation:

    a. Nausea and vomiting.

    b. Anorexia.

    c. Diarrhea.

    d. Acute enteritis.

    e. Fistulas.

C. Nutritional requirements of the patient receiving chemotherapy:

  1. Increased need for protein/calorie intake to aid in the repair of normal tissues.

  2. Nutritional status may influence the result of chemotherapy; a well-nourished patient can withstand a more aggressive treatment.

  3. Nutritional alterations are dependent on:

    a. Class of drug being given.

    b. Dose of drug.

    c. Combination of drugs.

    d. Combination of treatment modalities.

  4. Side effects of chemotherapy that may alter nutritional status (see Tables 26–1 and 26–2 for specific nursing interventions):

    a. Nausea and vomiting (most common side effect of chemotherapy).

    b. Anorexia.

    c. Diarrhea.

Table 26–2. NUTRITIONAL COMPLICATIONS OF CHEMOTHERAPY

Side Effect	Chemotherapeutic Agents	Nursing Management
Nausea and vomiting	All major classes of chemotherapeutic agents have potential	Give antiemetic prior to, during, and on a regular schedule after chemotherapeutic agent is administered
Anorexia	All chemotherapeutic agents may cause some degree of anorexia	See Table 26–1
Diarrhea	*Most common* 5-fluorouracil, actinomycin D, methyl glyoxal bisguanylhydrazone *May occur* with methotrexate, hydroxyurea, BCNU, CCNU, Methyl CCNU, 5-azacytidine, Adriamycin, 6-Mecaptapurine, cyclophosphamide, procarbazine	See Table 26–1
Stomatitis	Antimetabolites (Methotrexate, 5-fluorouracil) Antibiotics (anthracyclines, bleomycin, actinomycin)	See Table 26–1
Taste alterations	Methotrexate, cyclophosphamide, nitrogen mustard, Actinomycin D	See Table 26–1

    d. Stomatitis.

    e. Taste alterations (methotrexate, cyclophosphamide, nitrogen mustard, actinomycin D).

NUTRITIONAL ASSESSMENT

A. Nutritional assessment is the first step in the detection and treatment of malnutrition. There remains a controversy as to the value of each specific measurement; however, when all nutritional parameters are considered, a reliable picture of the nutritional status becomes evident.

B. Parameters to evaluate nutritional status:

    1. Assessing somatic protein compartment (body mass).

        a. Patient's weight is evaluated based on height by comparing it to a standard height/weight table (ideal weight).

        b. Percentage of ideal body weight is calculated by:

$$\% \text{ ideal body weight} = \text{actual weight/ideal weight} \times 100$$

        c. Present body weight compared to usual body weight (weight prior to cancer diagnosis):

$$\% \text{ usual weight} = \text{actual weight/usual weight} \times 100$$

        If patient has lost greater than 10% of usual body weight, this is significant.

        d. Changes in fit of clothing.

    2. Diet history.

        a. Usual daily diet (24 hour recall of food).

        b. Food preferences.

    c. Recent cancer treatments.
    d. Food intake problems due to side effects of treatment (see Tables 26–1 and 26–2).
    e. Problems with dentures or teeth.
    f. Current medications.
3. Anthropometric measurements.
    a. Mid-arm circumference to assess muscle mass.
    b. Tricep skinfold thickness to assess fat stores.
4. Visceral protein stores.
    a. Serum albumin to assess protein status.
    b. Serum transferrin to assess protein status.
    c. Total lymphocyte count to assess immunosuppression, which may be secondary to protein malnutrition.
    d. Cell-mediated immunity to assess the function of the immune system via a battery of skin tests.
    e. Nitrogen balance to assess energy balance. Protein ingested should be greater than that excreted; it is measured via a 24-hour urine specimen.
5. Somatic protein stores.
    a. Creatinine height index to assess somatic protein stores via a 24-hour urine specimen.
6. Other laboratory measurements.
    a. Hemoglobin and hematocrit. Anemia usually accompanies protein deficiency.

NUTRITIONAL SUPPORT MODALITIES

A. If aggressive anticancer therapy is indicated, then the person should aggressively be supported nutritionally using the appropriate modality. The goal is to maintain optimal nutritional status so that surgery, chemotherapy, and/or radiation therapy can be undertaken and tolerated with maximal benefit.
B. Selecting the appropriate nutritional modality.
  1. Oral route.
    a. Side effects of disease or treatment may alter nutritional intake via oral route (see Tables 26–1 and 26–2).

Table 26–3. NURSING INTERVENTIONS FOR COMPLICATIONS OF PPN

Complication	Nursing Intervention
Thrombophlebitis	Infuse fat emulsion and dextrose/amino acid solution simultaneously to decrease osmolarity of the solution Infuse products through separate infusion pumps or controllers Rotate I.V. site and change peripheral dressing per hospital procedure, noting signs and symptoms of redness, tenderness, or swelling
Fluid overload	Carefully monitor infusion using a volumetric pump or controller Average rate of infusion: 1,500 cc. over 12–24 hours Maintain accurate record of intake and output and daily weights
Hyperglycemia	Although rare, test patient's urine q 6 h for sugar and acetone Observe patient for signs and symptoms of hyperglycemia Monitor serum glucose levels

   b. Nursing interventions for oral route:
      (1) Relax dietary restrictions.
      (2) Emphasize high protein, high calorie diet.
      (3) Fortify diet with natural or commercial food sources.
      (4) Conduct patient teaching regarding high protein, high calorie diet.
      (5) Complete daily calorie counts with nutritional assessment.
   c. If oral route is not tolerated, another method of nutritional support must be explored.
2. Peripheral parenteral nutrition (PPN).
   a. Indicated if oral intake is interrupted temporarily (5–7 days).
   b. PPN solution.
      (1) 5% dextrose and water, 4.5% amino acid electrolytes and vitamins provides protein and calories.
      (2) Fat emulsion 10% or 20% provides fat source and major calorie source.
      (3) Solutions are administered simultaneously via peripheral vein.
   c. Complications (see Table 26–3).
3. Enteral route (tube feedings).
   a. Indications—if oral intake is not regained in 5–7 days and gastrointestinal tract is functional.

Table 26–4. NURSING INTERVENTIONS FOR
COMPLICATIONS OF ENTERAL FEEDING

Complication	Nursing Intervention
Nasogastric	
Malpositioned tube	Verify proper placement via chest x-ray
	Check placement each time before using by:
	Injecting air and auscultating over the stomach
	Aspirating gastric contents
	Observing for air bubbles by placing distal end of tube in water
	Tape tube securely to nose
Aspiration	Give bolus feeding rather than continuous feeding
	No more than 350–400 ml over 20 minutes q 3–4 hours while patient is awake. Initial volume is 240 ml
	Keep head of bed elevated 30° during and 1 hour after infusion
Contaminated equipment	Change feeding bag and tubing daily
Clogged tube	Flush NG tube with 30 ml of water or cranberry juice after each feeding
	If tube is clogged, flush with 30 ml cranberry juice with 1/4 tsp meat tenderizer
Abdominal distention, vomiting, cramping, diarrhea	Regulate infusion accurately over 20 minutes
	Give formula at room temperature
	May need to decrease volume of formula being given
Nasoduodenal	
Aspiration	Decreased risk of this occurring since tube is in the small bowel
	Should give continuous feeding rather than bolus
	Small bowel is sensitive to osmolarity; therefore, initial rate is 30–50 ml/hr of isotonic formula and increase by 25 ml/hr every 12 hours until desired volume is reached
Contaminated equipment	Amount of formula in the bag should not exceed what can be administered in 8 hours. Change entire administration set q 24 hours

Table 26–5. NURSING INTERVENTIONS FOR
COMPLICATIONS OF TPN

Complication	Nursing Intervention
Technical or Mechanical	
Pneumothorax	May occur during insertion of subclavian catheter
	Observe patient during insertion for chest pain, dyspnea, cyanosis
	Chest x-ray should be done after insertion to verify placement
	Blood return should be verified before connecting I.V. tubing to catheter
	$D_{10}W$ solution should be administered at 30 ml/hr until chest x-ray confirms placement
Arterial puncture	May occur during insertion
	Observe for bright red blood pulsating from catheter
	Patient may complain of pain at site
	Apply pressure to site for 15 minutes
Malpositioned catheter	Catheter may migrate from the superior vena cava to another vein. Patient may complain of neck and shoulder pain, swelling in the surrounding area
	Catheter placement should be confirmed by chest x-ray
Clotted catheter	Unable to infuse solution through catheter and unable to obtain blood return
	Declot catheter following hospital procedure
	Infuse $D_{10}W$ peripherally at the same rate as TPN to prevent hypoglycemia
Fluid overload	Infusion should be regulated on a volumetric pump for accuracy
	Time tape bottle, checking volume infused every hour
	Obtain daily weights
Air emboli	Secure all I.V. tubing connections with tape to prevent disconnection
	If air emboli are suspected, clamp tubing immediately and place patient on left side in Trendelenburg position
Metabolic	
Hyperglycemia	Increase rate of infusion gradually
	Check urine for sugar and acetone q 6 h
	Monitor serum glucose levels daily
Hypoglycemia	Observe for signs and symptoms of hypoglycemia
	Monitor serum glucose levels
	If sudden cessation of TPN occurs, infuse $D_{10}W$ peripherally at same rate as TPN
	Per physician's order, administer 50 ml of 50% dextrose I.V.
Infections	
Contaminated solution	Solution should not be left unrefrigerated for longer than 4 hours
	Check each bottle before and during infusion for color and clarity of solution
	Check bottle for cracks
Contaminated equipment	Change all I.V. tubing per hospital procedure, using aseptic technique
	Do not interrupt TPN for other infusions or blood-drawing
Local site infection	Change dressing using aseptic technique, following hospital procedure
	Observe site for redness, tenderness, swelling, and exudate
Fever	Monitor vital signs q 4 h
	Both peripheral and central line blood cultures should be obtained to identify source of infection

   b. Advantages:
      (1) Tube feeding maintains integrity of gastrointestinal tract.
      (2) More cost effective than PPN or TPN.
      (3) Patient comfort is enhanced owing to smaller, more pliable tubes.
   c. Common feeding routes (see Table 26–4):
      (1) Nasogastric—appropriate for short-term nutritional support.
      (2) Nasoduodenal—if patient cannot tolerate bolus feeding, is unable to remain elevated at 30°, or is susceptible to aspiration.
      (3) Gastrostomy—appropriate for long-term nutritional support or if a section of the gastrointestinal tract above stomach is obstructed. Bokes feeding may be given.
      (4) Jejunostomy—appropriate for long-term nutritional support or if a section of gastrointestinal tract above the jejunum is obstructed. Continuous 12–24 hour infusion must be administered rather than bolus.
   d. If patient's gastrointestinal tract is nonfunctional, total parenteral nutrition (TPN) should be considered.
4. Total parenteral nutrition (TPN).
   a. TPN solution.
      (1) Final concentration 25% dextrose and water, 4.25% amino acid, vitamins, trace elements, and electrolytes.
      (2) 1 liter provides approximately 1,200 calories.
      (3) Fat emulsion 10% or 20% may provide extra calories or prevent fatty acid deficiency.
   b. Complications associated with TPN (see Table 26–5):
      (1) Technical or mechanical problems.
      (2) Metabolic complications.
      (3) Infectious complications.

STUDY QUESTIONS

1. It is known that the effects of cancer treatment may alter the nutritional status. For each of the three major treatment modalities, surgery, radiation, and chemotherapy, choose one side effect and develop a brief nursing care plan of nutritional interventions to alleviate the side effect.
2. List and describe at least two nutritional assessment parameters.
3. What is the indication for selecting the enteral route as a nutritional modality?
4. Mr. C. has had his nasogastric tube in place for 2 days. After administration of his bolus feeding, he complained of abdominal fullness and cramping. What nursing interventions would you institute to alleviate this problem?

Bibliography

Carter, S.: Nutritional problems associated with cancer chemotherapy. *In* Newell, G. and Ellison, N. (eds.): Nutrition and Cancer: Etiology and Treatment. New York, Raven Press, pp. 301–318, 1981.

Donoghue, M., Nunnally, C., and Yasko, J.: Nutritional Aspects of Cancer Care. Reston, VA, Reston Publishing Co., 1982.

Gildea, J., Motz, K., Costlow, N., et al.: A systematic approach to providing nutritional care to cancer patients. Nutritional Support Services, 2(9):24–30, 1982.

Heber, D., Byerly, L., and Chlebowski, R.: Metabolic abnormalities in the cancer patient. Cancer, 55(1):225–229, 1985.

Kisner, D. and Dewys, W.: Anorexia and cachexia in malignant disease. *In* Newell, G. and Ellison, N. (eds.): Nutrition and Cancer: Etiology and Treatment. New York, Raven Press, pp. 355–366, 1981.

Rosenbaum, E., Stitt, C., Drasin, H., and Rosenbaum, I.: Daily nutritional care for cancer patients. *In* Newell, G. and Elllison, N. (eds.): Nutrition and Cancer: Etiology and Treatment. New York, Raven Press, pp. 339–354, 1981.

Stuart, R.: Nutritional support. *In* Abeloff, M. (ed.): Complications of Cancer. Baltimore, Johns Hopkins University Press, pp. 17–57, 1979.

27

Unproven Methods of Cancer Treatment

NANCY KANE, RN, MSN

CHARACTERISTICS OF UNPROVEN METHODS

A. Credentials of promoter.
   1. Lack of formal oncology training.
   2. Alternative degrees (e.g., chiropractor, naturalist, naprapathist).
   3. Meaningless letters after name.
B. Lack of controlled studies.
   1. Reports prevalent in mass media, not scientific publications.
   2. Use of testimonials and anecdotal reports.
   3. Disregard nonresponders, blaming patient rather than treatment for failures.
C. Unscientific data base.
   1. No proven, reproducible data.
   2. Special nutritional alterations often required.
   3. Claims of treatment being harmless, painless, and nontoxic.
D. Classified information.
   1. "Secret cure" known only to promoter.
   2. Claims of conspiracy to keep cure of cancer from public.
   3. Attacks on medical and scientific establishment.
E. Emphasis on freedom of choice and emotional support.
   1. Promotion of a caring environment.
   2. Focus on hope.

CLASSIFICATION OF UNPROVEN METHODS

A. Machines and devices.
   1. Less prevalent currently.
   2. May be used for diagnosis as well as treatment of cancer.
   3. Examples: oscillolast, Hubbard E Meter.
B. Drugs and chemicals.
   1. Include: herbs, drugs, vaccines, and chemical preparations.

    2. Based on unfounded concepts of carcinogenesis.
    3. Examples: Koch treatment, Hoxsey treatment, Krebiozen, Laetrile.
  C. Nutritional approaches.
    1. Often contradictory to known nutritional needs of people with cancer.
    2. Emphasis on dietary manipulation and intestinal purification.
    3. May include vitamins, minerals, enzymes.
    4. Often discourage concomitant use of drugs and radiation.
    5. Includes emphasis on positive mental outlook.
    6. Examples: Gerson's method, macrobiotic diet.
  D. Psychological techniques.
    1. Based on intense faith and promotion of hope.
    2. Examples: psychic surgery, Simonton method.

CURRENTLY AVAILABLE UNPROVEN METHODS

  A. Laetrile (amygdalin, Vitamin B_{17}).
    1. May be promoted as a drug or a vitamin.
    2. No proven anticancer effect as shown by N.C.I. studies.
    3. Symbolic of the category of unproven methods.
    4. Toxicities:
      a. Cyanide poisoning.
      b. Hypotension.
      c. Gastrointestinal disturbances.
      d. Rash.
      e. Agranulocytosis.
    5. Nursing assessment should focus on signs and symptoms of toxicity.
  B. Simonton method.
    1. Developed by physician and psychologist team.
    2. Major components include relaxation and visual imagery.
    3. Proponents emphasize combining it with conventional therapy.
    4. May increase person's feelings of personal control.
    5. No proven anticancer effect.
    6. May stimulate guilt feelings if person feels he or she has failed in gaining control over the disease.
  C. Macrobiotic diet.
    1. Based on balancing yin and yang foods in diet.
    2. Proponents do describe some patient groups who will not respond to diet.
    3. Multiple types of diets exist under this classification.
    4. No proven anticancer effect.
    5. Mineral, vitamin, and protein deficiencies associated with diet.
    6. Promotes weight loss.
  D. Immune-augmentative treatment (IAT).
    1. Purported to bolster the immune system.
    2. No antitumor activity found.

NURSING ROLE RELATED TO UNPROVEN METHODS

  A. Assess presence of psychosocial pressures on person with cancer.
    1. Pressure from family and friends to try every option.

2. Feelings of helplessness and hopelessness.
3. Difficulty in confronting poor prognosis.
B. Foster open communication with persons with cancer and their families.
  1. Many people who seek unproven methods feel lack of caring from health care team.
  2. People who feel emotional support from health care team are less likely to seek alternatives.
C. Promote exchange of information.
  1. Include client and family in decision making whenever possible.
  2. Use terminology client and family can understand.
  3. Maintain nonjudgmental, accepting attitude.
D. Recognize characteristics of unproven methods.
  1. Assist person seeking treatment in identifying characteristics.
  2. Avoid inducing guilt in person for inquiring about methods.
E. Community education.
  1. Increase public's awareness of dangers of unproven methods.
  2. Education about advances in cancer management to address "cancerphobia."

STUDY QUESTIONS

1. Identify descriptive characteristics of unproven methods of cancer treatment.
2. Identify reasons why people pursue treatment with unproven methods.
3. Describe nursing interventions that can assist individuals to make medically sound decisions concerning treatment.

Bibliography

Holland, J.: Why patients seek unproven remedies: A psychological perspective. Clinical Bulletin, 2(11):102–105, 1981.

Howard-Ruben, J. and Miller, N : Unproven methods of cancer management. Part II: Current trends and implications for patient care. Oncology Nursing Forum, 11(1):67–74, 1984.

Miller, N. and Howard-Ruben, J.: Unproven methods of cancer management. Part I: Background and historical perspectives. Oncology Nursing Forum, 10(4):46–54, 1984.

Patrick, P.: Cancer quackery: Information issues, responsibility, action. In Marino, L. B. (Ed.): Cancer Nursing. St. Louis, C. V. Mosby Co., pp. 357–370, 1981.

SECTION SEVEN

Cancer Nursing Practice

Section Editor
SUSAN McMILLAN, RN, PhD

28

Outcome Standards for Cancer Nursing Practice

CHRISTINE A. MIASKOWSKI, RN, MS

OVERVIEW OF STANDARDS

A. Definition of a *standard*—A standard is a level of performance considered acceptable by some authority or by the individual or individuals engaged in performing or maintaining such performance levels or conditions.
B. Types of standards:
  1. *Structure standards*—include statements of the conditions or mechanisms established to facilitate the provision of care. Components of structure standards include:
    a. Physical facilities.
    b. Environmental considerations.
    c. Organizational characteristics.
    d. Management characteristics.
    e. Philosophical considerations.
    f. Staffing.
    g. Equipment.
    h. Qualifications of health care personnel.
  2. *Process standards*—define the quality of implementation of the nursing care. They describe a series of actions, changes, or functions in providing care to patients.
  3. *Outcome standards*—define the expected change in the health status of the patient after he or she has received nursing care. They define the ends to be achieved.

COMPONENTS OF THE ONS OUTCOME STANDARDS FOR CANCER NURSING PRACTICE

A. Definition of the *ONS Outcome Standards for Cancer Nursing Practice*—the standards reflect primarily the high incidence problem areas of clients in any stage of their disease, regardless of the care setting.

1. Essential elements of the ONS Outcome Standards for Cancer Nursing Practice:
   a. Standards reflect high incidence problems.
   b. The problems affect patients at any stage of the disease process.
   c. These problems are dealt with in a variety of care settings.
   d. The standards focus on the client's and family's ability to function optimally. Care is seen as occurring on a continuum from the time of diagnosis and potential cure through to death.
   e. Standards include a prevention focus.
   f. The focus of the standards is threefold:
      (1) Client.
      (2) Family.
      (3) Community.
2. Format of the standards—the standards are written in an *Outcome* format
B. Components of the *ONS Outcome Standards for Cancer Nursing Practice*:
   1. *Standard*—is defined as the desired level of attainment consistent with the individual client's and family's intellectual, physical, and psychosocial capacity.
   2. Rationale for the standard:
      a. Provides current information pertinent to the specific standard.
      b. Explains why the standard is important.
      c. Explains any scientific rationale important to the standards interpretation.
      d. Provides additional information that needs to be considered prior to implementing the standard.
   3. Outcome criteria:
      a. *Criteria* are defined as statements that are measurable and that represent the intent of the standard.
      b. The *outcome criteria* are written as measurable and observable behaviors in the client and family that can be used in measuring and evaluating attainment of the standard.
      c. The criteria are general enough to allow the development of more specific criteria reflecting local practices and cultural values.

SPECIFIC STANDARDS

A. There are ten specific *ONS Outcome Standards for Cancer Nursing Practice.*
   1. Prevention and detection standard—the client and family possess adequate information about cancer prevention and detection.
      a. Rationale:
         (1) Epidemiologic trends can be used to determine which individuals and groups are at high risk for cancer.
         (2) Cancer incidence may be decreased through appropriate prevention measures, and the extent of the disease may be limited by early detection.
         (3) The client and family have a right to information about environmental and personal carcinogenic risk factors.
         (4) Values and attitudes may affect the use of resources for the prevention and early detection of cancer.
      b. Outcome criteria—the client and family:

(1) Recognize factors that place an individual at risk and may lead to cancer, such as the use of tobacco, improper nutrition, and therapy with immunosuppressive agents.
(2) State cancer's warning signs.
(3) Identify a plan for seeking health care assistance whenever any alteration in health status occurs.
(4) Describe applicable cancer self-detection measures.

2. Information standard—the client and family possess knowledge about the disease and therapy in order to attain self-management, participation in therapy, optimal living, and peaceful death.
   a. Rationale:
      (1) The client and family have the right to accurate information about the disease, options for treatment, consequences of treatment, potential oncologic emergencies, alternative care settings, and resources.
      (2) The rate and level of information provided to the client and family is determined by their intellectual capacity and emotional resources.
      (3) Securing adequate information is a prerequisite to development of functional coping.
   b. Outcome criteria—the client and family:
      (1) Describe the state of the disease and therapy at a level consistent with their intellectual and emotional states.
      (2) Participate in the decision making process pertaining to the plan of care and life activities.
      (3) Identify appropriate community and personal resources that would provide information and services.
      (4) Describe appropriate actions for highly predictable problems, oncologic emergencies, and major side effects of disease or therapy.
      (5) Describe the schedule when ongoing therapy is predicted.
      (6) Describe plans for integrating valued activities into daily life.

3. Coping standard—while living with cancer, the client and family manage stress within their individual physical, psychological, and spiritual capacities and their values systems.
   a. Rationale:
      (1) In American society, cancer connotes a stressful situation that has different implications for different people.
      (2) The client and family may experience a variety of stressors brought about by either the nature or the perception of the disease and its treatment; stressors may include loss of function, altered body image, fear of death, or fear of social isolation.
      (3) Cancer's chronic nature with acute episodes may require periodic alterations in coping strategies.
      (4) Physical, psychosocial, spiritual, and economic resources available to the client and family influence their ability to cope.
      (5) A functional coping process can be facilitated.
   b. Outcome criteria—within a level consistent with physical, psychosocial, and spiritual capacities and their value system, the client and family:
      (1) Use appropriate resources for support in coping.
      (2) Communicate feelings about living with cancer.

      (3) Participate in care and ongoing decision making.

      (4) Identify alternative resources when present coping strategies do not provide support.

      (5) State accomplishable goals.

4. Comfort standard—the client and family identify and manage factors that influence comfort. (Comfort is defined as the minimizing of psychobiologic distress.)

   a. Rationale:

      (1) The client and family have a right to information pertaining to interventions that promote psychobiologic comfort.

      (2) Discomfort may be experienced as a result of pathologic changes or psychologic distress.

      (3) Alterations in comfort may be an indication of a change in disease state.

      (4) Pain:

         (a) Is a protective mechanism; its occurrence, intensity, and duration may vary throughout the disease and treatment.

         (b) Is influenced by such variables as cultural, social, or ethnic orientation; anxiety; guilt; and fear of the unknown.

         (c) Is often a major disability.

      (5) Effective pain and sleep management are available for most patients.

   b. Outcome criteria—the client and family:

      (1) Report alterations in comfort level.

      (2) Identify measures to modify psychosocial, environmental, and physical factors that influence comfort and enhance the continuance of valued activities and relationships.

      (3) State the source of pain, the treatment, and the expected outcome of the proposed intervention.

      (4) Describe appropriate interventions for potential or predictable problems of the pain and sleep management program.

5. Nutrition standard—the client and family manage nutrition and hydration, which facilitates optimal health and comfort in the presence of disease and treatment.

   a. Rationale:

      (1) Optimal nutritional status favorably influences tolerance of and response to treatment.

      (2) The nutritional needs of patients with cancer are increased because of the disease process, recuperative demands following surgery, radiation therapy, and chemotherapy, and stimulation by immunotherapy.

      (3) Food intake and retention may be altered by cancer therapy or the disease process; common problems include taste changes, anorexia, mucosal irritation, and obstruction of the gastrointestinal tract.

      (4) Cultural, social, and ethnic influences affect the attitudes individuals have toward eating.

      (5) Adjustment of eating schedules, types and amounts of food, and quality and quantity of fluids enhance the client's control over his or her nutritional state.

   b. Outcome criteria—the client and family:

    (1) Identify foods that are tolerated and those that cause discomfort or aversion.

    (2) State measures that enhance food intake and retention.

    (3) Select appropriate dietary alternatives to provide sufficient nutrients when usual foods are not tolerated.

    (4) State methods of modifying consistency, flavor, or amounts of nutrients to ensure adequate nutrient intake.

    (5) State dietary modifications compatible with cultural, social, and ethnic practices.

    (6) State foods and fluids that provide optimal comfort during the terminal stage of illness.

6. Protective mechanisms standard—the client and family possess the knowledge to prevent or manage problems related to alterations in protective mechanisms (immune, hematopoietic, integumentary, and sensory-motor systems).

  a. Rationale:

    (1) Protective mechanisms can be compromised by disease and treatment.

    (2) Morbidity and mortality in persons with cancer are often related to alterations in protective mechanisms.

    (3) Clinical signs of compromised protective mechanisms can be absent or greatly modified by disease or therapy.

  b. Outcome criteria—the client and family:

    (1) List measures to prevent skin breakdown, mucosal trauma, infection, and bleeding.

    (2) Identify signs and symptoms of infection, bleeding, or sensory-motor dysfunction.

    (3) Contact an appropriate health team member when initial signs and symptoms of infection, bleeding, or sensory-motor dysfunction occur.

    (4) State measures to manage infection, bleeding, or sensory-motor dysfunction.

7. Mobility standard—the client and family maintain an optimal mobility level of the client consistent with the disease and therapy.

  a. Rationale:

    (1) Decreased mobility may be caused by the cancer itself or by complications of the disease and its treatment.

    (2) Decreased mobility can lead to many physiologic dysfunctions.

    (3) Passive or active muscle movement is necessary to maintain skin integrity, full range of motion of all joints and muscles, and adequate circulation.

    (4) The level of mobility influences longevity.

  b. Outcome criteria—the client and family:

    (1) State the cause of the immobility, the treatment, and the outcome of the treatment.

    (2) Describe the appropriate management plan to optimally integrate the alteration in mobility into the lifestyle.

    (3) Describe optimal level of activities of daily living in keeping with disease state and treatment.

    (4) Identify health services and community resources available for managing changes in mobility.

(5) Use measures to aid or improve mobility.

(6) Demonstrate measures to prevent the complications of decreased mobility.

8. Elimination standard—the client and family manage alterations in elimination to be consistent with activities of daily living. (Alterations in elimination may include fecal and urinary diversions, fistulas, diarrhea, constipation, bladder insufficiencies, incontinence, or fecal or urinary obstruction.)

    a. Rationale:

        (1) Cancer therapy or disease can result in changes in elimination.

        (2) Altered elimination is often an indicator of a change in disease state.

        (3) There are social, cultural, and ritualistic behaviors surrounding the process of elimination.

        (4) A change in elimination poses a threat to the client's anatomic-physiologic integrity, personality, or sexual function.

        (5) Factors other than the disease or its specific treatment can affect elimination.

    b. Outcome criteria—the client and family:

        (1) State appropriate actions if changes in elimination patterns occur.

        (2) Describe the relationship between adequate elimination and physiologic integrity.

        (3) Identify and manage factors that may affect elimination, such as diet, stress, physical activity, and neurogenic conditions.

        (4) Develop a plan for managing an altered elimination route within personal lifestyle.

9. Sexuality standard—the client and partner can identify aspects of sexuality that may be threatened by disease and can enumerate ways of maintaining sexual identity.

    a. Rationale:

        (1) Anatomic, physiologic, or psychosocial dimensions altered by cancer therapy or disease may temporarily or permanently affect behavior used to express sexual identity.

        (2) Sexuality is expressed by patterns of behavior both prescribed by mores of society and subscribed to in order to meet the needs of the individual personality.

        (3) There are alternate modes of sexual behavior and expression that the client and partner may choose to exercise.

        (4) Attention to problems regarding sexual activity is often neglected, avoided, or overlooked by health professionals.

    b. Outcome criteria—the client and partner:

        (1) Identify potential or actual alterations in perception of sexuality or sexual function.

        (2) Identify alternate methods of expressing sexuality.

10. Ventilation standard—the client and family recognize factors that may impair ventilatory function and can intervene with measures that may enhance optimum ventilatory capacity.

    a. Rationale:

        (1) Impaired ventilatory function, e.g., effusions, obstruction, or pulmonary fibrosis, may be caused by the cancer therapy or the disease.

      (2) Psychologic factors may potentiate respiratory distress.

      (3) Ventilatory problems can be distressing and limiting factors to optimum lifestyle.

      (4) Through environmental, mechanical, and activity modifications, respiratory function can be enhanced.

  b. Outcome criteria—the client and family:

      (1) State plans for daily activity that demonstrate maximum conservation of energy.

      (2) List measures to reduce or modify pulmonary irritants from the environment, such as smoke, dry air, powders, and aerosols.

      (3) Describe the effect of environmental extremes on ventilatory function and oxygen utilization.

      (4) State effective measures to maintain a patent airway.

      (5) Identify reasons for altered ventilation, such as decreased hemoglobin, infection, anxiety, effusion, and obstructed airway.

      (6) Identify an appropriate plan of action should altered ventilation occur.

      (7) Develop a plan for managing an altered airway.

B. Purpose of the *ONS Outcome Standards for Cancer Nursing Practice.*

  1. They reorient the focus of cancer nursing care toward a more explicit reflection of the fact that cancer is increasingly a chronic illness with intermittent acute episodes, rather than an acute process that brings immediate death.

  2. They emphasize education of clients and families.

  3. They establish oncology nursing as a distinct subspecialty.

  4. They provide recognition that cancer is a major health problem.

  5. They define the high incidence problem areas of clients in any stage of the cancer process.

USE OF THE STANDARDS IN THE EVALUATION OF PATIENT CARE

A. Implementation using the nursing process:

  1. Standards are meaningless unless they are utilized in practice.

  2. One of the best examples of how the standards have been implemented using a nursing process framework is the *Guidelines for Cancer Nursing Practice* by McNally and associates.

  3. The guidelines are intended to provide direction for the nurse in the care of cancer patients and their families.

  4. The guidelines are structured using the four steps in the nursing process:

    a. Assessment.

    b. Planning.

    c. Intervention.

    d. Evaluation.

B. Evaluation of patient care:

  1. The standards can be used as a framework to tailor quality assurance activities.

  2. The standards can be used to conduct chart audits.

  3. The standards can be used for direct patient evaluation of how well or how poorly the specified outcomes within the standards were achieved.

NEED FOR NURSING RESEARCH FOR REVISION AND EXPANSION

A. The ONS and ANA state that these standards and criteria reflect the most current knowledge. As the specialty of cancer nursing develops, nursing research will mandate periodic revision and expansion.
B. Researchable questions must be defined.
C. Research must be conducted in the clinical setting.

STUDY QUESTIONS

1. Describe the three types of nursing standards.
2. Utilizing the nursing process as a framework, describe a plan for implementing one of the *ONS-ANA Outcome Standards for Cancer Nursing Practice.*

Bibliography

Cantor, M. M.: Achieving Nursing Care Standards: Internal and External. Wakefield, Massachusetts, Nursing Resources, Inc., 1978.
Hyman, R., Nielsen, B., and Miaskowski, C.: The Nielsen-Hyman oncology case study rating scale. Oncology Nursing Forum, *10*(3):40–44, 1983.
McNally, J. C., Stair, J. C., and Somerville, E. T. (eds.): Guidelines for Cancer Nursing Practice. Orlando, Grune & Stratton, 1985.
Oncology Nursing Society: ONS-ANA Outcome Standards for Cancer Nursing Practice. Kansas City, Missouri, American Nurses' Association, 1979.

29

Nursing Management of Outcomes of Disease, Psychological Response, Treatment, and Complications

JANE CLARK RN, MSN, OCN
LORI LANDIS RN, MN
ROSE McGEE RN, PhD

ALOPECIA

A. Definition—The temporary or permanent loss of hair (scalp, facial, axillary, pubic, body).
B. Assessments.
  1. Risk factors:
    a. Treatment that has an affinity for rapidly dividing cells will damage hair follicles.
      (1) Radiation therapy of greater than 4500 rads may cause permanent hair loss in the area being treated.
      (2) Chemotherapy generally results in temporary hair loss.
    b. Duration and dose of therapy.
      (1) Location of radiation field.
      (2) Total dose/fractionation of radiation dose, e.g., increased dose over decreased number of treatments, increases hair loss within radiated field.
      (3) Additive toxic effects of chemotherapeutic agent with combination therapy.
      (4) Dose of chemotherapeutic agents, e.g., increased dose increases severity of hair loss.
  2. History:
    a. Previous patterns of hair growth.
    b. Usual hair care practices.
      (1) Frequency of shampooing.

    (2) Frequency of permanents, color, and rinses.
    (3) Use of blow dryers, heated rollers, and curling irons.
  c. Perceptions of client prior to and after hair loss.
    (1) Self concept.
    (2) Body image.
    (3) Perceived sexuality.
    (4) Responses of significant others and social and/or work acquaintances to hair loss.
  3. Physical findings:
    a. Decreased thickness of hair.
    b. Changes in texture of hair.
  4. Psychological findings:
    a. Anxiety.
    b. Decreased social interaction.
  5. Sequelae of hair loss:
    a. Increased heat loss via scalp.
    b. Impaired self concept.
    c. Decreased sexual and social interaction.
C. Interventions:
  1. Provide anticipatory guidance related to hair loss.
    a. Provide information related to hair loss and regrowth.
      (1) Loss occurs over a period of days to weeks.
      (2) Regrowth usually occurs 6 to 8 weeks after completion of therapy.
      (3) Color and texture of regrown hair may be different from hair growth prior to loss.
    b. Encourage client to obtain scarves, turbans, caps, and/or wigs prior to hair loss.
    c. Identify community and personal resources for financial assistance with wigs, e.g., insurance, American Cancer Society.
    d. Encourage discussion of responses to alopecia among client, significant others, and members of the health care team.
  2. Institute measures to decrease hair loss.
    a. Wash hair less frequently with a mild shampoo or a dry shampoo.
    b. Avoid the use of permanents, hair coloring, excessive use of blow dryers, curling irons, heated rollers, and brushing.
  3. Institute medical orders as indicated.
    a. Scalp hypothermia.
    b. Scalp tourniquet.
D. Evaluation. The client and/or significant other will:
  1. Define alopecia.
  2. Identify personal risk factors for alopecia.
  3. Describe patterns of hair loss and potential hair regrowth.
  4. Discuss potential effects of alopecia on self concept, body image, sexuality, and social interaction.
  5. Participate in measures to prevent, minimize, and/or adapt to alopecia.
  6. Identify community resources and insurance benefits available.

ANEMIA

A. Definition—A quantitative or qualitative deficiency in circulating red blood cells.

B. Assessments.
 1. Risk factors:
  a. Nutritional deficiencies.
   (1) Decreased iron and vitamin K intake, absorption, and/or utilization.
   (2) Decreased folic acid and/or vitamin B_{12} intake, absorption, and/or utilization.
  b. Treatment effects:
   (1) Chemotherapy—most cytotoxic agents affect the bone marrow, resulting in a decrease in the number of red blood cells and precursors.
   (2) Radiation therapy—treatment fields that include areas of increased hematopoietic activity (e.g., pelvis, sternum, and proximal ends of the long bones) result in a decrease in red cell production.
  c. Disease effects:
   (1) Primary disease of bone marrow, e.g. leukemia, may decrease actual numbers of mature red cells and/or inhibit red cell maturation.
   (2) Secondary disease of bone marrow by tumor infiltration will decrease the number of red blood cells and platelets produced.
   (3) Autoimmune disorders associated with malignancies may cause an increase in red blood cell destruction and/or sequestration of cells.
  d. Renal disease.
   (1) Red cell production depends on the release of erythropoietin from the kidneys.
   (2) In acute and chronic renal disease, erythropoietin production and release are impaired.
  e. Deficiencies in clotting factors resulting in hemorrhage are caused by:
   (1) Primary tumors of the liver.
   (2) Metastatic disease of liver.
   (3) Treatment-related hepatic toxicity.
  f. Decreased bone marrow function because of:
   (1) Aging.
   (2) Exposure to toxic substances, e.g., benzene, antibiotics.
 2. Physical findings:
  a. Vital signs—increased pulse, respirations, and pulse pressure and decreased blood pressure.
  b. Pallor (skin, nailbeds, conjunctivae, circumoral) weakness, fatigue, and listlessness.
  c. Headache, vertigo, tinnitus, palpitations, hypersensitivity to cold, dyspnea or exertion, and insomnia.
  d. Acute or chronic blood loss via stool, urine, emesis, menses, or sputum.
  e. Active bleeding from operative site, nasophraynx, or site of invasive procedure.
 3. Laboratory findings:
  a. Decreased hemoglobin and hematocrit.
  b. Decreased red blood cell indices.
  c. Decreased reticulocyte and erythrocyte counts.
  d. Changes in associated tests, e.g., total iron binding capacity (TIBC), iron, and vitamin B_{12}.

4. Psychological responses to anemia:
   a. Depression.
   b. Apathy.
C. Interventions:
   1. Report presence of signs and symptoms of anemia and its complications to physician.
   2. Institute measures to minimize potential complications of anemia.
      a. Safety precautions.
         (1) Avoid sudden position changes.
         (2) Assist with ambulation as indicated.
         (3) Avoid driving if syncopal.
      b. Nutritionally balanced diet and/or supplements, especially high protein and iron intake.
   3. Set priorities for activities to minimize energy expenditure.
      a. Observe safety precautions.
      b. Assist with activities of daily living.
      c. Use devices to assist with ambulation and work.
      d. Schedule rest periods throughout the day.
   4. Institute medical orders as indicated.
      a. Administer red blood cell transfusions.
         (1) Whole blood for volume replacement.
         (2) Packed cells for quantitative red cell replacement.
      b. Monitor administration of oxygen therapy.
      c. Provide supplemental minerals and vitamins.
D. Evaluation. The client and/or significant other will:
   1. Define anemia.
   2. Describe risk factors for development of anemia.
   3. Report signs and symptoms and/or potential complications of anemia.
   4. Participate in measures to:
      a. Minimize complications of anemia.
      b. Minimize potential complications of treatment for anemia.
      c. Conserve energy.
   5. Identify foods high in protein, iron, vitamin B_{12}, and folic acid.
   6. Identify situations that require professional intervention:
      a. Acute increase in fatigue.
      b. Acute bleeding.
      c. Syncope and/or palpitations.
   7. Identify community resources to meet needs resulting from anemia, e.g., Red Cross.

BLEEDING DUE TO THROMBOCYTOPENIA

A. Definition—A quantitative decrease in the number of circulating platelets.
B. Assessments.
   1. Risk factors:
      a. Disease effects.
         (1) Primarily disease of bone marrow; it may decrease production of and inhibit maturation of platelets.
         (2) Invasion of marrow from tumor may decrease number of platelets produced through competition for nutrients.

   (3) Autoimmune thrombocytopenia associated with malignancy may result in an increased destruction of platelets.
   (4) Disseminated intravascular coagulation results in an increased consumption of platelets.
   (5) Bacterial or viral interaction with platelets results in platelet damage and aggregation.
   (6) Genetically transmitted platelet deficiency diseases result in platelet deficits.
   b. Treatment effects:
   (1) Chemotherapy—hematopoietic toxicity of cancer chemotherapeutic agents results in a decrease in the production of platelet precursors and ultimately mature platelets.
   (2) Radiation therapy—treatment fields that include areas of increased hematopoietic activity (e.g., pelvis, sternum, and proximal ends of the long bones) result in a decrease in platelet production.
   (3) Massive blood transfusions, extracorporeal circulation, and exchange transfusions may result in dilutional thrombocytopenia.
   c. Pharmacologic effects on platelet function and production:
   (1) Aspirin decreases adhesiveness of platelets.
   (2) Thiazides, alcohol, and estrogens inhibit platelet production.
2. Physical findings:
   a. Anemia.
   b. Petechiae, bruising, and ecchymosis.
   c. Active bleeding from body orifices, operative sites, and sites of invasive procedures.
   d. Signs and symptoms of intracranial hemorrhage:
   (1) Changes in level of consciousness.
   (2) Restlessness.
   (3) Headache.
   (4) Change in pupillary response.
   (5) Seizures.
   (6) Widening of pulse pressure.
   (7) Focal changes—visual changes, ataxia, and affective changes.
3. Laboratory values:
   a. Platelet count $<150,000 \text{ mm}^3$
   b. Prolonged bleeding times.
4. Sequelae of bleeding due to thrombocytopenia.
   a. Hemorrhage.
   b. Anemia.
   c. Interference with activities of daily living, e.g., work, leisure, sexual relations.
C. Interventions:
   1. Notify physician of platelet count $<50,000 \text{ mm}^3$ or presence of active bleeding.
   2. Initiate measures to decrease risk of bleeding.
      a. Bleeding precautions notification.
      b. Apply direct pressure for 5 minutes to needle puncture sites.
      c. Avoid invasive procedures, e.g., catherizations, enemas, IM injections, rectal temperatures.
      d. Avoid activities that increase vasodilatation, e.g., hot showers.

e. Avoid Valsalva maneuver, e.g., straining with bowel movement, blowing nose.
f. Use soft toothbrushes, toothettes.
g. Elevate site of bleeding and apply cold if applicable.
3. Initiate safety measures to decrease risk of injury.
   a. Side rails at night.
   b. Assistance with ambulation as needed.
   c. Avoid sharp objects, such as razors or knives.
   d. Increased lubrication is needed for intercourse.
   e. Initiate bowel program to minimize constipation.
4. Initiate measures to increase constriction at bleeding site.
   a. Apply pressure.
   b. Use cold compresses and rinses.
5. Institute medical orders as indicated.
   a. Administer platelet transfusions.
   b. Apply topical thrombin to sites of bleeding.
   c. Avoid drugs that inhibit platelet production and/or function, if possible, e.g., aspirin, vasodilators.
   d. Stool softeners.
D. Evaluation. The client and/or significant other will:
   1. Define thrombocytopenia.
   2. Describe personal risk factors for thrombocytopenia.
   3. Participate in activities to decrease risks of bleeding due to thrombocytopenia.
   4. Report signs and symptoms and complications of thrombocytopenia.
   5. Identify situations that require professional intervention.
   6. Identify resources in the community and the health care system for management of bleeding emergencies.

CONSTIPATION

A. Definition—Passage of hard, infrequent stool, which is often associated with abdominal and rectal pain.
B. Assessments.
   1. Risk factors.
      a. Disease related:
         (1) Obstruction of bowel by tumor.
         (2) Fluid and electrolyte imbalances.
             (a) Dehydration.
             (b) Hypercalcemia.
             (c) Hypokalemia.
         (3) Immobility.
      b. Treatment related:
         (1) Manipulation of intestines during surgery.
         (2) Surgical trauma to neurogenic pathways to intestines and/or rectum.
         (3) Neurotoxic effects of cancer chemotherapeutic agents, e.g., vincristine, velban.
         (4) Nutritional deficiencies, e.g., decreased fiber and/or roughage intake.
      c. Side effects of pharmacologic agents.

(1) Narcotics.
(2) Anticholinergics.
(3) Antacids.
(4) Iron.
   d. Failure to respond to defecation reflex bacause of pain or fatigue.
2. History:
   a. Usual patterns of bowel elimination, e.g., frequency, character of stool, type and frequency of use of laxatives.
   b. Recent changes in factors contributing to bowel elimination:
      (1) Activity level.
      (2) Fluid intake.
      (3) Roughage and fiber in diet.
3. Physical findings:
   a. Decreased or absent bowel sounds.
   b. Nausea.
   c. Anorexia.
   d. Flatus.
   e. Abdominal distention.
   f. Abdominal cramping.
   g. Fecal impaction.
C. Interventions:
1. Notify physician of signs and symptoms of constipation.
2. Institute measures to maintain bowel elimination patterns.
   a. Provide at least 3000 cc fluid intake each day.
   b. Modify diet as tolerated to include high fiber and roughage—fresh fruits, vegetables, whole grains, dried beans.
   c. Maintain or increase physical activity level, including bed mobility.
   d. Establish a daily bowel program.
3. Implement interventions normally used by client to alleviate constipation.
4. Check for impaction if indicated.
5. Implement medical orders as indicated.
   a. Enemas.
   b. Laxatives.
   c. Stool softeners.
   d. Suppositories.
D. Evaluation. The client and/or significant other will:
1. Define constipation.
2. Identify usual bowel pattern and practices.
3. Describe personal risk factors for constipation.
4. Participate in measures to decrease risk of constipation.
5. Establish a daily bowel program.
6. Report signs and symptoms of constipation to health care team.
7. List situations related to constipation that require professional intervention.
   a. Constipation unrelieved by usual methods.
   b. Severe pain or bleeding with bowel movement.

DIARRHEA

A. Definition—Passage of loose, fluid stools more frequently than usual pattern of bowel elimination.

B. Assessments.
  1. Risk factors:
    a. Disease related, e.g., obstruction.
    b. Treatment related:
      (1) Cancer chemotherapeutic agents, e.g., 5-fluorouracil and methotrexate.
      (2) Radiation therapy to fields that include the bowel.
      (3) Effects of resection of significant portions of bowel.
      (4) Graft-versus-host disease in bone marrow transplantation.
    c. Medications, e.g., antibiotics, antacids.
    d. Diet modifications, e.g., tube feedings, dietary supplements, food intolerances.
    e. Inflammation or infection of the bowel.
    f. Increased stress with inadequate coping strategies.
  2. History:
    a. Usual bowel pattern.
      (1) Frequency.
      (2) Character of stool:
        (a) Color.
        (b) Amount.
        (c) Odor.
        (d) Consistency.
      (3) Type and frequency of laxatives used.
    b. Recent changes in factors contributing to adequate bowel elimination.
      (1) Activity level.
      (2) Fluid intake.
      (3) Roughage and fiber in diet.
      (4) Food intolerances.
      (5) Increased levels of stress.
  3. Physical findings:
    a. Flatus.
    b. Cramping.
    c. Abdominal pain.
    d. Hyperactive bowel sounds.
    e. Urgency to defecate.
    f. Weight loss.
    g. Output of 500 cc more than intake.
  4. Signs and symptoms of persistent diarrhea:
    a. Dehydration.
    b. Electrolyte imbalance.
    c. Impaired skin integrity in perineal area.
    d. Weakness or fatigue.
    e. Decreased social interaction.
C. Interventions:
  1. Notify physician of persistent diarrhea unrelieved by usual methods of management.
  2. Modify diet to decrease risks of diarrhea:
    a. Avoid food the client cannot tolerate.
    b. Decrease fiber and roughage in diet.
    c. Provide a clear liquid diet during episodes of diarrhea.

d. Serve foods at room temperature.
e. Advance diet as tolerated.
3. Institute measures to decrease risks of complications of diarrhea.
   a. Offer foods high in sodium and potassium.
   b. Maintain fluid intake of 300 cc per day.
   c. Initiate perineal hygiene measures after each bowel movement.
4. Teach strategies to modify stress response:
   a. Relaxation.
   b. Distraction.
   c. Imagery.
   d. New coping strategies.
5. Implement associated medical interventions:
   a. Antidiarrheal medications.
   b. Fluid and electrolyte replacement.
   c. Nutritional supplements.
   d. Tranquilizers.
   e. Steroids.
D. Evaluation. The client and/or significant other will:
1. Define diarrhea.
2. Describe usual bowel pattern and characteristics of stool.
3. Identify personal risk factors for diarrhea.
4. Participate in measures to decrease risks and minimize complications of diarrhea.
5. Report signs and symptoms of diarrhea to health care team.
6. List situations related to diarrhea that require professional intervention.
   a. Persistant diarrhea unrelieved by usual measures.
   b. Signs and symptoms of complications of diarrhea.

DYSPHAGIA

A. Definition—Difficulty in swallowing, usually with a sensation of material sticking in the esophagus.
B. Assessments.
1. Risk factors:
   a. Tumor infiltration or impingement on the esophagus by tumor or edema.
   b. Stomatitis resulting from chemotherapy and/or radiation therapy to fields that include the esophagus.
   c. Long-term sequelae of radiation therapy to fields including the esophagus:
     (1) Stenosis.
     (2) Fibrosis.
   d. Surgical procedures that impair ability to hold food in mouth, lateralize, masticate, form a bolus, move bolus through the oropharynx, or move bolus through the esophagus.
   e. Loss of vocal cord sphincter control.
   f. Loss of innervation to esophagus.
   g. Emotional responses to disease or treatment.
2. Ability of client to swallow food or liquids.
   a. Ability to hold food in mouth and lateralize food for chewing.

      b. Mastication.

      c. Propulsion of food to oropharynx by tongue.

  3. Objective responses to attempts to swallow:

      a. Drooling.

      b. Gagging.

      c. Pain.

      d. Aspiration.

      e. Regurgitation.

  4. Subjective responses to attempts to swallow:

      a. Fear.

      b. Anxiety.

  5. Signs and symptoms of complications of dysphagia:

      a. Fluid and electrolyte imbalance.

      b. Decreased nutritional intake.

      c. Inability to control secretions.

      d. Avoidance of attempts to swallow.

C. Interventions:

  1. Institute measures to decrease pain with swallowing:

      a. Provide soft foods, foods cut in small pieces or pureed.

      b. Serve foods at extreme temperatures to initiate sensation.

  2. Institute measures to decrease fear and anxiety with attempts to swallow:

      a. Relaxation exercises.

      b. Be physically present when client is attempting to swallow.

      c. Provide explanation of measures to manage difficulties in swallowing prior to occurrence.

  3. Institute measures designed to increase ease and effectiveness of swallowing:

      a. Position client in upright position.

      b. Tilt head forward, chin pointing to chest.

      c. Stimulate steps in swallowing that client is unable to initiate independently.

        (1) Opening mouth:

          (a) Apply light pressure on chin.

          (b) Stroke digastric muscle beneath the chin.

          (c) Touch lips with a spoon.

        (2) Bring lips together:

          (a) Stroke lips with spoon or finger.

          (b) Apply manual pressure to close the upper and lower lips.

        (3) Stimulate saliva secretion:

          (a) Allow client to see food.

          (b) Stimulate salivary glands with application of ice.

        (4) Swallowing:

          (a) Ice sternal notch and rub the back of the neck.

          (b) Provide an environment free of distractions.

          (c) Encourage multiple swallows with each attempt.

        (d) Provide with appropriate assistive devices.

          (1) Straws.

          (2) Plunger spoon to place food in pharynx.

          (3) Asepto syringe or pastry tube.

  4. Request referral to speech pathologist for additional rehabilitation if problem is unresolved.

5. Implement associated medical interventions:
   a. Self-intubation for supplemental feedings.
   b. Prepare for surgical insertion of feeding tube.
   c. Prosthetic devices.
   d. Medications to decrease pain and anxiety.
D. Evaluation. The client and/or significant other will:
   1. Define dysphagia.
   2. Identify risk factors that contribute to development of dysphagia.
   3. Report signs and symptoms of dysphagia and complications of dysphagia to health care team.
   4. Participate in methods to minimize dysphagia and its potential complications.
   5. List resources in the community to assist with rehabilitation.

DEHYDRATION

A. Definition—the loss of or deprivation of water from body tissues.
B. Assessments.
   1. Risk factors:
      a. Disease related:
         (1) Primary tumor of the pituitary or adrenal gland, kidney, or gastrointestinal tract.
         (2) Metastatic disease resulting in a fluid shift to extravascular space, e.g., edema, ascites, effusions.
         (3) Hemorrhage related to invasion by tumor.
      b. Treatment related:
         (1) Excessive water losses.
            (a) Surgical procedures resulting in trauma.
            (b) Wound or fistula drainage.
            (c) Nausea or vomiting resulting from radiation therapy or chemotherapy.
            (d) Gastrointestinal suctioning.
            (e) Diarrhea.
            (f) Diaphoresis with fever.
            (g) Drainage of extravascular space, e.g., paracentesis.
            (h) Therapeutic hyperthermia.
            (i) Excessive enemas.
         (2) Decreased water intake.
            (a) Decreased motivation to drink.
            (b) Anorexia related to radiation and/or chemotherapy.
            (c) Functional deficit in swallowing liquids.
            (d) NPO.
            (e) Decreased thirst sensation.
            (f) Decreased level of consciousness and/or neuromuscular control.
         (3) Redistribution of water to extravascular space.
            (a) Edema.
            (b) Ascites.
            (c) Effusions.
      c. Drugs, e.g., diuretics, laxatives, antibiotics, tranquilizers, antiepileptics.

2. Physical findings:
   a. Changes in output, e.g., decreased or excessive urine output, output greater than intake.
   b. Changes in integument, e.g., dry skin and mucous membranes, furrowed tongue, decreased skin turgor.
   c. Cardiovascular changes, e.g., decreased blood pressure, increased pulse rate, decreased pulse volume/pressure, postural hypotension.
   d. Anorexia, nausea, vomiting, weight loss.
   e. Weakness, lethargy.
3. Laboratory findings:
   a. Increased specific gravity of urine.
   b. Electrolyte imbalances.
4. Sequelae of dehydration:
   a. Electrolyte imbalances.
   b. Impairment of skin and mucous membrane integrity.
   c. Decreased level of consciousness.
   d. Circulatory collapse.
   e. Renal failure.
   f. Coma.
   g. Death.
C. Interventions:
   1. Report signs and symptoms of dehydration and/or complications of dehydration to physician.
   2. Institute measures to minimize loss. See information on:
      a. Nausea and vomiting.
      b. Diarrhea.
      c. Fever.
   3. Institute measures to prevent decreased water intake:
      a. Encourage minimum of 3000 cc oral intake each day (small amounts at frequent intervals).
      b. Provide assistance as needed with oral intake.
         (1) Manage dysphagia.
         (2) Offer ice chips, popsicles.
         (3) Provide assistive devices for moving liquids from container to mouth.
   4. Institute measures to protect client from injury in presence of weakness or postural hypotension.
   5. Institute medical orders as indicated.
      a. Fluid volume and electrolyte replacement.
      b. Administration of albumin.
      c. Hydration prior to chemotherapy and/or therapeutic hyperthermia.
D. Evaluation. The client and/or significant other will:
   1. Describe personal risk factors for development of dehydration.
   2. Report signs and symptoms of dehydration to health care team.
   3. Participate in measures to decrease risks of dehydration.
   4. Identify situations that require professional intervention.
      a. Marked decrease or increase in urine output.
      b. Inability of client to take oral fluids.
      c. Sudden confusion or change in level of consciousness.

EDEMA

A. Definition—Generalized or localized accumulation of excess fluid in interstitial spaces.
B. Assessments.
    1. Risk factors:
        a. Increased capillary pressure.
            (1) Blood clots that prevent return of blood flow to the heart.
            (2) Allergic reactions with release of histamine, resulting in relaxed arteriole and venule constriction, e.g., local edema (hives).
            (3) Emotional response mediated by the autonomic nervous system, e.g., laryngeal edema resulting in hoarseness.
        b. Decreased plasma proteins.
            (1) Abnormal protein losses in renal dysfunction.
            (2) Inadequate dietary intake of proteins.
            (3) Liver disease.
        c. Lymphatic obstruction.
            (1) Blockage of lymphatic channels by external compression and/or tumor infiltration.
            (2) Excision of lymphatic channels during surgery.
        d. Increased capillary permeability.
            (1) Allergic reactions.
            (2) Bacterial infections.
        e. Retention of fluids by the kidney.
        f. Secretion of fluid by tumor cells; fluid becomes trapped in fluid spaces, e.g., peritoneal, pericardial, and/or pleural spaces.
        g. Medications, e.g., estrogens, ACTH.
    2. Laboratory values:
        a. Increased blood urea nitrogen (BUN).
        b. Increased creatinine.
        c. Decreased serum protein/albumin.
        d. Abnormal serum electrolytes.
    3. Physical findings:
        a. Patterns of edema.
            (1) Generalized.
            (2) Localized.
         b. Swelling of tissues in dependent areas:
            (1) Extremities.
            (2) Sacrum.
            (3) Periorbital area.
            (4) Abdomen.
        c. Responses to fluid shift to interstitial spaces:
            (1) Decreased blood pressure, increased pulse, increased respirations.
            (2) Decreased urine output.
            (3) Increased weight.
            (4) Decreased comfort.
        d. Site specific responses:
            (1) Pulmonary edema.
                (a) Shortness of breath on exertion.
                (b) Increased respirations.

           (c) Adventitious breath sounds.

           (d) Dullness on percussion of lungs.

      (2) Ascites.

           (a) Increased abdominal girth.

           (b) Increased, shallow respirations.

           (c) Presence of abdominal fluid wave.

           (d) Dependent edema in lower extremities.

           (e) Increased weight.

           (f) Fullness, bloating, abdominal pressure.

      (3) Pericardial edema.

           (a) Jugular venous distention.

           (b) Narrowing pulse pressure.

  4. Sequelae of edema:

    a. Changes in self concept and body image.

    b. Anxiety related to meaning of edema in relation to disease and/or treatment.

    c. Changes in mobility, performance of activities of daily living, social interactions.

C. Interventions

  1. Notify physician of edema and/or complications of prolonged edema.

  2. Institute measures to minimize severity of edema:

    a. Offer a high protein, low salt diet.

    b. Limit fluid intake.

    c. Elevate edematous extremities while at rest.

    d. Avoid restrictive clothing in edematous areas.

  3. Institute measures to minimize occurrence of complications of edema:

    a. Institute skin care protocols for edematous areas.

    b. Place client in an upright position to facilitate expansion of diaphragm and lungs with pulmonary edema.

    c. Assist with activities of daily living (grooming, bathing, toileting) to maintain and/or improve self concept and body image.

    d. Encourage discussion of perceptions of meaning and effects of edema among the client, significant others, and health care team.

  4. Institute medical orders as indicated.

    a. Treatment of underlying pathology.

    b. Diuretics.

    c. Oxygen therapy.

    d. Albumin replacement.

    e. Assist with thoracentesis, paracentesis, and/or pericardiocentesis and monitor for complications of procedures.

    f. Electrolyte replacement.

    g. Tranquilizers.

D. Evaluation. The client and/or significant other will:

  1. Identify personal risk factors for development of edema and complications of edema.

  2. Participate in measures to decrease risk for and complications of edema.

  3. Report signs and symptoms of edema and its complications to health care team.

  4. List situations related to edema that require professional assistance.

    a. Acute change in symptom distress.

    b. Skin breakdown in edematous areas.

HYPERKALEMIA

A. Definition—Serum potassium levels greater than 5.5 mEq/L.
B. Assessments.
   1. Risk factors:
      a. Inadequate excretion or metabolism of potassium.
         (1) Acute renal failure.
         (2) Chronic renal failure with oliguria.
         (3) Liver metastasis.
         (4) Addison's disease.
         (5) Potassium sparing diuretics.
      b. Increased release of potassium from damaged cells.
         (1) Lymphoproliferative diseases, e.g., leukemia, lymphomas, Hodg-kins's disease.
         (2) Cancer therapy.
      c. Shifts in cellular distribution of potassium.
         (1) Metabolic acidosis.
         (2) Respiratory acidosis.
      d. Spurious plasma elevations.
         (1) Release of potassium from platelets, e.g., thrombocytosis.
         (2) Release of potassium from white blood cells, e.g., chronic leukemia.
   2. Physical findings:
      a. Cardiovascular: arrhythmias, EKG changes.
      b. Neuromuscular: weakness, flaccid paralysis.
   3. Sequelae of marked hyperkalemia:
      a. Paralytic ileus.
      b. Respiratory arrest.
      c. Cardiac arrest.
C. Interventions:
   1. Report elevations of serum potassium to physician, especially in high risk clients.
   2. Institute measures to minimize occurrence of complications of hyperkalemia.
      a. Follow safety precautions with respect to clients with muscle weakness.
      b. Avoid fluid overload; monitor intake and output.
      c. Limit foods high in potassium.
   3. Report symptoms or complications of hyperkalemia to physician.
   4. Institute medical orders as indicated:
      a. Intravenous calcium, hypertonic glucose or saline, and sodium bicarbonate.
      b. Cation-exchange resins by mouth or enema.
      c. Dialysis.
D. Evaluation. The client and/or significant other will:
   1. Describe personal risk factors for hyperkalemia.
   2. Report signs, symptoms, and complications of hyperkalemia to health care team.
   3. Participate in measures to decrease risks and complications of hyperkalemia.
   4. Identify community resources for chronic and/or emergency care.

HYPOKALEMIA

A. Definition—A serum potassium level less than 3.0 mEq/L.
B. Assessments.
   1. Risk factors:
      a. Decreased intake of potassium.
         (1) Anorexia.
         (2) NPO.
         (3) Knowledge deficit of foods rich in potassium.
      b. Increased loss of potassium.
         (1) Vomiting.
         (2) Diarrhea.
         (3) Draining fistulas.
         (4) Gastric suctioning.
         (5) Villous adenoma of rectum.
         (6) Carcinoid syndrome.
         (7) Renal disease.
      c. Medications.
         (1) Potassium depleting diuretics.
         (2) Antibiotics and/or antifungal agents, e.g., Ticarcillin, amphotericin.
         (3) Chemotherapy, e.g., AMSA.
      d. Hyperaldosteronism.
         (1) Primary.
         (2) Inappropriate ADH syndrome.
   2. Physical findings:
      a. Neuromuscular
         (1) Weakness.
         (2) Decreased deep tendon reflexes.
         (3) Paresthesias.
      b. Cardiovascular changes:
         (1) EKG changes.
         (2) Arrhythmias, especially if client is taking digitalis.
      c. Renal dysfunction.
         (1) Polyuria.
         (2) Polydipsia.
   3. Sequelae of hypokalemia:
      a. Digitalis intoxication.
      b. Paralytic ileus.
      c. Respiratory arrest.
      d. Cardiac arrest.
C. Interventions:
   1. Report decrease in serum potassium levels to physician, especially in high risk clients.
   2. Institute measures to prevent and/or minimize hypokalemia:
      a. Offer potassium rich foods, e.g., bananas, oranges, potatoes, nuts, potato chips.
      b. Offer potassium rich fluids, e.g., fruit juices, broth, colas, Gatorade.
   3. Institute measures to protect from injury secondary to neuromuscular weakness and decreased reflexes.
   4. Report signs and symptoms of complications of hypokalemia to physician.

    5. Institute medical orders as indicated:
       a. Oral potassium supplements.
       b. Intravenous potassium chloride.
D. Evaluation. The client and/or significant other will:
    1. Describe personal risk factors for development of hypokalemia.
    2. Report signs and symptoms and complications of hypokalemia to health care team.
    3. Report signs and symptoms of intolerance to oral potassium supplements.
    4. Identify community resources available to assist in dietary management and/or supervision.

FEVER/CHILLS

A. Definition:
    1. Fever—an elevation in the body temperature above the normal temperature for the individual.
    2. Chills—quivering and shaking as if cold.
B. Assessments.
    1. Risk factors:
       a. Decreased absolute granulocyte count (SEGS + BANDS) × WBC = AGC
       b. Transfusions.
       c. Drugs, e.g., amphotericin.
       d. Exposure to bacteria, viruses, and fungi.
       e. Therapeutic hyperthermia.
       f. Paraneoplastic syndrome.
       g. Tumor necrosis.
    2. Physical findings:
       a. Increased temperature, pulse, and respirations, and decreased blood pressure.
       b. Verbal complaints of fever, chills, and discomfort.
       c. Signs and symptoms of infection and inflammation at sites of:
          (1) Impaired skin integrity.
            (a) Venous access.
            (b) Surgical incisions.
            (c) Lesions.
            (d) Fistula.
          (2) Body orifices.
            (a) Ears, nose, mouth, and throat.
            (b) Urethra, vagina, and rectum.
          (3) Organ systems.
            (a) Gastrointestinal.
            (b) Pulmonary.
            (c) Urinary.
            (d) Neurologic.
    3. Sequelae of increased temperature:
       a. Dehydration.
       b. Increased metabolic needs.
       c. Fatigue.
       d. Confusion.
       e. Organ damage.

C. Interventions:
  1. Report signs and symptoms of increased temperature to physician.
     a. Chills.
     b. Flushing.
     c. Increased temperature of skin.
     d. Measured temperature.
  2. Institute measures to decrease temperature when febrile:
     a. Increase fluid intake.
     b. Remove excess clothing and/or linen.
     c. Cool or tepid bath/compresses with water or alcohol.
     d. Ice packs.
     e. Cooling blanket.
  3. Institute measures to increase comfort:
     a. Warm blankets with chilling.
     b. Change wet linen and clothing with diaphoresis.
     c. Cool room.
     d. Provide for rest period.
     e. Offer fluids rich in electrolytes (Na^+ and K^+).
     f. Explain potential etiology and treatment of chills and fever.
  4. Offer high caloric and high protein foods.
  5. Institute medical orders as indicated:
     a. Antipyretics without aspirin.
     b. Antibiotic therapy.
     c. Steroids and antihistamines.
     d. Tepid enemas.
     e. Fever work-up.
D. Evaluation. The client and/or significant other will:
  1. Identify chills and fever as warning signals.
  2. Describe factors that increase risks for fever/chills.
  3. List possible complications of an increased temperature.
  4. Report signs and symptoms of an increased temperature and sequelae to health care team.
  5. Participate in measures to decrease fever and improve comfort.
  6. Participate in preventive measures to decrease risks of infection and drug/transfusion reactions.
  7. Demonstrate techniques for:
     a. Taking a temperature.
     b. Reading a thermometer.

FATIGUE

A. Definition—A feeling of weariness, tiredness, or temporary loss of physical or emotional energy to respond to sensory or motor stimuli.
B. Assessments.
  1. Risk factors:
     a. Anemia.
     b. Sleep disturbances.
        (1) Decreased concentration and memory.
        (2) Irritability.
        (3) Impaired problem solving ability.
        (4) Restlessness.
        (5) Increased hours of sleep without feeling rested and revitalized.

  c. Decreased emotional energy.
   (1) Depression.
   (2) Withdrawal.
   (3) Apathy.
   (4) Helplessness.
   (5) Hopelessness.
   (6) Powerlessness.
  d. Inadequate nutritional intake for metabolic needs.
  e. Increased metabolic processes.
   (1) Fever.
   (2) Disease progression.
  f. Increased cellular destruction.
   (1) Surgery.
   (2) Chemotherapy.
   (3) Radiation therapy.
   (4) Tumor necrosis.
   (5) Metastasis.
  g. Hypokalemia.
 2. History:
  a. Site and stage of disease.
  b. Type of therapy.
  c. Comparisons of previous and present levels of activity.
C. Interventions:
 1. Prioritize activities of daily living to allow for independence in client valued activities, pacing of activity, and rest periods.
 2. Provide assistance with activities of daily living as needed:
  a. Bathing.
  b. Grooming.
  c. Toileting.
  d. Feeding.
  e. Mobility.
  f. Problem solving/decision making.
 3. Institute measures to minimize effects of associated conditions:
  a. Physiologic conditions:
   (1) Anemia.
   (2) Sleep disturbances.
    (a) Allow for periods of uninterrupted sleep during day (naps) and night.
    (b) Institute nursing measures to decrease associated symptoms: pain, nausea, vomiting, and anxiety.
    (c) Teach methods to elicit the relaxation response.
   (3) Inadequate nutritional intake for metabolic needs.
  b. Psychological conditions.
   (1) Depression.
   (2) Changes in mood.
 4. Institute medical orders as indicated:
  a. Blood components.
  b. Sedatives.
  c. Antidepressants.
  d. Professional counseling.
D. Evaluation. The client and/or significant other will:
 1. Describe factors that place client at increased risk for fatigue.

2. Describe expected duration of fatigue.
3. Report signs and symptoms of fatigue to health care team.
4. List possible consequences of fatigue on physical, psychological, and social responses.
5. Participate in measures to conserve energy, achieve adequate rest, and participate in valued activities.
6. Identify resources within the health care system and community to assist with activities of daily living.

GRIEF AND LOSS

A. Definition—Changes in thinking, feelings, and behaviors that occur as a direct consequence of an actual or perceived loss of a loved person and/or a valued object.
B. Assessment.
   1. Anticipated, actual, or perceived losses, which may precipitate a grief response.
      a. Developmental losses, e.g., aging.
      b. Loss of persons, e.g., divorce, death, or separation.
      c. Loss of "part" of self, e.g., surgery, illness, functional change.
      d. Loss of external objects, e.g., pets, home.
      e. Loss of status, e.g., failures, demotion, firing, retirement.
      f. Loss of social organization and/or support.
      g. Loss of lifestyle, e.g., bankruptcy, illness.
   2. Previous losses and patterns of resolution.
   3. Sociocultural factors that influence the grief response.
   4. Potential strengths and weaknesses that may facilitate or impede the grief process:
      a. Personality traits.
      b. Coping patterns.
      c. Spiritual beliefs.
      d. Patterns of family interaction.
      e. Availability of resources.
   5. Presence of cognitive, affective, and behavioral patterns associated with components of the grief process.
      a. Shock and disbelief.
         (1) Emotional and physical immobility.
         (2) Denial of loss.
      b. Developing awareness.
         (1) Crying, angry outbursts.
         (2) Subjective distress, e.g., shortness of breath, choked feelings, sighing.
         (3) Flashes of anguish.
         (4) Retelling the story.
         (5) Painful dejection.
         (6) Changes in eating and sleeping patterns.
         (7) Decrease in libido.
      c. Bargaining and restitution.
         (1) Idealizing the loss.
         (2) Contracting for reprieval or deliverance.
      d. Accepting the loss.

       (1) Reliving past experiences.

       (2) Preoccupation with the lost object.

       (3) Crying.

       (4) Somatic symptoms.

       (5) Fight or flight responses.

       (6) Dreams and nightmares.

   e. Resolving the loss.

       (1) Establishing new relationships.

       (2) Planning for the future.

       (3) Recalling rich memories of past experiences.

       (4) Affirming oneself.

       (5) Resuming previous roles.

  6. Presence of signs and symptoms of a dysfunctional grief response.

   a. Failure to complete the normal grief response within a year or a time span proportional to the meaning of the lost object.

   b. Anticipatory grief responses that result in resolution prior to the actual loss.

   c. Behavioral disorders such as manic-depressive states, hysteria, obsessive-compulsive behavior, and suicidal ideation.

   d. Abnormal social behavior such as drug or alcohol addiction, juvenile delinquency, or excessive generosity.

C. Interventions:

  1. Use interpersonal relationship skills appropriate to the stage of the grief process.

   a. Encourage verbalization of perceived loss(es).

   b. Actively listen to subjective responses to loss.

   c. Provide nonjudgmental atmosphere to facilitate expression of negative emotions and minimize feelings of guilt.

   d. Validate perceptions of responses.

   e. Facilitate verbalization of personal goals.

   f. Give permission to grieve and to resolve the loss.

  2. Institute measures to facilitate coping:

   a. Relaxation techniques.

   b. Participation in support groups.

   c. Counseling referrals.

   d. Give permission to resume past roles and establish new relationships.

  3. Advocate avoidance of conditions that block resolution of the grief process:

   a. Oversedation.

   b. Closed communications.

   c. Social isolation.

  4. Report signs and symptoms of dysfunctional grief to physician.

  5. Identify means to channel energy constructively.

  6. Institute associated medical orders.

   a. Antidepressants.

   b. Counseling referrals.

D. Evaluation. The client and/or significant other will:

  1. Identify losses that precipitate the grief response.

  2. List stages of the normal grief response.

  3. Identify changes in cognition indicative of a normal grief response.

   a. Decreased concentration.

     b. Shortened attention span.
     c. Dreams and nightmares.
     d. Preoccupation with self and/or lost person or object.
     e. Viewing the world as empty.
     f. Idealizing the lost object.
4. Identify affective responses associated with normal grief:
     a. Sadness.
     b. Crying.
     c. Anger.
     d. Guilt.
     e. Hostility.
     f. Aloofness.
     g. Emotional lability.
     h. Social withdrawal.
5. Identify physical changes associated with normal grief:
     a. Loss of appetite.
     b. Inactivity.
     c. Purposeless activity.
     d. Attachment behavior.
     e. Fatigue.
     f. Sleep disturbances.
     g. Tenseness.
     h. Anxiety attacks.
     i. Decreased libido.
6. Demonstrate positive coping strategies:
     a. Diversional activities.
     b. Open communications.
     c. Use of support systems.
7. Report signs and symptoms of dysfunctional grief to health care team.
8. Identify resources to deal with responses to loss.
     a. Counseling services.
     b. Support groups.

IMMOBILITY

A. Definition—Inability of a person to move purposefully within the environment.
B. Assessments.
  1. Risk factors:
     a. Disease related:
        (1) Primary tumor of musculoskeletal or neurologic system.
        (2) Metastatic disease involving the skeletal system or neurologic system, e.g., spinal cord compression.
     b. Treatment related:
        (1) Inadequate treatment of symptoms related to therapy, e.g., pain, nausea, fluid and electrolyte imbalances.
        (2) Amputation.
        (3) Intracavitary radiation therapy.
     c. Aging.
     d. Altered level of consciousness.

2. History:
   a. Comparison of previous and present levels of activity and mobility.
   b. Decreased range of motion in extremities.
   c. Decreased level of consciousness.
   d. Symptoms produced with mobility.
   e. Effects of immobility on activities of daily living, role performance, self-concept.
   f. Use of assistive devices for ambulation.
3. Physical findings:
   a. Decreased range of motion in extremities.
   b. Pain on movement.
   c. Neuromuscular impairment.
   d. Impaired skeletal integrity.
4. Psychological findings:
   a. Fear.
   b. Dependence.
   c. Decreased self-esteem.
   d. Powerlessness.
5. System sequelae of immobility:
   a. Cardiovascular—thrombophlebitis, postural hypotension.
   b. Gastrointestinal—anorexia, constipation, fecal impaction.
   c. Urinary—infection, calculi.
   d. Integumentary—ischemia, necrosis, ulceration.
   e. Pulmonary—emboli, infection, decreased diaphragmatic excursion.
   f. Musculoskeletal—decreased muscle tone, muscular atrophy, contractures, osteoporosis.
   g. Sensory nervous system—sensory losses, changes in orientation.
   h. Psychosocial responses—anxiety, depression, suicidal ideations, conflict with family or significant others.
C. Interventions:
   1. Report signs and symptoms and complications of immobility to physician.
   2. Institute measures to minimize potential sequelae of immobility:
      a. Perform active/passive range of motion and isometric exercises.
      b. Maintain body alignment with appropriate support.
      c. Assist with mobilization as needed.
      d. Provide with assistive devices for mobilization.
      e. Initiate a bowel program to prevent constipation.
      f. Encourage turning, coughing, deep breathing during periods of decreased mobility.
      g. Keep bony prominances supported.
      h. Keep skin over prominences clean, dry, and well lubricated.
      i. Pace activities to allow rest periods.
      j. Encourage independence in self-care activities.
   3. Institute medical orders as indicated:
      a. Referrals to occupational and physical therapy, social service, vocational rehabilitation, dietary.
      b. Antiembolic hose.
      c. Stool softeners, laxatives.
      d. Respiratory therapy.
      e. Low pressure devices, e.g., Clinitron beds, water mattresses.
      f. Splints, braces, corsets.

D. Evaluation. The client and/or significant other will:
1. Describe personal risk factors for immobility.
2. Discuss potential sequelae of immobility.
3. Report signs and symptoms and complications of decreased mobility.
4. Participate in measures to decrease risks of immobility and maintain range of motion, muscle tone, and strength.
5. Identify community resources to assist with coping with consequences of immobility, e.g., American Cancer Society, Visiting Nurses Association.

INFECTION DUE TO NEUTROPENIA OR LYMPHOPENIA

A. Definition—The process by which microbes from either exogenous or endogenous sources enter a susceptible site in the body and multiply, resulting in disease.
B. Assessments.
1. Risk factors:
   a. Decrease in the ability of the body to resist infection.
      (1) Decreased quantity of neutrophils and lymphocytes.
         (a) Tumor infiltration of bone marrow.
         (b) Nutritional deficiencies.
         (c) Exposure to toxic substances.
         (d) Genetically acquired immune deficiency syndromes.
         (e) Immunosuppressive therapy, e.g., antirejection agents, chemotherapy, and radiation therapy.
         (f) Age.
         (g) Steroid therapy.
      (2) Decrease in the quantity and/or maturity of neutrophils and lymphocytes.
         (a) Primary malignancy of blood-forming tissues, e.g., leukemia and lymphoma.
         (b) Autoimmune diseases that result in premature destruction of neutrophils and lymphocytes.
      (3) Alteration in natural protective barriers to microorganisms.
         (a) Decreased secretions in eyes, ears, nose, mouth, and throat.
         (b) Loss or impaired function of hair or cilia, e.g., absence of eyelashes, absence of cilia movement in bronchial tree after smoking.
         (c) Impaired skin integrity, e.g., I.V. sites, surgery, cutaneous lesions, mucosal lesions.
   b. Exposure to altered microorganisms.
      (1) Antibiotic-resistant organisms in the hospital environment.
      (2) Suprainfections resulting from antibiotic therapy.
   c. Creation of a favorable environment for microorganism proliferation.
      (1) Immunosuppression.
      (2) Effects of tumor growth, e.g., invasion, obstruction, necrosis.
2. Physical findings:
   a. Localized symptoms of infection, e.g., redness, swelling, pain, and pus. *Note:* may not be present with neutropenia or lymphopenia.

  b. Fever or hypothermia.
  c. Generalized symptoms of infection, e.g., fatigue, malaise.
  d. Increased pulse and respirations.
  e. Decreased blood pressure.
  f. Site-specific symptomatology, e.g., cough, abnormal breath sounds, back pain, burning and/or pain on urination, frequent urination, rectal discomfort with bowel movements.
 3. Laboratory values:
  a. White blood count <3000 mm^3.
  b. Absolute granulocyte count <500 mm^3.
 4. Sequelae of infection:
  a. Septicemia.
  b. Suprainfection.
  c. Septic shock.
  d. Organ system damage.
  e. Death.
C. Interventions:
 1. Report signs and symptoms of infection or septicemia to physician.
 2. Institute measures to decrease risks from endogenous organisms.
  a. Handwashing.
  b. Personal hygiene measures.
   (1) Bathing.
   (2) Oral care protocols.
   (3) Perineal care.
 3. Institute measures to decrease risks from exogenous organisms.
  a. Plan nursing care assignments to decrease risks of cross-contamination (private rooms, isolation as recommended).
  b. Instruct all persons in contact with client in handwashing techniques.
  c. Limit exposure to large crowds within closed environment.
  d. Avoid contact with persons with communicable and/or infectious diseases.
  e. Avoid immunizations.
  f. Limit exposure to children, pets, raw foods that may have high numbers of microbes, and freshly cut flowers.
  g. Maintain aseptic technique when caring for open wounds or lesions.
 4. Institute medical orders as indicated:
  a. Fever work-up, e.g., blood, urine, stool cultures, site specific evaluation.
  b. Antibiotic therapy.
  c. Prophylactic antifungal therapy.
  d. Granulocyte transfusions.
  e. Treatment of symptoms associated with infection, e.g., pain, fever, changes in integument.
D. Evaluation. The client and/or significant other will:
 1. Describe personal risk factors for development of infection.
 2. Report signs and symptoms of infection to health care team.
 3. Participate in measures to decrease risk of infection from endogenous and exogenous sources.
 4. Identify situations that require professional intervention:
  a. Temperature >101°F.
  b. Localized symptoms without fever.

    c. Exposure to communicable diseases, e.g., chickenpox, measles.
    d. Changes in level of consciousness.
  5. Identify community resources available for management of emergency situations.

INSOMNIA

A. Definition—Inability to go to sleep, stay asleep, or sleep long enough, uninterrupted, to feel rested and relaxed on awakening.
B. Assessments.
  1. Risk factors:
    a. Disease factors:
      (1) Paraneoplastic syndromes with increased steroid production.
      (2) Symptomatology associated with tumor invasion, e.g., obstruction, pain, fever, shortness of breath, pruritus, fatigue.
    b. Treatment factors:
      (1) Symptomatology related to surgery, e.g., pain, frequent monitoring, narcotics.
      (2) Chemotherapy, e.g., exogenous corticosteroids.
      (3) Symptomatology related to chemotherapy administration and/or supportive therapy, e.g., frequent voiding with increased I.V. fluid administration for hydration prior to chemotherapy and dilution of antibiotics.
    c. Drugs, e.g., narcotics, caffeine, sedatives, steroids.
    d. Changes in sleep environment, e.g., hospitalization.
    e. Increased physical and/or psychological stress.
    f. Decrease in physical exercise.
    g. Depression.
  2. History:
    a. Usual patterns of sleep.
      (1) Usual time to retire.
      (2) Routine prior to retiring, e.g., bath, food, warm milk, drugs to help sleep.
      (3) Length of time to fall asleep.
      (4) Awaking episodes during the night and/or early morning.
        (a) Perceived causes, e.g., noises, nightmares, voiding.
        (b) Difficulty in falling asleep again.
      (5) Usual time to awaken.
      (6) Subjective responses to sleep/rest periods.
      (7) Quantity and quality of rest periods during day.
    b. Changes since diagnosis, treatment, and/or hospitalization.
    c. Perceptions of significant others related to quantity and quality of sleep of client (client perceptions may be exaggerated).
  3. Physical findings:
    a. Restlessness.
    b. Irritability.
    c. Lethargy.
    d. Fatigue.
    e. Apathy.
    f. Decreased concentration and attention span and/or loss of train of thought.
    g. Inability to solve problems.

4. Psychological findings:
   a. Anxiety.
   b. Depression.
C. Interventions:
   1. Report signs and symptoms of sleep disturbances to physician.
   2. Institute measures to increase relaxation prior to bedtime.
      a. Bath.
      b. Snack and/or warm milk.
      c. Back rub.
      d. Positioning.
      e. Reading, watching television.
      f. Relaxation techniques.
      g. Avoid stimulants prior to bedtime.
   3. Institute measures to promote a restful sleep environment.
      a. Straighten or provide clean bed linens.
      b. Encourage use of usual clothing worn at bedtime, e.g., gowns, pajamas, underwear, no clothing.
      c. Decrease/increase environmental stimuli according to client preference, e.g., lighting, music, presence of significant other.
      d. Preferred room temperature.
   4. Institute measures to decrease physical and psychological stress.
   5. Institute measures to decrease interruption of sleep by occurrence of symptoms (see specific symptom section).
   6. Plan care during night and/or day to decrease interruptions during sleep periods.
   7. Institute medical orders as indicated:
      a. Administer drugs or treatments to control physical symptoms of disease or treatment, e.g., anxiety, depression, nausea, vomiting, pain, pruritus.
      b. Administer sedative-hypnotics to induce and maintain sleep.
D. Evaluation. The client and/or significant other will:
   1. Describe personal risk factors for insomnia.
   2. Report signs and symptoms of insomnia to health care team.
   3. Participate in measures to:
      a. Increase relaxation prior to bedtime.
      b. Control symptoms of disease or treatment that interfere with sleep.
      c. Maintain and/or improve the sleep environment.
      d. Induce and maintain sleep.
   4. Report side effects of pharmaceutical drugs used to induce and/or maintain sleep or control symptoms.

LOSS OF PERSONAL CONTROL

A. Definition—Perception of the individual that one's own actions will not affect significantly the course and/or outcome of a situation or happening.
B. Assessments.
   1. Risk factors:
      a. Disease factors:
         (1) Diagnosis with poor prognosis.
         (2) Progression of disease.
         (3) Recurrence of disease.

   (4) Multiple health problems.
   (5) Failure to respond to therapy.
  b. Health care system factors:
   (1) Professional dominance.
   (2) Ineffective communications.
   (3) Depersonalization of care.
   (4) Complexity of health care system and environment.
  c. Personal and social factors:
   (1) Ineffective coping strategies.
   (2) Cumulative losses.
   (3) Lack of social support.
   (4) Depletion of financial resources.
 2. Verbalization of loss of control.
  a. Attributes control to chance, luck, fate, and/or powerful others.
  b. Expresses lack of confidence in treatment or preventive measures to control symptoms and disease.
  c. Gives up.
  d. Expresses interest in unproven methods of therapy.
 3. Behavioral responses to loss of control:
  a. Dependency.
  b. Nonparticipation in activities of daily living.
  c. Inability to solve problems or make decisions.
  d. Impaired ability to learn and use information about health problems.
  e. Failure to participate in or adhere to treatment plan.
 4. Psychological responses to loss of control:
  a. Withdrawal.
  b. Pessimism.
  c. Decreased interpersonal interaction.
  d. Submissiveness.
  e. Apathy.
  f. Self doubt.
 5. Perceived outcomes of health care professional intervention in disease or treatment.
C. Interventions:
 1. Modify health care environment to provide increased client control.
  a. Acknowledge client as primary participant in health care team.
   (1) Inform client of Patient's Bill of Rights.
   (2) Clarify rights relative to informed consent, second opinions, right to refuse treatment.
  b. Orient to hospital or clinic environment.
  c. Describe situations in which client is able to control activities, timing, and outcomes of the plan of care:
   (1) Activities of daily living.
   (2) Teaching sessions.
   (3) Time of clinic appointments.
  d. Coach client in information seeking behaviors.
  e. Explain medical terminology, rationale for procedures, tests, and treatment regimen.
 2. Assist client to set realistic goals.
  a. Consensually validate problems and goals with client and family.
  b. Discuss personal strengths with client and significant others.

c. Identify goals client wishes to achieve.
d. Determine the order in which realistic, short-term goals should be accomplished.
e. Define client's perception of assistance needed from health care team to achieve goals.
f. Review goal achievement with client and family at predetermined time intervals.
3. Encourage information seeking behaviors.
a. Review client concerns prior to visit with health care team.
b. Assist in generation of questions to address concerns identified.
c. Evaluate client's perception of information shared by health care team.
d. Assist client in problem solving and decision making activities based on new information.
e. Evaluate client's satisfaction with abilities to seek and use health care information.
f. Increase sensitivity of health care team and significant others to sense of loss of control.
D. Evaluation. The client and/or significant other will:
1. Describe factors that place client at risk for a perceived loss of control.
2. Identify personal strengths in problem solving and decision making.
3. Report signs and symptoms of loss of control to members of health care team.
4. Describe potential consequences of a sense of loss of control.
5. Participate in measures to decrease risks of loss of control and increase a sense of personal control.

LYMPHEDEMA

A. Definition—An accumulation of fluids in the subcutaneous tissues due to venous obstruction, damage of lymphatic vessels, or lymph node dissection.
B. Assessments.
1. Risk factors:
a. Venous obstruction, e.g., tumor compression, infection, thrombophlebitis.
b. Damage to lymphatic vessels, e.g., tumor infiltration, inflammation, and fibrosis due to radiation therapy.
c. Dissection of lymph nodes.
2. History:
a. Patterns of lymphedema.
b. Impact of lymphedema on activities of daily living.
3. Physical findings:
a. Local changes:
(1) Swelling, i.e., circumference of involved extremity 4 cm greater than that of uninvolved extremity at a specified body landmark.
(2) Warmth or coolness of skin.
(3) Sensory changes, e.g., tingling, numbness, pain.
b. Motor changes, e.g., limited range of motion.
c. Circulatory changes:
(1) Diminished pulses in involved extremity.
(2) Discoloration.
(3) Nail blanching.

4. Psychological findings:
   a. Anxiety related to meaning of lymphedema.
   b. Changes in body image.
   c. Fear regarding use of extremity.
5. Sequelae of lymphedema:
   a. Increased risk of infection.
   b. Impaired skin integrity.
   c. Increased risk of injury related to sensory changes.
   d. Impaired physical mobility.
   e. Changes in self concept, body image, and sexuality.

C. Interventions:
1. Report signs and symptoms of lymphedema to physician.
2. Monitor changes in lymphedema, i.e., serial measurements of extremity at a specified body landmark.
3. Institute measures to decrease lymphedema:
   a. Elevation of extremity above the apex of the heart.
   b. Progressive exercises of involved extremity.
   c. Avoid constrictive clothing or jewelry on involved extremity.
4. Institute measures to decrease risks of complications of lymphedema:
   a. Use of loose protective clothing on extremity, e.g., gloves, long-sleeved shirts, slacks.
   b. Avoid contact with irritants to skin, e.g., allergic substances.
   c. Follow skin care protocols.
   d. Test temperatures with uninvolved extremity prior to contact with involved extremity, e.g., bath water, cooking utensils.
   e. Avoid invasive and/or constrictive procedures in involved extremity, e.g., venipunctures, blood pressure measurements.
   f. Provide assistive devices to minimize limitations imposed by restricted range of motion.
   g. Encourage discussion of impact of lymphedema on self concept, body image, and sexuality among client, significant others, and health care team.
5. Institute medical orders as indicated:
   a. Diuretics.
   b. Lymphedema sleeve.
   c. Mechanical pumps.
   d. Consults with occupational and physical therapy departments.
   e. Provide referrals to support groups, e.g., Reach to Recovery.

D. Evaluation. The client and/or significant other will:
1. Describe personal risk factors for development of lymphedema.
2. Report signs and symptoms and complications of lymphedema to health care team.
3. Participate in measures to decrease risks of and complications of lymphedema.
4. Identify situations that require professional intervention.
   a. Infection in involved extremity.
   b. Acute changes in the severity of lymphedema or its impact on activity.

MOOD ALTERATION: DEPRESSION

A. Definition—A state of being sad, discouraged, and in low spirits.
B. Assessments.

1. Risk factors:
    a. Disease effects:
        (1) Diagnosis.
        (2) Prognosis.
        (3) Anticipatory effects of treatment.
    b. Treatment effects:
        (1) Surgery—loss of body part and/or function.
        (2) Radiation therapy–induced symptomatology, e.g., weakness, fatigue, nausea, and vomiting.
        (3) Chemotherapy, e.g., hormones, unrelieved somatic responses.
    c. Situational factors:
        (1) Increased financial burden of disease and treatment.
        (2) Loss of personal control.
        (3) Social isolation of hospitalization and illness.
        (4) Cumulative crises and past losses.
        (5) Age.
        (6) Associated debilitating conditions.
        (7) Inadequate social support and financial resources.
2. History:
    a. Mood swings prior to diagnosis and treatment.
    b. Predominant mood.
    c. Accompanying behavioral components to mood.
    d. Changes in mood in times of stress and/or crisis.
    e. Reactions of significant others to changes in mood.
    f. Impact of mood swings, especially depression, and responses of significant others on client.
3. Physical findings:
    a. Fatigue, decreased energy.
    b. Loss of appetite.
    c. Sleep disturbances.
    d. Decreased physical activity.
    e. Slowing of responses to stimuli.
    f. Inability to concentrate.
    g. Decreased libido.
4. Psychological findings:
    a. Hopelessness.
    b. Irritability.
    c. Emotional lability.
    d. Lack of trust of others.
    e. Apathy.
    f. Guilt.
    g. Feelings of worthlessness.
5. Behavioral findings:
    a. Withdrawal.
    b. Decreased social interaction.
    c. Indecisiveness.
    d. Slowed cognitive processes.
    e. Regression and/or dependency.
6. Sequelae of depression:
    a. Decreased or increased nutritional intake.
    b. Decreased or increased physical activity.
    c. Decreased social interaction and/or support.

    d. Inadequate use of personal, social, professional, and economic resources.

    e. Suicidal ideation and/or attempt.

C. Interventions:

    1. Report signs and symptoms of depression to physician.

    2. Institute measures to prevent depression related to disease or treatment.

        a. Clarify perceptions of client and/or significant others regarding diagnosis, prognosis, control of symptoms, and rehabilitation.

        b. Encourage expression of feelings regarding situational factors among client, significant others, and health care team.

    3. Institute measures to prevent complications of depression.

        a. Facilitate nutritional intake.

            (1) Present personal food and fluid preferences attractively.

            (2) Arrange for social interaction during meal time.

            (3) Reinforce improved food intake.

        b. Increase physical activity.

            (1) Negotiate an activity program with client or significant other.

                (a) Progressive independence with activities of daily living.

                (b) Increased exercise and/or ambulation.

                (c) Increased participation in diversional activities, e.g., reading, watching TV, hobbies.

            (2) Return to previous home or work environment responsibilities as feasible.

        c. Improve personal sense of control.

        d. Increase social interaction.

            (1) Encourage participation in support and self help groups.

            (2) Encourage participation in pre-illness client valued activities, e.g., school, shopping, church.

        e. Encourage use of resources.

            (1) Assist client in identifying personal strengths to meet crises of cancer.

            (2) Identify areas in which client and significant others need assistance in management of personal, social, and economic factors.

            (3) Assist client as needed in problem solving to meet identified needs.

        f. Respond to suicidal ideation and/or attempts.

            (1) Provide safety measures to prevent risks of personal injury.

            (2) Report signs and symptoms of suicidal ideation to physician.

            (3) Refer client for psychiatric intervention.

    4. Institute medical orders as indicated:

        a. Treatment of underlying condition.

        b. Strategies to control symptoms associated with treatment, e.g., narcotics, sedatives, hypnotics, tranquilizers.

        c. Tricyclic antidepressants.

D. Evaluation. The client and/or significant other will:

    1. Describe personal risk factors for development of depression.

    2. Participate in strategies to decrease risk or complications of depression.

    3. Use personal, family, community, and professional resources to meet crises of cancer experience.

    4. List situations that require professional intervention.

        a. Acute changes in ability to control physical and/or psychological symptoms.

   b. Rapid deterioration of physical status.

   c. Verbalization of suicidal ideation.

NAUSEA AND VOMITING

A. Definitions:
  1. Nausea—An unpleasant sensation associated with an inclination to vomit.
  2. Vomiting—A forceful expulsion of gastric contents through the mouth.
B. Assessments.
  1. Risk factors:
    a. Disease effects:
      (1) Primary and/or secondary malignancy of the central nervous system.
      (2) Consequence of increased intracranial pressure resulting from intracranial bleeding.
      (3) Obstruction of gastrointestinal tract by tumor.
      (4) Consequence of food toxins, infection, or motion sickness.
    b. Treatment effects:
      (1) Cancer chemotherapy, e.g., cisplatin, nitrogen mustard, doxorubicin, dacarbazine.
      (2) Radiation therapy with stomach, intestines, esophagus, and/or brain included in treatment fields.
      (3) Waste products from increased cellular destruction.
      (4) Irritation of gastrointestinal tract.
    c. Drugs, e.g., digitalis, morphine, antibiotics, vitamins, iron.
    d. Pain.
    e. Concentrated supplemental feedings.
    f. Electrolyte imbalances, e.g., hypercalcemia, hyponatremia.
    g. Renal dysfunction.
    h. Psychogenic factors:
      (1) Anticipatory nausea prior to therapy or contact with health care system and personnel.
      (2) Tension, anxiety.
      (3) Noxious visual and/or olfactory stimuli.
  2. History:
    a. Patterns of nausea and vomiting.
    b. Associated factors, timing, and duration.
  3. Physical findings:
    a. Nausea.
      (1) Increased pulse and depth of respiration, and decreased blood pressure.
      (2) Circumoral pallor, weakness.
      (3) Warmth of skin, sweating.
      (4) Increase in oral secretions.
    b. Vomiting.
      (1) Decreased pulse, increased depth of respiration and blood pressure.
      (2) Coolness of skin.
      (3) Emesis—color, character, volume.
  4. Psychological findings:
    a. Increased stress.
    b. Conditioning to adversive stimuli.

5. Sequelae of prolonged nausea and vomiting:
   a. Fluid and electrolyte imbalance, e.g. dehydration, hypokalemia, decreased H^+ and Cl^-.
   b. Nutritional deficiencies resulting in weight loss.
   c. Decreased activity level.
   d. Weakness, lethargy, apathy, anxiety.
   e. Esophageal trauma.
   f. Aspiration pneumonia.
C. Interventions:
   1. Institute measures to minimize occurrence of nausea or vomiting.
      a. Decrease environmental stimuli, e.g., noise, smells, lighting.
      b. Provide well-ventilated, cool environment.
      c. Avoid sudden movement and surges of movement.
      d. Restructure daily activities to minimize activity during times of increased nausea.
      e. Modify diet to include cool, bland foods.
      f. Teach relaxation or distraction techniques.
   2. Institute measures to minimize potential complications of nausea or vomiting.
      a. Replace fluids lost via emesis with high caloric, electrolyte-rich, cool liquids, e.g., Gatorade, popsicles, soft drinks.
      b. Allow for rest periods during times of increased nausea.
      c. Plan activities to conserve physical energy while maintaining maximal level of independence.
      d. Position patient during vomiting episode to decrease risks of aspiration.
   3. Institute comfort measures when vomiting subsides.
      a. Wash face with cool cloth.
      b. Allow rest periods.
      c. Provide or encourage mouth care.
      d. Provide diversional activities.
   4. Report signs and symptoms of nausea and vomiting and complications of nausea and vomiting to physician.
   5. Institute medical orders as indicated:
      a. Administer antiemetics on a round-the-clock basis during periods of high incidence of nausea or vomiting.
      b. Replace fluids and electrolytes.
D. Evaluation. The client and or significant other will:
   1. Describe personal risk factors for nausea and vomiting.
   2. Report patterns of nausea and vomiting to health care team.
   3. Participate in activities to decrease risks of nausea and vomiting.
   4. Report signs, symptoms, and complications of nausea and vomiting to health care team.

PAIN

A. Definition—An unpleasant, uncomfortable, distressing subjective sensation experienced by an individual in response to noxious stimuli.
B. Assessments.
   1. Risk factors:
      a. Disease related:
         (1) Infiltration of nerves by tumor.

     (2) Compression of tissues and nerves by tumor.

     (3) Localized tissue necrosis resulting from tumor invasion.

     (4) Metastatic disease of the musculoskeletal system.

     (5) Effusions and edema resulting from disease that distends normal tissues that are sensitive to pain.

  b. Treatment related:

     (1) Diagnostic and surgical procedures.

     (2) Long-term consequences of radiation therapy, e.g., fibrosis of tissues and compression of nerves.

     (3) Long-term consequences of surgery, e.g., adhesions.

     (4) Complications of cancer therapy, e.g., stomatitis, localized infection, inflammation of tissues in radiation field, opportunistic infections, phantom limb pain.

  c. Pre-existing diseases or conditions, e.g., arthritis, dysmenorrhea, musculoskeletal disease.

  d. Overactivity.

  e. Immobility and/or improper body alignment.

  f. Anxiety precipitated by impact of diagnosis of cancer on activities of daily living, role performance, relationships, communication patterns, and economic factors.

2. History:

  a. Patterns of pain.

  b. Responses of client or significant others to pain experience.

  c. Perceived relationship of pain to the cancer experience.

  d. Past experiences with pain and degree of success in management.

3. Physical findings are listed in Table 29–1.

4. Behavioral findings are listed in Table 29–1.

5. Affective findings are listed in Table 29–1.

  a. Anxiety.

  b. Depression.

  c. Fear.

6. Sequelae of unrelieved pain:

  a. Depression, anger, social withdrawal.

  b. Failure to participate in activities of daily living and treatment plan, impairment of role performance and self concept.

  c. Distrust of health care professionals.

  d. Immobility.

  e. Substance abuse, e.g., drugs, alcohol.

  f. Use of pain for secondary gains.

C. Interventions:

1. Institute measures to promote physical comfort and relaxation.

  a. Positioning.

  b. Turning.

  c. Application of heat or cold.

  d. Minimize noxious environmental stimuli.

  e. Relaxation therapy.

  f. Splinting.

  g. Cutaneous stimulation, e.g., massage, back rubs.

2. Institute measures to provide distraction.

  a. Imagery of pleasant or exciting experiences.

  b. Touch, if acceptable.

  c. Humor, as appropriate.

Table 29–1. DIFFERENTIATION BETWEEN ACUTE
AND CHRONIC PAIN

	Acute	Chronic
Characteristics of Pain	Sharp, localized sensation	Dull, generalized aching
	Occurs suddenly, subsides quickly with intervention	Continuous and occurs regularly for an undetermined period of time
	Associated with diagnostic and surgical procedures	Most commonly occurs with advanced or terminal illness
	Associated with acute effects of cancer therapy	Associated with long-term sequelae of cancer and/or therapy
Physical findings	Increased blood pressure, pulse rate, and respirations	No significant changes in pulse rate, respirations, or blood pressure
	Muscle spasms	Muscle spasms
	Tense body posture	Tense body posture
	Evidence of inflammation	May not have evidence of inflammation
	Peripheral vasoconstriction	Reflex abnormalities
	Sleep disturbances	Insomnia
	Anorexia	Anorexia or weight loss
		Nausea and vomiting
Behavioral Findings	Heightened awareness	Withdrawal, lethargy
	Guarding	Guarding
	Restlessness	Inactivity
	Agitation	Decreased participation in activities of daily living
	Increased personal interactions	Decreased personal interactions
	Decreased ability to solve problems	Decreased ability to work, solve problems
Affective Findings	Apprehension	Depression
	Anxiety	Fear
	Fear	Inability to enjoy life
		Flat affect
		Hopelessness
		Helplessness

      d. Diversional activities, e.g., reading, occupational therapy.
      e. Encourage expression of feelings regarding cancer diagnosis and re-
         actions of significant others.
      f. Music therapy.
   3. Institute measures to manage potential side effects of drug regimen for
     pain control.
      a. Changes in level of consciousness.
      b. Respiratory depression.
      c. Constipation.
   4. Institute measures to promote psychological comfort.
      a. Reassurance.
      b. Trusting relationship.

      c. Positive reinforcement of efforts to manage own pain.

      d. Negative reinforcement of maladaptive coping behaviors.

      e. Advocate use of sedatives, antidepressants, and/or tranquilizers as ordered.

  5. Institute measures to promote a team approach to pain management.

      a. Include client or significant other in planning strategies for pain management.

      b. Serve as a client advocate in encouraging behaviors that convey the pain experience to the health care team.

      c. Suggest administration of combinations of narcotic and non-narcotic drugs when feasible.

      d. Suggest changes in dosage or frequency, not both, when adjusting pain regimen to meet client needs.

      e. Assess components of pain experience and adequacy of relief measures systematically.

  6. Institute measures to decrease exacerbation of pain response.

      a. Administer analgesics early in the pain experience to avoid severe pain.

      b. Administer pain medications on a regularly scheduled basis, determined by the duration and peak action of drugs, needs of client, and physician's orders.

      c. Schedule pain-inducing activities or procedures to occur during peak analgesic effect.

      d. Advocate an adequate trial period of a regimen prior to adjusting ineffective analgesic plan.

  7. Institute associated medical orders:

      a. Analgesics.

      b. Antidepressants, sedatives, hypnotics, and/or tranquilizers.

      c. Neural stimulators, e.g., transcutaneous nerve stimulation.

      d. Client-controlled analgesia.

      e. Referrals for behavior modification, physical therapy, occupational therapy, and/or chronic pain management.

      f. Prepare client for surgical procedures to relieve pain, e.g., nerve blocks, cordotomy, neurectomy.

D. Evaluation. The client and/or significant other will:

  1. Describe personal risk factors for development of pain.

  2. Describe characteristics of pain experience.

  3. Identify impact of client's or significant other's perceptions and attitudes about pain and its relationship to the cancer experience.

  4. Participate in measures to eliminate or modify the pain experience to tolerable limits for the individual client.

  5. Participate in measures to minimize the effects of pain on activities of daily living, role performance, work or home maintenance, and self concept.

  6. Discuss the goals of professional intervention in pain management.

  7. Participate in measures to minimize the potential complications of pain medication.

  8. Identify situations that require professional intervention.

      a. Pain unrelieved with usual pain management regimen.

      b. Acute changes in the severity, location, and/or duration of pain.

      c. Unrelieved complications of pain management regimen.

PRURITUS

A. Definition—Itching.
B. Assessments.
  1. Risk factors:
     a. Disease related:
        (1) Hematologic malignancies, e.g., lymphomas, leukemias, myeloma, Hodgkin's disease.
        (2) Solid tumors, e.g., melanomas, inflammatory breast cancer.
     b. Treatment related:
        (1) Surgery, e.g., wound healing.
        (2) Radiation therapy, e.g., local skin reaction in treatment field.
        (3) Chemotherapy, e.g., allergies to cancer drugs, fluid and electrolyte imbalances related to side effects of drugs (dehydration, hypercalcemia).
        (4) Immunotherapy, e.g., local skin reactions at present or previous injection sites, allergic response.
        (5) Graft-versus-host disease.
     c. Aging.
     d. Dry atmospheric conditions.
     e. Allergic reactions to foods, clothing, drugs, and so forth.
     f. Liver and/or kidney dysfunction.
     g. Anxiety.
  2. History:
     a. Patterns of pruritus.
     b. Impact of pruritus on activities of daily living, life style, and comfort.
  3. Physical findings:
     a. Scratch marks on skin.
     b. Erythema.
     c. Thickening of skin.
     d. Dryness of skin.
     e. Deposits of urea and/or bilirubin on skin surface.
  4. Presence of complications of pruritus.
     a. Impaired skin integrity.
     b. Infection.
C. Interventions:
  1. Institute measures to maintain hydration of skin.
     a. Adequate fluid intake, > 3000 cc/day.
     b. Water-soluble skin emollients on damp skin.
     c. Humidified environment.
  2. Institute measures to protect the skin integrity.
     a. Short, smooth fingernails and handwashing.
     b. Alternative methods of skin stimulation:
        (1) Pressure.
        (2) Massage.
        (3) Vibration.
        (4) Cool temperature.
     c. Avoidance of allergic foods, materials, and drugs.
     d. Avoidance of tight clothing made of irritating fabrics (corduroy, wool).
  3. Institute measures to prevent vasodilation.
     a. Cool environment.

      b. Cool baths or showers.

      c. Avoidance of alcoholic beverages and caffeine.

      d. Decrease anxiety.

        (1) Distraction.

        (2) Relaxation.

    4. Institute associated medical treatment as ordered:

      a. Treatment of underlying disease.

      b. Antihistamines.

      c. Tranquilizers.

      d. Steroids.

      e. Topical agents.

D. Evaluation. The client and/or significant other will:

    1. Describe personal risk factors for development of pruritus.

    2. Discuss potential complications of pruritus.

    3. Report signs and symptoms and complications of pruritus to health care team.

    4. Participate in measures to decrease pruritus, prevent complications, and promote comfort.

RENAL DYSFUNCTION

A. Definition—Decreased ability of the kidney to perform normal functions of filtration, secretion, and excretion of fluids, electrolytes, and waste products of cellular metabolism.

B. Assessments.

    1. Risk factors:

      a. Disease related:

        (1) Primary tumor involving the kidney.

        (2) Increased production of cellular waste products resulting from effects of tumor growth, i.e., invasion, obstruction, necrosis, altered metabolism.

        (3) Tubular damage resulting from fever.

      b. Treatment related:

        (1) Rapid tumor cell lysis resulting from radiation therapy, chemotherapy, and/or immunotherapy.

        (2) Increased cellular metabolism resulting from therapeutic hyperthermia and/or fever.

        (3) Renal toxicities of cancer chemotherapeutic agents.

      c. Renal toxicities of drugs, e.g., antibiotics.

    2. History:

      a. Changes in character of urine, e.g., amount, color, odor.

      b. Dietary intake.

      c. Pre-existing renal dysfunction.

      d. Perception of client or significant other regarding etiology, significance, and prognosis of renal dysfunction.

    3. Physical findings:

      a. Increased pulse, respirations, blood pressure.

      b. Dependent edema, e.g., extremities, periorbital area.

      c. Increased weight.

      d. Anorexia.

      e. Weakness and fatigue.

      f. Flank pain.

      g. Pruritus.

      h. Urea crystals on skin.

   4. Behavioral findings:

      a. Apathy.

      b. Listlessness.

      c. Confusion.

      d. Decreased ability to solve problems.

   5. Laboratory findings:

      a. BUN > 20 mg/100 ml.

      b. Creatinine > 1.6 gm/24 hours.

      c. Uric acid > 8.5 mg/100 ml.

      d. Electrolyte imbalances.

      e. Decreased hemoglobin.

   6. Sequelae of renal dysfunction:

      a. Fluid and electrolyte imbalances. See material on:

         (1) Edema.

         (2) Dehydration.

         (3) Hyperkalemia.

         (4) Hypokalemia.

         (5) Syndrome of inappropriate antidiuretic hormone (see Chapter 30).

      b. Renal failure.

      c. Convulsions.

      d. Coma.

      e. Death.

C. Interventions:

   1. Report signs and symptoms of renal dysfunction to physician.

   2. Institute measures to promote comfort.

      a. Skin care.

      b. Paced activities.

      c. Discussion of client's or significant other's responses to renal dysfunction.

      d. Provide information related to renal status as indicated.

   3. Institute measures to decrease risks of injury in the presence of confusion or weakness.

   4. Institute medical orders as indicated.

      a. Food and fluid modifications.

      b. Diuretics.

      c. Allopurinol in the presence of increased cellular destruction related to disease and/or treatment.

      d. Dialysis.

      e. Hydration prior to administration of nephrotoxic chemotherapeutic agents.

D. Evaluation. The client and/or significant other will:

   1. Describe personal risk factors for development of renal dysfunction.

   2. Report signs and symptoms of renal dysfunction to the health care team.

   3. Participate in measures to decrease the risk of complications of renal dysfunction.

   4. Identify resources available to assist with management of renal dysfunction, e.g., dietary management and supervision, home dialysis programs.

   5. Identify situations that require professional intervention.

    a. Acute, marked decrease in urine output.
    b. Changes in sensorium.
    c. Convulsions.

SECONDARY MALIGNANCY

A. Definition—The occurrence of a second primary malignancy presumably related to exposure to cancer therapy, e.g., chemotherapy and/or radiation therapy.
B. Assessments.
  1. Treatment related changes in normal tissues at the cellular level that may result in malignant growth:
    a. Chromosome breaks.
    b. Translocation of genetic material.
    c. Incorporation of faulty substances in RNA/DNA structure.
  2. Exposure to alkylating agents appears to lead to the greatest risk of secondary malignancy.
  3. Additive effects of combination chemotherapy or radiation therapy.
  4. Physical findings:
    a. Symptomatology usually consistent with malignancies of hematopoietic or immune system.
    b. Tumors may arise at the sites of previous radiation fields.
  5. Psychological findings:
    a. Anxiety.
    b. Fear
    c. Powerlessness.
    d. Hopelessness.
  6. Perceptions of client/significant others regarding risks of cancer therapy
C. Interventions:
  1. Report signs and symptoms of malignancy to physician.
  2. Institute measures to alert client or significant other to potential side effects of therapy.
    a. Teaching.
    b. Informed consent.
  3. Institute measures to assist client or significant other in coping with potential risks of therapy.
    a. Discuss risk/benefit ratio of therapy.
    b. Allow expression of feelings regarding risks of therapy.
    c. Teach self-evaluation techniques for monitoring health status.
    d. Encourage routine follow-up medical care.
D. Evaluation. The client and/or significant other will:
  1. Describe personal risk factors for secondary malignancy.
  2. Participate in routine follow-up medical care activities.
  3. Report signs and symptoms of malignancy to health care team.

SEXUAL AND REPRODUCTIVE DYSFUNCTION

A. Definition—Inability to express sexual behaviors, attitudes, and functions satisfactorily and consistently with personal needs and preferences.
B. Assessments (Client and partner, if available).

1. Risk factors:
   a. Disease related:
      (1) Primary tumors of reproductive organs and/or organs closely associated with masculinity or feminity.
      (2) Invasion of reproductive organs by tumor resulting in hemorrhage, obstruction, or necrosis.
      (3) Inadequate control of symptoms of tumor growth.
      (4) Prolonged hospitalizations.
      (5) Forced dependency.
      (6) Role reversals.
      (7) Lack of privacy.
   b. Treatment related:
      (1) Structural deficits, e.g., vaginectomy, pudendal nerve damage, vulvectomy.
      (2) Reproductive deficits, e.g., anovulation, oligospermia, spontaneous abortions.
      (3) Functional deficits, e.g., impotence, retrograde ejaculation, vaginal fibrosis, amenorrhea.
      (4) Genetic changes, e.g., mutations of ova and/or sperm, teratogenetic effects of chemotherapy or radiation therapy.
      (5) Impaired self concept, body image, feelings of attractiveness as a sexual being, e.g., masculinization or feminization or obesity resulting from hormone therapy, role reversal.
      (6) Inadequate control of symptoms resulting from cancer therapy.
2. History:
   a. Previous sexual patterns and preferences.
      (1) Sexual roles.
      (2) Perceptions of self as sexual being.
      (3) Perceived perceptions of others as to self as a sexual being.
      (4) Sexual behaviors.
         (a) Frequency.
         (b) Satisfaction.
   b. Previous reproductive history.
      (1) Number, sex, and ages of children.
      (2) Difficulty or complications of impregnation, pregnancy, and delivery.
      (3) Type and length of use of contraceptives.
      (4) Menstrual history (females).
3. Psychological responses to disease and treatment:
   a. Changes in libido.
   b. Anxiety.
   c. Fear.
   d. Depression.
   e. Mood swings.
   f. Anticipatory grief.
   g. Loss of control.
   h. Loss of intimacy.
4. Drugs:
   a. Antidepressants.
   b. Antihypertensives.
   c. Narcotics.

C. Interventions:
   1. Institute measures to provide information related to effects of disease and/or treatment on sexuality.
      a. Validate specific concerns with client and partner.
      b. Evaluate meaning of terms used in describing sexual concerns, e.g., orgasm, erection, impotence, infertility, sterility.
   2. Institute measures to provide specific suggestions on strategies to adapt to changes in sexuality imposed by disease and/or treatment.
      a. Lubrication.
      b. Changes in position.
      c. Modifications of daily activities to decrease fatigue prior to intimacy.
      d. Methods to increase stimulation prior to coitus.
      e. Discussion of sexuality concerns with partner.
      f. Resumption of previous roles and responsibilities.
      g. Support groups, e.g., I Can Cope, Reach to Recovery, Make Today Count.
      h. Use of wigs, turbans, hats for alopecia.
   3. Institute measures to assist client and partner to solve problems and identify resources to deal with marked changes in sexuality.
   4. Institute medical orders as indicated.
      a. Referrals for professional counseling.
      b. Preparation for reconstruction, e.g., breast, vagina.
      c. Assistive devices to promote satisfactory sexual function, e.g., use of lubricants, penile implants, vibrators.
      d. Preparation for salvage of reproductive function, e.g., sperm banking, protection of ovary by tacking behind uterus.
      e. Referrals for genetic counseling.
      f. Birth control during therapy.
      g. Control of symptomatology related to disease and/or treatment, e.g., pain, nausea, fatigue.
      h. Hormone replacement.
D. Evaluation. The client and/or significant other will:
   1. Describe personal risk factors for sexual dysfunction related to disease and/or treatment.
   2. Discuss perceived changes in sexual behaviors, attitudes, and function with significant other and health care team.
   3. Participate in measures to decrease the impact of disease and therapy on sexuality and sexual function.
   4. Participate in measures to maintain a positive self concept, body image, and a sense of control.
   5. Identify community resources available to assist in coping with sexual dysfunction.

STOMATITIS, ESOPHAGITIS, OR MUCOSITIS

A. Definitions:
   1. Mucositis—Generalized inflammation of mucous membranes.
   2. Esophagitis—Inflammation of mucous membranes of the esophagus.
   3. Stomatitis—Inflammation of the mucous membranes of the oral cavity.
B. Assessments.

1. Risk factors:
    a. Disease effects via infiltration of mucous membranes by tumor.
    b. Treatment effects:
        (1) Local reaction of mucous membranes to surgical manipulation.
        (2) Cancer chemotherapeutic agents that destroy normal rapidly dividing cells, e.g., mucous membranes, and result in inflammation.
            (a) Antimetabolites, e.g., methotrexate.
            (b) Antibiotics.
        (3) Radiation therapy that includes head and neck, chest, abdomen, and pelvis in treatment fields.
        (4) Graft-versus-host disease.
    c. Pre-existing disease states.
        (1) Poor oral hygiene.
        (2) Dehydration.
        (3) Immunosuppression.
    d. Exposure to chemical irritants:
        (1) Mouthwashes.
        (2) Tobacco.
        (3) Alcohol.
    e. Exposure to physical irritants:
        (1) Extreme temperatures in foods.
        (2) Coarse, high fiber foods.
        (3) Poorly fitting dentures.
        (4) Repeated enemas.
2. Physical findings:
    a. Redness, swelling, tenderness of mucous membranes.
    b. Diminished taste sensations.
    c. Burning sensation.
    d. Pain.
    e. Changes in the character of the stool.
3. Psychosocial findings:
    a. Decreased verbal communication.
    b. Social isolation.
    c. Apathy.
4. Sequelae of mucositis:
    a. Impaired integrity of mucous membranes.
    b. Infection.
    c. Difficulty swallowing.
    d. Difficulty speaking.
    e. Inadequate nutritional intake or absorption.
    f. Diarrhea.
    g. Pain.
C. Interventions:
    1. Institute measures to decrease inflammation of mucous membranes.
        a. Avoid exposure to chemical and/or physical irritants.
        b. Encourage oral hygiene measures prior to and after each meal and before bedtime.
        c. Encourage adequate fluid intake (> 3000 ml/day).
    2. Institute measures to increase comfort:
        a. Topical protective agents, e.g., antacids, kaolin-containing substances, Orabase.
        b. Sitz baths.

3. Institute measures to minimize complications of mucositis:
   a. Modify dietary intake, e.g., bland, soft, liquid, high caloric, high protein foods.
   b. Encourage oral and perineal hygiene measures.
   c. Develop alternate means of communication, e.g., Magic slate, cards, and direct, short response questions.
   d. Encourage participation in activities of daily living, especially hygiene.
4. Institute medical orders as indicated:
   a. Prophylactic antibacterial, antifungal, and antiviral agents.
   b. Systematic and/or topical analgesics, e.g., viscous xylocaine, benadryl, Tucks compresses, Sitz baths.
   c. Topical protective agents.
   d. Dietary and vitamin supplements.
   e. Systematic and/or local anti-inflammatory agents, e.g., steroid enemas.
   f. Antidiarrheal medications.
D. Evaluation. The client and/or significant other will:
   1. Describe personal risk factors for mucositis.
   2. Report signs and symptoms and complications of mucositis to health care team.
   3. Participate in measures to minimize complications of mucositis.
   4. List situations that require professional assistance in management.
      a. Temperature > 101°F.
      b. Significant changes in nutritional intake.
      c. Poorly controlled symptom management, e.g., discomfort, diarrhea.

TASTE ALTERATIONS

A. Definition—Actual or perceived changes in taste sensations.
B. Assessments.
   1. Risk factors:
      a. Disease effects:
         (1) Invasion of oral cavity or tongue by tumor.
         (2) Excretion of noxious substances by the tumor, which increase the bitter taste sensation.
         (3) Volume of tumor.
      b. Treatment effects:
         (1) Surgical removal of tongue, interruption of olfactory nerve, variation of normal breathing pathway, e.g., tracheostomy.
         (2) Radiation-induced destruction of taste buds (> 1000 rads), dryness of mouth, loss of taste for food.
         (3) Chemotherapy-induced changes in taste buds:
            (a) Lowered threshold for bitter tastes.
            (b) Increased threshold for sweet tastes.
            (c) Metallic or medicine taste.
      c. Aging induced degeneration of taste buds.
      d. Poor oral hygiene or infection.
      e. Decreased levels of zinc.
   2. Physical findings:
      a. Patterns of taste changes, e.g., aversion to red meat.
      b. Impact taste changes have on dietary intake.

   3. Sequelae of prolonged alterations in taste:
      a. Anorexia.
      b. Decreased dietary intake.
      c. Weight loss.
C. Interventions:
   1. Institute measures to increase sensitivity of taste buds.
      a. Increase use of flavorings and spices in foods.
      b. Serve foods warm to increase aroma.
      c. Increase fluid intake with meals.
      d. Encourage oral hygiene prior to and after meals.
   2. Institute measures to decrease aversiveness of selected foods or food groups:
      a. Add increased sweeteners to foods.
      b. Marinate red meats in sweet juices.
      c. Offer meat protein substitutes, e.g., peanut butter, eggs, cheese.
   3. Institute measures to decrease risks of and detect sequelae of prolonged taste alterations:
      a. Weigh at regular intervals.
      b. Supplement diet with high calorie, high protein foods, e.g., milkshakes, pudding.
D. Evaluation. The client and/or significant other will:
   1. Describe personal risks for changes in taste sensations.
   2. Report signs and symptoms and complications of taste changes to health care team.
   3. Participate in measures to minimize the effects of taste changes on the joy of eating and nutritional status.

XEROSTOMIA

A. Definition—Dryness of the mouth.
B. Assessments.
   1. Risk factors:
      a. Disease related effects on salivary gland function, e.g., primary or secondary tumor involvement.
      b. Treatment effects:
         (1) Surgical removal of salivary gland.
         (2) Radiation therapy fields that include the salivary glands.
         (3) Medical management of chemotherapy-induced symptoms, e.g., phenothiazines for nausea and vomiting.
      c. Administration of drugs, e.g., antihistamines, atropine.
      d. Alcohol or nicotine ingestion.
      e. Other diseases, e.g., diabetes, infection.
   2. Physical findings:
      a. Dry, shiny oral mucous membranes.
      b. Thick, scanty saliva.
      c. Decreased pH of oral secretions.
      d. Difficulty in swallowing.
   3. Psychological factors affecting the occurrence of xerostomia:
      a. Fear.
      b. Anxiety.

4. Sequelae of prolonged xerostomia:
   a. Inadequate digestion of starches.
   b. Impaired mucous membrane integrity.
   c. Dental caries.
C. Interventions:
   1. Report signs and symptoms and complications of xerostomia to physician.
   2. Institute measures to increase saliva flow:
      a. Offer selected foods, e.g., tart, sugar-free candy, or hot tea with lemon.
      b. Suggest chewing Gatorgum.
      c. Apply pressure to sternal notch.
      d. Massage back of neck.
   3. Institute measures to provide moisture in the oral cavity.
      a. Use of artificial saliva.
      b. Sip liquids with meals.
      c. Moisten foods with liquids and sauces, e.g., gravy, cream, soups, beverages.
      d. Keep container with preferred fluids near client.
   4. Institute measures to decrease risks of sequelae of xerostomia:
      a. Increase fluid intake with meals.
      b. Encourage strict oral hygiene before and after meals.
      c. Avoid use of loose dentures, alcohol, hard, coarse or spicy foods, lemon-glycerin swabs.
      d. Encourage routine dental examinations.
   5. Institute medical orders as indicated:
      a. Fluoride treatments.
      b. Properly fitting dentures.
D. Evaluation. The client and/or significant other will:
   1. Describe personal risk factors for xerostomia.
   2. Report signs and symptoms and complications of xerostomia to health care team.
   3. Participate in measures to decrease the risks and complications of xerostomia.
   4. List situations that require professional assistance in management.
      a. Impaired integrity of oral mucosa.
      b. Dental caries.

STUDY QUESTIONS

1. Identify appropriate assessment data in each of the following categories for common problems experienced by clients/significant others facing cancer:
   a. risk factors
   b. history
   c. physical findings
   d. psychological findings
2. Select relevant nursing interventions for common problems experienced by clients with cancer.
3. Formulate client-centered goals to use as evaluation criteria for clients experiencing common oncologic problems.

Bibliography

American Cancer Society: Cancer: A Manual for Practitioners, 5th ed., Boston, American Cancer Society, 1978.

American Cancer Society: Cancer Management. Philadelphia, J. B. Lippincott Company, 1968.

American Cancer Society: Unproven Methods of Cancer Management. New York, American Cancer Society, 1971.

Berger, K. and Bostwick, J.: A Woman's Decision. St. Louis, C. V. Mosby Company, 1984.

Bouchard, R.: Nursing Care of the Cancer Patient. St. Louis, C. V. Mosby Company, 1967.

Burkhalter, P. and Donley, D.: Dynamics of Oncology Nursing. New York, McGraw-Hill Book Company, 1978.

Burns, N.: Nursing and Cancer. Philadelphia, W. B. Saunders Company, 1982.

Carpenito, L.: Nursing Diagnosis: Application to Clinical Practice. Philadelphia, J. B. Lippincott Company, 1983.

Chernecky, C. and Ramsey, P.: Critical Nursing Care of the Client With Cancer. Norwalk, CT, Appleton-Century-Crofts, 1984.

Corbett, N. and Beveridge, P.: Clinical Simulations in Nursing Practice. Philadelphia, W. B. Saunders Company, 1980.

Craytor, J. and Fass, M.: The Nurse and the Cancer Patient: A Programmed Textbook. Philadelphia, J. B. Lippincott Company, 1970.

DeVita, V., Hellman, S., and Rosenberg, S. (eds.): Cancer: Principles and Practice of Oncology. Philadelphia, J. B. Lippincott Company, 1982.

Dohrenwend, B. S. and Dohrenwend, B. P. (eds.): Stressful Life Events and Their Contexts. New York, Neale Watson Academic Publications, Inc, 1981.

Donoghue, M., Nunnally, C., and Yasko, J.: Nutritional Aspects of Cancer Care. Reston, VA, Reston Publishing Company, 1982.

Donovan, M.: Cancer Care: A Guide for Patient Education. New York, Appleton-Century-Crofts, 1981.

Donovan, M. and Girton, S.: Cancer Care Nursing, 2nd ed. Norwalk, CT, Appleton-Century-Crofts, 1984.

Gonnella, C., Parker, D., Hollender, J., et al.: Normative Criteria for Cancer Rehabilitation. Atlanta, Emory University, 1978.

Gormican, A.: Influencing food acceptance in anorexic cancer patients. Postgraduate Medicine, 68:145–152, 1980.

Groer, M. and Pierce, M.: Guarding against cancer's hidden killer: Anorexia-cachexia. Nursing, 11:39–43, 1981.

Guyton, A.: Textbook of Medical Physiology, 7th ed. Philadelphia, W. B. Saunders Company, 1986.

Handbook of Clinical Nutrition. Columbus, OH, Ross Laboratories, 1979.

Haskell, C. (ed.): Cancer Treatment. Philadelphia, W. B. Saunders Company, 1980.

Jones, D., Dunbar, C., and Jirovec, M.: Medical-Surgical Nursing: A Conceptual Approach. New York, McGraw-Hill Book Company, 1978.

Kellogg, C. and Sullivan, B. (eds.): Current Perspectives in Oncologic Nursing (Vol. 2). St. Louis, C. V. Mosby Company, 1978.

Kruse, L., Reese, J., and Hart, L. (eds.): Cancer: Pathophysiology, Etiology, and Management. St. Louis, C. V. Mosby Company, 1979.

Kubler-Ross, E.: On Death and Dying. New York, Macmillan Company, 1969.

Laszlo, J. (ed.): Antiemetics and Cancer Chemotherapy. Baltimore, Williams & Wilkins, 1983.

Leaby, I., St. Germain, J., and Varricchio, C.: The Nurse and Radiotherapy: A Manual for Daily Care. St. Louis, C. V. Mosby Company, 1979.

Lee, P., Brown, N., and Red, I. (eds.): The Nation's Health. San Francisco, Boyd & Fraser Publishing Company, 1981.

Little, D. and Carnevali, D.: Nursing Care Planning, 2nd ed. Philadelphia, J. B. Lippincott Company, 1976.

Marino, L.: Cancer Nursing. St. Louis, C. V. Mosby Company, 1981.

McCaffery, M.: Nursing Managemennt of the Patient With Pain. Philadelphia, J. B. Lippincott Company, 1972.

McCaffery, M. and Meinhart, N.: Pain: A Nursing Approach to Assessment and Analysis. Norwalk, CT, Appleton-Century-Crofts, 1983.

McIntire, S. and Cioppa, A. (eds.): Cancer Nursing: A Developmental Approach. New York, John Wiley & Sons, 1984.

Mechanic, D. (ed.): Symptoms, Illness Behavior, and Help-Seeking. New York, Neale Watson Academic Publications, Inc, 1982.

Miller, J.: Coping With Chronic Illness: Overcoming Powerlessness. Philadelphia, F. A. Davis Company, 1983.

Ostchega, Y.: Preventing . . . and treating . . . cancer chemotherapy's oral complications. Nursing, 10:47–52, 1980.

Petersdorf, R., Adams, R., Braunwald, E., et al.: Harrison's Principles of Internal Medicine, 10th ed. New York, McGraw-Hill Book Company, 1983.

Peterson, B. and Kellogg, C.: Current Practice in Oncologic Nursing (Vol. 1). St. Louis, C. V. Mosby Company, 1976.

Plumer, A.: Principles and Practices of Intravenous Therapy. Boston, Little, Brown & Company, 1982.

Rosenbaum, E. and Rosenbaum, I.: A Comprehensive Guide for Cancer Patients and Their Families. Palo Alto, CA, Bull Publishing Company, 1980.

Simko, M., Cowell, C., and Gilbride, J.: Nutrition Assessment: A Comprehensive Guide for Planning Intervention. Rockville, MD, Aspen Systems Publications, 1984.

Snetselaar, L.: Nutrition Counseling Skills. Rockville, MD, Aspen Systems Publications, 1983.

Werner-Beland, J.: Grief Responses to Long-Term Illness and Disability. Reston, VA, Reston Publishing Company, 1980.

Yasko, J.: Guidelines for Cancer Care: Symptom Management. Reston, VA: Reston Publishing Company, 1983.

30

Nursing Management of Common Oncologic Emergencies

JOANNE PETER FINDLEY, RN, MS

CARDIAC TAMPONADE

A. Pathophysiology.
   1. Intrapericardial pressure increases secondary to:
      a. An accumulation of fluid from direct tumor invasion, metastatic tumor, or infection.
      b. Constriction due to the pericardial thickening caused by radiation therapy or the tumor itself.
   2. Increased intrapericardial pressure results in compression of the heart and decreased diastolic filling.
   3. Decreased diastolic filling of the ventricles results in decreased stroke volume and cardiac output.
B. Etiology.
   1. Malignancies:
      a. Primary—rarely owing to a tumor of the pericardium.
      b. Metastatic.
         (1) Lung—most common cause.
         (2) Breast.
         (3) Lymphomas and leukemias.
         (4) Melanomas.
   2. Radiation therapy—pericardial thickening occurs at greater than or equal to 4,000 rads.
C. Assessment.
   1. Signs and symptoms:
      a. Dyspnea, cough, chest pain.
      b. Anxiety and apprehension.

   c. Jugular venous distention, muffled heart sounds, cyanosis, edema, rales, pulsus paradoxus.
   d. Decreased systolic blood pressure, narrowed pulse pressure, increased central venous pressure (CVP).
  2. Diagnostic tests:
   a. EKG—low voltage, elevated ST, sinus tachycardia, ventricular electrical alternans.
   b. Chest x-ray—cardiomegaly, or tumor may be visualized.
   c. Echocardiogram—two echoes are seen instead of one.
   d. Cytology of pericardial fluid—usually serosanguineous.
D. Intervention.
  1. Prepare for medical procedures:
   a. Pericardiocentesis—emergency treatment; immediate, temporary relief with removal of 50–100 ml of fluid.
   b. Pericardial window—surgical opening to drain fluid to pleural space; used for prolonged palliation.
   c. Chemotherapy—instillation of an agent such as mechlorethamine (nitrogen mustard), triethylene thiophosphoramide (thiotepa), fluorouracil, radioactive isotopes, tetracycline, or talc through an indwelling pericardial catheter to induce fibrosis.
   d. Radiation therapy—treatment of choice if radiation pericarditis is not the cause; dose of 2,000–3,000 rads.
   e. Total pericardiectomy—not usually indicated unless the cause is radiation constrictive pericarditis.
  2. Monitor vital signs and EKG.
  3. Administer hemodynamic support such as intravenous fluids, blood, and vasopressor agents per physician's order.
  4. Administer oxygen and pain medications as ordered.
  5. Encourage periods of rest.
E. Evaluation.
  1. Hemodynamic stablization.
  2. Adequate oxygenation.
  3. Minimal anxiety.
  4. Absence of pain or discomfort.

DISSEMINATED INTRAVASCULAR COAGULATION (DIC)

A. Pathophysiology.
  1. Imbalance of normal coagulation; always secondary to an underlying cause.
  2. Internal and/or external pathway of the clotting cascade is uncontrollably triggered, resulting in accelerated coagulation and the formation of excessive thrombin.
  3. Fibrinolytic system is activated as long as coagulation occurs.
  4. Clotting and bleeding continue at a life-threatening pace if the cause is untreated and remains a stimulus.
  5. Clotting factors are consumed.
B. Etiology.
  1. Obstetrical complications are the most common cause.

2. Cancer-related causes include:
   a. Tissue thromboplastin released from tumor cells, such as lung and prostate and during leukemia (especially acute progranulocytic leukemia).
   b. Sepsis—Gram negative and positive organisms.
   c. Infections.
   d. Hemolytic transfusion reactions or multiple whole blood transfusions.
   e. Hepatic failure.
C. Assessment.
   1. Signs and symptoms:
      a. Systemic bleeding ranging from petecchiae to hematuria to an acute gastrointestinal bleed.
      b. Organ dysfunction, e.g., renal failure, pulmonary emboli, thromboemboli in extremities.
      c. Decreased blood pressure and heart rate, cool, clammy skin.
      d. Anemia, pallor, shortness of breath.
   2. Diagnostic tests:
      a. Prolonged thrombin time.
      b. Prolonged prothrombin time (PT) and partial thromboplastin time (PTT).
      c. Decreased platelets.
      d. Decreased fibrinogen.
      e. Elevated fibrin split products—most indicative of DIC.
D. Intervention.
   1. Institute medical orders:
      a. Antibiotics if sepsis is the cause.
      b. Chemotherapy if cancer is the cause.
      c. Heparin is effective in acute progranulocytic leukemia; its use is controversial in other etiologies.
      d. Blood products such as red blood cells, platelets, and fresh frozen plasma (FFP). FFP may aggravate the problem since it contains clotting factors.
      e. EACA (Epsilon-aminocaproic acid) inhibits fibrinolysis; its use is controversial (Table 30–1).
   2. Monitor sites and amount of bleeding.
   3. Assess tissue perfusion.
   4. Monitor laboratory values.
   5. Minimize or prevent bleeding.
E. Evaluation.
   1. Decreased or absent bleeding.
   2. Adequate tissue perfusion as evidenced by:
      a. Alert and oriented state.
      b. Pink, warm skin.
      c. Urine output greater than 30 cc/hour.
      d. Stable vital signs.

HYPERCALCEMIA

A. Pathophysiology.
   1. Serum calcium greater than 11 mg/100 ml.

Table 30–1. MANAGEMENT OF DISSEMINATED
INTRAVASCULAR COAGULATION

Therapy	Action	Dose	Nursing Implications
Heparin	Interferes with thrombin production	10–15 units per kg. per hour via continuous infusion	Monitor signs and symptoms of bleeding, PT, and PTT
Epsilon-amino-caproic acid (EACA or Amicar)	Anti-fibrinolytic, slows clot lysis	5 grams slow IVP followed by 2 grams every 1–2 hours for 24 hours	Monitor signs and symptoms of tissue ischemia: decreased urine output, thrombi
Fresh Frozen Plasma	Contains clotting factors necessary for coagulation	1 unit = 150 to 250 ml of plasma plus 400 mg of fibrinogen and 1 unit activity per ml of other clotting factors	Monitor signs and symptoms of transfusion reaction and fluid overload
Platelets	Necessary for the coagulation process	Per clinical condition and platelet count: less than 20,000 requires a platelet transfusion of about 2 to 5 units per day	Monitor signs and symptoms of transfusion reaction

    2. Normal regulation of calcium level via parathyroid hormone (increases serum calcium) and calcitonin (decreases serum calcium); calcium and phosphorus levels are inversely proportional.
    3. 99% of calcium is in the bones and teeth; 1% is in the blood.
    4. Cancer is the most common cause of hypercalcemia.
    5. 20–30% incidence in persons with cancer.
    6. Abnormal increase in serum calcium is largely due to bone resorption (demineralization).
    7. Kidneys are unable to excrete increased calcium.
B. Etiology.
    1. Metastatic bony disease:
       a. Breast cancer—incidence is 40–50%.
       b. Lung cancer.
       c. Renal cancer.
    2. Primary bony disease—multiple myeloma—incidence is 50%.
    3. Immobility causes increased calcium to be released from bones.
    4. Increased secretion of ectopic parathyroid hormone from squamous cell cancer of lung or head and neck.
    5. Prostaglandins produced by solid tumors.
C. Assessment.
    1. Signs and symptoms:
       a. Neurologic—fatigue, lethargy, irritability, weakness, depression, hyporeflexia.
       b. Gastrointestinal—nausea, vomiting, anorexia, constipation.
       c. Renal—polyuria, polydipsia, dehydration, calculi.
       d. Cardiovascular—arrhythmias, hypertension.
       e. Ocular—white crystals visible on cornea.

    2. Diagnostic tests:
      a. Elevated serum and urine calcium levels.
      b. BUN and creatinine may be elevated.
      c. EKG—prolonged P-R interval, shortened QT interval, changes in ST wave.
D. Intervention.
    1. Support during chemotherapy or radiation treatment for primary disease.
    2. Maintain hydration—3 liters of normal saline per day.
    3. Maintain accurate intake and output.
    4. Administer diuretics such as Furosemide to increase urine flow.
    5. Promote mobilization—ambulation, standing, isometric exercises.
    6. Administer medications as ordered:
      a. Mithramycin—25 mcg/kg every 24–48 hours IV—lowers serum calcium by inhibiting bone resorption; thrombocytopenia is a side effect.
      b. Oral phosphates for treatment of mild, chronic hypercalcemia decrease reabsorption of calcium from gastrointestinal tract; diarrhea is a side effect.
    7. Monitor EKG.
    8. Monitor laboratory values, especially calcium, potassium, BUN, and creatinine.
    9. Exercise safety precautions because of patient's confusion, weakness, and susceptibility to fractures.
    10. Educate patient and family in the signs and symptoms of hypercalcemia.
E. Evaluation.
    1. Absence of symptoms and a normal serum calcium level.
    2. Knowledge of potential signs and symptoms of hypercalcemia.
    3. Maintenance of skeletal integrity.

SYNDROME OF INAPPROPRIATE ANTIDIURETIC HORMONE (SIADH)

A. Pathophysiology.
    1. Antidiuretic hormone (ADH) is normally released from the posterior pituitary in response to increased plasma osmolarity or decreased plasma volume.
    2. ADH causes water retention at the renal tubules.
    3. ADH may be abnormally produced or stimulated, resulting in excessive water retention and hyponatremia.
    4. Hyponatremia occurs secondary to the dilutional effect of increased vascular water.
    5. Urinary sodium excretion increases due to the increased plasma volume and subsequent increase in urine output.
B. Etiology.
    1. Secretion by tumor, especially small cell lung cancer, also lymphoma and pancreatic and prostatic cancers.
    2. Stimulation by drugs such as cyclophosphamide, vincristine, and thiazide diuretics.
    3. Pulmonary infections, viral or bacterial pneumonia, abscess.
    4. Neurologic trauma.
C. Assessment.

1. Signs and symptoms:
   a. Neurologic—confusion, irritability, weakness, lethargy, headache, hyporeflexia.
   b. Gastrointestinal—nausea, vomiting, anorexia, diarrhea.
   c. Weight gain without edema.
2. Diagnostic tests:
   a. Serum sodium < 130 mEq/L.
   b. Serum osmolality <280 mOsm/kg H_2O.
   c. Urine sodium >20 mEq/L.
D. Intervention.
   1. Institute medical orders as indicated:
      a. Chemotherapy for tumor.
      b. Antibiotics for pulmonary infections.
      c. Discontinue causative agents.
      d. Hypertonic saline (3–5% sodium chloride).
      e. Diuretics to eliminate excess water.
      f. Demeclocycline (900–1200 mg) interferes with action of ADH.
   2. Restrict fluids; maintain strict intake and output record.
   3. Monitor neurologic status.
   4. Monitor fluid and electrolyte balance.
   5. Institute safety measures if patient is confused and weak.
E. Evaluation.
   1. Normal serum and urine sodium levels and normal serum and urine osmolality.
   2. Appropriate fluid balance.
   3. Protective environment.

SEPSIS

A. Pathophysiology.
   1. Exemplified by decreased tissue perfusion secondary to the effects of bacterial invasion of the circulatory system.
   2. Gram-negative bacteria release endotoxin from their cell walls.
   3. Endotoxin causes increased capillary permeability and leakage, resulting in stagnation of blood and lactic acidosis.
   4. A decrease in circulating volume of blood results in a decrease in cardiac output.
   5. Most common cause of death in neutropenic patients who are very susceptible to infection.
   6. May cause DIC.
B. Etiology.
   1. Gram-negative bacterial invasion is the most common cause.
   2. Other causes include:
      a. Fungal infection.
      b. Parasitic invasion.
      c. Viral infection.
C. Assessment.
   1. Signs and symptoms:
      a. Fever, chills.
      b. Neurologic—change in level of consciousness, restlessness, confusion.

c. Cardiac—tachycardia, hypotension, decreased pulses, cool, clammy skin.

d. Renal—decreased urine output.

e. Bleeding from any site. It may be due to DIC.

2. Diagnostic tests:

a. Blood cultures—positive for Gram-negative organisms.

b. Chest x-ray—infiltrates.

c. Complete blood count—depressed or elevated white blood cell level.

d. Arterial blood gas—metabolic acidosis.

e. PT/PTT—prolonged.

D. Intervention.

1. Monitor vital signs, arterial blood gas values, and hemodynamic stability.

2. Perform blood cultures and physical assessment for fever >101°F (>38°C).

3. Administer antibiotics on schedule as ordered.

4. Reduce temperature as needed with antipyretics, ice packs, hypothermia blanket.

5. Administer volume replacements as ordered.

E. Evaluation.

1. Adequate tissue perfusion:

a. Alert and oriented.

b. Pink, warm skin.

c. Urine output >30 cc/hour.

d. Stable vital signs.

2. Absence of pain or discomfort.

SPINAL CORD COMPRESSION

A. Pathophysiology.

1. Compression is due to direct tumor invasion of spinal canal or vertebral collapse due to tumor invasion.

2. Tumors can be primary or, more commonly, metastatic in nature.

3. Damage to the cord is a result of tumor infiltration or ischemia.

4. Tumors are generally anterior to the cord in the epidural space (Fig. 30–1).

5. 70% of tumors occur in the thoracic region of the spine.

B. Etiology.

1. Most commonly caused by tumors that arise in or metastasize to bone such as breast, lung, prostate, kidney.

2. Lymphomas also have a high incidence secondary to lymph node extension into the epidural space.

C. Assessment—early diagnosis is very important to patient's prognosis.

1. Signs and symptoms:

a. Pain is the most common presenting symptom (95% of cases). Pain can be localized in the back or referred to the chest, abdomen, or extremities.

b. Muscular weakness—degree depends upon level of compression; may range from unsteadiness to foot drop to paralysis.

c. Sensory impairment—numbness and paralysis, tingling in extremities, loss of bowel and bladder control, diminished pain or temperature sensation, paraplegias, sexual dysfunction.

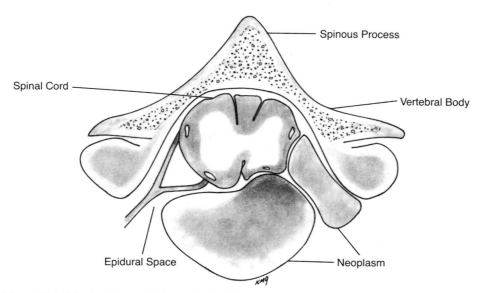

Figure 30–1. *Spinal cord tumor. (Redrawn from Yasko, J.: Guidelines for Cancer Care: Symptom Management. Reston, V.A., Reston Publishing Co., Inc., 1983.)*

   2. Diagnostic tests:
     a. Spinal films—bony abnormalities.
     b. Myelogram—extradural mass.
     c. Lumbar puncture—performed at time of myelogram to decrease morbidity.
D. Intervention.
   1. Preparation for treatments.
     a. Laminectomy—decompresses spinal cord. With the posterior approach it may be difficult to locate tumor, which is usually anterior.
     b. Radiation therapy, alone or postoperatively. 3,000–4,000 rads are given over 2–4 weeks.
   2. Administer medications as ordered:
     a. Steroids—high doses to decrease edema.
     b. Chemotherapy—as adjuvant treatment if tumor is chemosensitive.
     c. Analgesics.
   3. Institute safety measures if motor-sensory loss is present.
   4. Perform skin care; this is especially important if bedrest is necessary.
E. Evaluation.
   1. Maintenance or improvement of sensory and motor function at time of diagnosis
   2. Absence of pain or discomfort.
   3. Maintenance of optimal bowel and bladder function.
   4. Maintenance of skin integrity.

SUPERIOR VENA CAVA SYNDROME (SVCS)

A. Pathophysiology.
   1. The superior vena cava is a thin-walled, low-pressure vessel located in a tight compartment, the bony thorax.

2. The superior vena cava may be obstructed externally by tumor or enlarged nodes or internally by a thrombus (Fig. 30–2).
3. Venous drainage from the head, upper thorax, and upper extremities is impeded, resulting in decreased venous return and increased venous pressure.
4. 95% of SVCS cases are related to cancer.

B. Etiology.
1. Lung cancer accounts for 75%
2. Lymphoma accounts for 15%.
3. Metastatic disease, such as breast cancer, accounts for a small percentage.

C. Assessment.
1. Signs and symptoms:
   a. Dyspnea, chest pain, cough, tachypnea.
   b. Facial, trunk, and arm edema, especially upon awakening.
   c. Thoracic and neck vein distention.
   d. Hypotension.
   e. Cyanosis.
   f. Headache, vision changes, lethargy.
2. Diagnostic tests:
   a. Chest x-ray may show mass.
   b. Superior vena cavogram is contraindicated due to increased venous pressure and potential for bleeding.

D. Intervention.
1. Preparation for treatments.

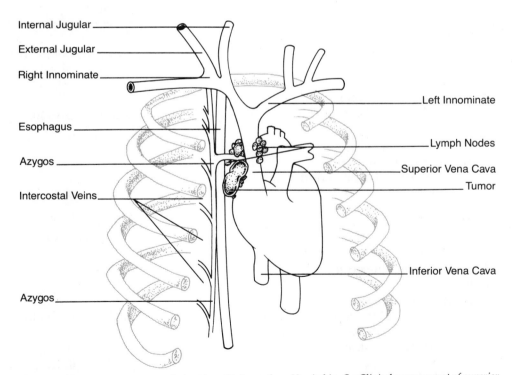

Figure 30–2. *Superior vena cava obstruction. (Redrawn from Varricchio, C.: Clinical management of superior vena cava syndrome. Heart Lung 14(4):411, 1985.)*

    a. Radiation therapy.
      (1) Treatment of choice (400 rads × 3 days initially).
      (2) Total dose of 3,000–5,000 rads.
      (3) Subjective response within 72 hours.
    b. Chemotherapy.
      (1) Especially effective in lymphomas or small cell lung cancer.
      (2) Treatment of choice if mediastinal radiation limit has been reached.
    c. Surgery is generally not indicated owing to high morbidity.
  2. Administer diuretics and steroids, as ordered, to reduce edema.
  3. Maintain airway.
  4. Promote gravity drainage of upper torso fluid, i.e., elevate head and upper extremities.
  5. Provide psychological support to decrease anxiety.
E. Evaluation.
  1. Maintenance of adequate ventilation and perfusion.
  2. Minimal anxiety.

TUMOR LYSIS SYNDROME

A. Pathophysiology.
  1. Metabolic imbalance due to the rapid release of intracellular components as a result of tumor kill.
  2. Components released from the tumor cells are potassium, phosphorus, and uric acid.
  3. Calcium is lowered secondary to the increase in phosphorus.
  4. Bulky tumors with a high growth fraction increase the risk of tumor lysis syndrome.
  5. The syndrome usually begins 1–5 days after the initiation of chemotherapy.
B. Etiology.
  1. Non-Hodgkin's lymphomas, especially undifferentiated.
  2. Leukemias, especially acute lymphoblastic and chronic leukemia in blast phase.
C. Assessment.
  1. Signs and symptoms:
    a. Renal—oliguria, anuria, urine crystals, flank pain, hematuria.
    b. Cardiac—dysrhythmias.
    c. Neuromuscular—cramps, tetany, confusion.
  2. Diagnostic tests:
    a. Elevated serum BUN, creatinine, potassium, phosphorus, and uric acid.
    b. Decreased serum calcium.
D. Intervention.
  1. Institute medical orders:
    a. Administer allopurinol—lowers uric acid concentration by inhibiting the enzyme xanthine oxidase. Dose is 300–800 mg/day.
    b. Maintain intravenous fluids with sodium bicarbonate for 3–5 days after start of chemotherapy to increase diuresis and alkalinize the urine. Use cautiously if hyperphosphatemia or hypocalcemia is present.
    c. Administer calcium supplements.

2. Preparation for hemodialysis—lowers uric acid, phosphorus, and potassium levels.

E. Evaluation.
1. Maintenance of adequate urine output of greater than 30 cc/hour.
2. Normal serum potassium, uric acid, phosphorus, and calcium levels.

STUDY QUESTIONS

1. Describe the probable clinical presentation of a patient with cardiac tamponade.
2. List three potential causes of DIC in the client with cancer.
3. Develop a nursing care plan for the client with hypercalcemia.
4. Identify two causes of SIADH in the client with cancer.
5. Develop a nursing plan of care for the client in septic shock.
6. Identify the most common presenting symptom of cord compression.
7. Identify the most common cause of SVCS.
8. Describe the signs and symptoms of SVCS.

Bibliography

Altman, A. J. and Schwartz, A. D.: Oncologic emergencies. *In* Altman, A. J. and Schwartz, A. D. (eds.): Malignant Diseases in Infancy, Childhood and Adolescence, 2nd ed. Philadelphia, W. B. Saunders Co., pp. 136–176, 1985.

Arseneau, J. D. and Rubin, P.: Oncologic emergencies. *In* Rubin, P. (ed.): Clinical Oncology—A Multidisciplinary Approach, 6th ed. Rochester, N. Y., American Cancer Society, pp. 516–525, 1983.

Bruckman, J. E. and Bloomer, W. E.: Management of spinal cord compression. Seminars in Oncology, 5(2):135–140, 1978.

Cannelos, G. P. and Stark, J. J.: Medical emergencies in oncology. *In* Cancer—A manual for Practitioners, 5th ed. Boston, American Cancer Society, pp. 300–306, 1978.

Carabell, S. C. and Goodman, R. L.: Superior vena caval syndrome. *In* DeVita, V. T. (ed.): Cancer—Principles and Practice of Oncology, 2nd ed. Philadelphia, J. B. Lippincott Co., pp. 1855–1860. 1985.

Chernecky, C. C. and Ramsey, P. W.: Critical Nursing Care of the Client With Cancer. Norwalk, CT, Appleton-Century-Crofts, 1984.

Concilus, E. M. and Bohachick, P. A.: Cancer: Pericardial effusion and tamponade. Cancer Nursing, 1(5):391–398, 1984.

Darovic, G.: Disseminated intravascular coagulation. Critical Care Nurse, 2(6):36–44, 1982.

Doogan, R. A.: Hypercalcemia of malignancy. Cancer Nursing, 4(4):299–304, 1981.

Eisert, D. R.: Respiratory emergencies in cancer patients. Your Patient and Cancer, 2(12):62–64, 1982.

Fields, A. L., Josse, R. G., and Bergsagel, D. E.: Metabolic emergencies. *In* DeVita, V. T. (ed.): Cancer—Principles and Practice of Oncology, 2nd ed. Philadelphia, J. B. Lippincott Co., pp. 1866–1881, 1985.

Franco, L. M.: Acute disseminated intravascular coagulation. Cardiovascular Nursing, 15(5):22–27, 1979.

Gilbert, I. and Henning, R. J.: Adenocarcinoma of the lung presenting with pericardial tamponade: Report of a case and review of the literature. Heart and Lung, 14(1):83–87, 1985.

Johndrow, P. D. and Thornton, S.: Syndrome of inappropriate antidiuretic hormone—A growing concern. Focus on Critical Care, 12(5):29–34, 1985.

Kirchner, C. W. and Reheis, C. E.: Two serious complications of neoplasia: Sepsis and disseminated intravascular coagulation. Nursing Clinics of North America, 17(4):595–605, 1982.

Morse, L. K., Heery, M. L., and Flynn, K. T.: Early detection to avert the crisis of superior vena cava syndrome. Cancer Nursing, 8(4):228–232, 1985.

Nissenblatt, M. J.: Oncologic emergencies. American Family Physician, 20(2):104–114, 1979.

Rooney, A. and Haviley, C.: Nursing management of disseminated intravascular coagulation. Oncology Nursing Forum, 12(1):15–22, 1985.

Sarna, G.: Oncologic emergencies and urgencies: Recognition and treatment. *In* Sarna, G. (ed.): Practical Oncology. Boston, Houghton Mifflin Professional Publishers, pp. 53–71, 1980.

Theologides, A.: Neoplastic cardiac tamponade. Seminars in Oncology, 5(2):181–191, 1978.

Valentine, A. S. and Steward, J. A.: Oncologic emergencies. American Journal of Nursing, 83(9):1283–1285, 1983.

Varricchio, C.: Clinical management of superior vena cava syndrome. Heart and Lung, 14(4):411–416, 1985.

Waterbury, L.: Hematologic problems. In Abeloff, M. D. (ed.): Complications of Cancer—Diagnosis and Management. Baltimore, Johns Hopkins University Press, pp. 121–145, 1979.

Yasko, J. M.: Guidelines for Cancer Care Management: Symptom Management. Reston, VA, Reston Publishing Co., Inc. 1983.

31

Nursing Administration of Chemotherapy

LINDA TENENBAUM, RN, MSN, OCN

PREPARATION, HANDLING AND DISPOSING OF CHEMOTHERAPEUTIC AGENTS

A. Qualifications: Only adequately prepared registered nurses who are skilled in administering chemotherapeutic agents should assume responsibility for their administration in order to assure quality of care and patient safety.

B. Nursing Interventions:

1. Check appropriate laboratory data prior to reconstituting chemotherapy.
2. Verify physician's written order for specific dosage, route, and mode of administration.
3. Calculate drug dosage appropriately. A nomogram (Figs. 31–1 and 31–2) is frequently used to calculate body surface area (BSA) from height and weight (mass).
4. Observe precautions in drug preparation and handling.
5. Wash hands before and after preparation and administration of chemotherapy.
6. Reconstitute medications under sterile conditions, according to information provided on package insert and agency policy.
7. Discard unused portion of drug in proper container for hazardous waste disposal.
8. Follow institutional policy and procedure should any of the following occur:
   a. Medication spill.
   b. Medication spray (aerosolization).
   c. Contact of medication with skin, eyes, or mucous membranes.
9. If medication is to be administered by the direct I.V. route, change needle after withdrawing medication from vial or ampule to prevent tissue irritation.

333

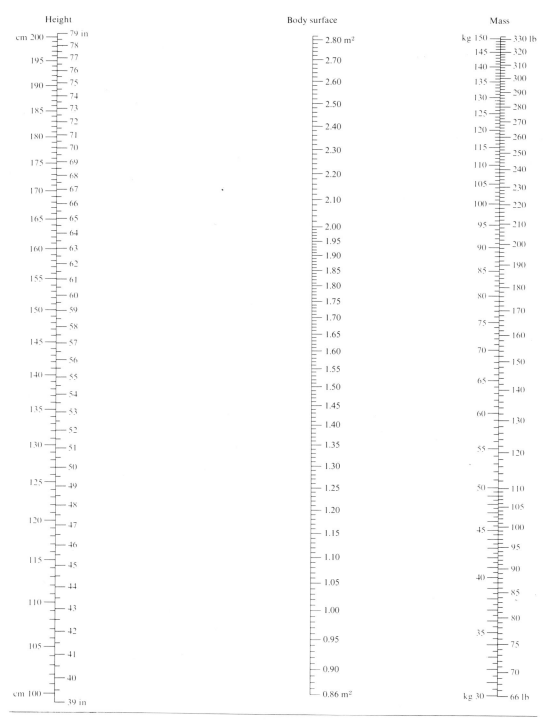

Height

cm 200 — 79 in
195 — 78
— 77
— 76
190 — 75
— 74
185 — 73
— 72
180 — 71
— 70
175 — 69
— 68
170 — 67
— 66
165 — 65
— 64
160 — 63
— 62
155 — 61
— 60
150 — 59
— 58
145 — 57
— 56
140 — 55
— 54
135 — 53
— 52
130 — 51
— 50
125 — 49
— 48
120 — 47
— 46
115 — 45
— 44
110 — 43
— 42
105 — 41
— 40
cm 100 — 39 in

Body surface

2.80 m²
2.70
2.60
2.50
2.40
2.30
2.20
2.10
2.00
1.95
1.90
1.85
1.80
1.75
1.70
1.65
1.60
1.55
1.50
1.45
1.40
1.35
1.30
1.25
1.20
1.15
1.10
1.05
1.00
0.95
0.90
0.86 m²

Mass

kg 150 — 330 lb
145 — 320
140 — 310
135 — 300
130 — 290
125 — 280
120 — 270
115 — 260
110 — 250
105 — 240
100 — 230
95 — 220
90 — 210
85 — 200
80 — 190
75 — 180
70 — 170
65 — 160
60 — 150
55 — 140
50 — 130
45 — 120
40 — 110
35 — 105
— 100
— 95
— 90
— 85
— 80
— 75
— 70
kg 30 — 66 lb

¹ From the formula of Du Bois and Du Bois. *Arch. intern. Med.,* **17**. 863 (1916): $S = M^{0.425} \times H^{0.725} \times 71.84$. or $\log S = \log M \times 0.425 + \log H \times 0.725 + 1.8564$ (S: body surface in cm², M: mass in kg, H: height in cm).

To determine Body Surface Area (BSA):

1. Place ruler or other straight edge item with one end crossing the left-hand scale at patient's height and the other end crossing the right hand scale at patient's weight (mass).
2. Draw a real or imaginary line from height to mass.
3. The point at which the line crosses the center scale indicates Body Surface Area (BSA), represented in meters squared (m²).
4. Chemotherapy medications are commonly calculated in mg (or units) per m².

334

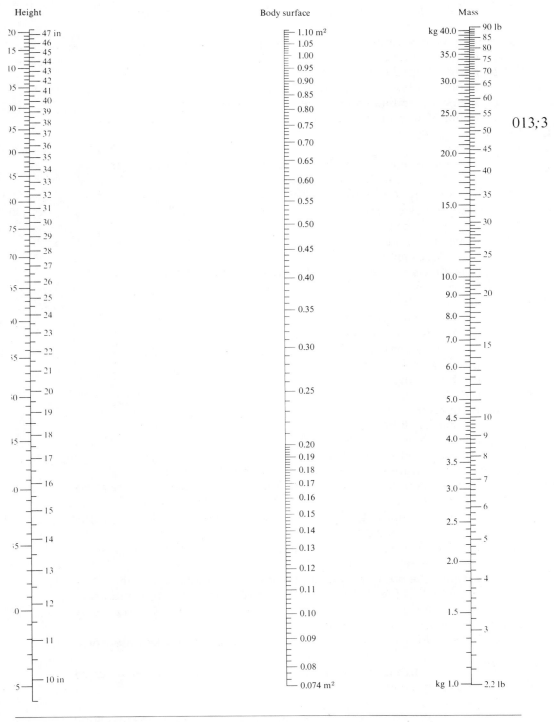

Height | Body surface | Mass

Height		Body surface	Mass
20	47 in	1.10 m²	kg 40.0 — 90 lb
15	46	1.05	— 85
	45	1.00	35.0 — 80
10	44	0.95	— 75
	43	0.90	30.0 — 70
)5	42	0.85	— 65
	41		— 60
)0	40	0.80	
	39		25.0 — 55
)5	38	0.75	— 50
	37	0.70	
)0	36		20.0 — 45
	35	0.65	
%5	34		— 40
	33	0.60	
	32		— 35
%0	31	0.55	15.0
	30	0.50	
75	29		— 30
	28	0.45	
70	27		— 25
	26	0.40	
%5	25		10.0
	24	0.35	9.0 — 20
)0	23		8.0
	22	0.30	7.0 — 15
%5	21		6.0
	20	0.25	
%0	19		5.0
	18		4.5 — 10
15	17	0.20	4.0 — 9
		0.19	— 8
	16	0.18	3.5
.0		0.17	3.0 — 7
	15	0.16	— 6
		0.15	2.5
%5	14	0.14	— 5
	13	0.13	2.0
		0.12	— 4
0	12	0.11	
		0.10	1.5
	11	0.09	— 3
		0.08	
5	10 in	0.074 m²	kg 1.0 — 2.2 lb

013;3

the formula of DuBois and Du Bois, *Arch. intern. Med.*, **17**, 863 (1916): $S = M^{0.425} \times H^{0.725} \times 71.84$.
$;S = \log M \times 0.425 + \log H \times 0.725 + 1.8564$ (S: body surface in cm²; M: mass in kg; H: height in cm).

Figure 31–2. *Nomogram for determination of body surface area of a child from height and mass. (From Lentner, C., Ed.: Geigy Scientific Tables. 8th edition, Volume 1. Basel, Ciba-Geigy, 1981.) See adult nomogram (Fig. 31–1) for directions for use.*

Figure 31–1. *Nomogram for determination of body surface area of an adult from height and mass. (From Lentner, C., Ed.: Geigy Scientific Tables. 8th edition, Volume 1. Basel, Ciba-Geigy, 1981.)*

10. Properly label syringe or I.V. bag with:
    a. Patient's name.
    b. Hospital number (if indicated).
    c. Room and bed numbers (if indicated).
    d. Medication name and dosage.
    e. Route of administration.

C. Handling.
   1. Outcome.
      a. The nurse and the environment should not be unnecessarily exposed to potentially hazardous substances.
      b. The sterility of the drug shall be maintained.
   2. Potential routes of exposure:
      a. Direct skin contact.
      b. Inhalation of aerosols.
      c. Direct eye contact.
   3. Possible effects of exposure to chemotherapeutic agents:
      a. Short-term:
         (1) Dermatitis.
         (2) Hyperpigmentation of exposed skin area.
         (3) Sores in nasal mucosa.
         (4) Burning of eyes.
         (5) Dizziness.
         (6) Headache.
         (7) Nausea.
      b. Long-term:
         (1) Partial alopecia.
         (2) Chromosomal abnormalities.
         (3) Increased risk of cancer.
   4. General procedure for safe handling of chemotherapeutic agents:
      a. Review literature (agency procedures, policies, package insert) before preparing or administering chemotherapeutic agent.
      b. Use sterile handling techniques and handwashing before and after mixing or administration.
      c. Do not eat, drink, smoke or apply makeup in the area in which chemotherapy is prepared.
      d. Prepare chemotherapeutic agent in a Class II (and preferably Type B) biologic safety cabinet (containment cabinet) for maximum protection. If this is not available, prepare in a quiet work space, away from heating or cooling vents.
      e. Protect the work area with a disposable, plastic-backed absorbent pad.
      f. Use protective garments (gown, gloves, goggles, mask), as indicated by agency policy.
         (1) Gown.
            (a) Should close in back and have elastic or knit cuffs long enough to fit under cuff of gloves.
            (b) Remove before leaving work area.
         (2) Gloves.
            (a) Use talc-tree, disposable surgical gloves when leakage of medication may result. This includes:

          i. Ejection of air from syringe or tubing containing a chemotherapeutic agent.

          ii. Injection of chemotherapeutic agent into I.V. bag or tubing.

          iii. Connection or disconnection of I.V. tubing.

    (b) Cuffs should be long enough to cover cuff of gown.

    (c) Current research indicates that surgical latex gloves are less permeable to cytotoxic agents than gloves made of PVC (polyvinyl chloride).

  (3) Mask and/or goggles should be used if indicated in agency policy.

g. Use syringes, tubing, and connectors with Luer-Lok attachments.

h. When opening ampules:

  (1) Clear all fluid from neck of the ampule.

  (2) Tilt tip of ampule away from yourself.

  (3) Wrap a sterile gauze or an alcohol pad around the neck of ampule before breaking.

  (4) Use a syringe that will be no more than $\frac{3}{4}$ full when desired amount is drawn up.

  (5) Inject excess solution from the ampule into a sealed waste vial, or dispose of material according to institutional policy.

i. Prevent aerosol generation from vials by:

  (1) Using an 18- or 19-gauge needle and a 0.2 micron hydrophobic filter.

  (2) Aspirating a volume of air slightly larger than the volume of diluent added to create negative pressure in the vial.

  (3) Adding diluent slowly, allowing it to run down the side of the vial.

  (4) Performing final dose measurement before removing needle from vial.

  (5) Allowing air pressure to equalize from vial to the syringe before removing needle from vial.

  (6) Using dispensing pins or filters.

  (7) Placing an alcohol swab over the bevel of needle as it is withdrawn from the vial.

j. When expelling air from a syringe or priming I.V. tubing with chemotherapy solution:

  (1) Do so slowly into a sterile gauze pad held at the tip of the needle.

  (2) Contain gauze pad within a sealable plastic bag whenever possible.

k. Assess I.V. tubing and pump for signs of leakage.

l. Clean all spills immediately, according to agency policies and procedures.

m. Should skin contact occur when preparing or administering chemotherapeutic agents, wash the involved area thoroughly with soap and water.

n. Should eye contact occur when preparing or administering chemotherapeutic agents:

  (1) Irrigate the involved eye(s) for 15 minutes.

  (2) Have the eye(s) evaluated by a physician.

D. Disposal of Cytotoxic Agents and Related Equipment.
  1. Outcome: The nurse and the environment should not be unnecessarily exposed to potentially hazardous substances.
  2. Nursing measures:
     a. Place sharp objects in a puncture-resistant and leakproof container.
     b. Dispose of needles intact—do not break them.
     c. Leave unused portions of antineoplastic agents in vial or ampule and dispose of in a plastic bag lined with absorbent material.
     d. Dispose of I.V. bags and tubing used for administration of chemotherapeutic agents according to agency policy.
     e. Place all gowns, masks, absorbent pads, and other materials used in proper bag and discard according to agency policy.
     f. Mark or label the outside of containers and disposal bags "Caution Chemotherapy," or "Biohazard."
     g. Discard gloves after each use, or after a medication spill. Avoid skin contact when removing.
     h. Wash hands thoroughly after removing gloves.
     i. Report accidental contact with chemotherapeutic agents according to agency policy.
     j. Destroy hazardous waste containers by proper incineration or burial in a landfill.

ADMINISTRATION TECHNIQUES FOR CYTOTOXIC AGENTS

A. Outcome.
  1. The patient will receive the drug(s) in a safe and appropriate manner.
  2. Potential extravasations are avoided.
B. Nursing Measures.
  1. Verify medication and dose.
  2. Review patient's allergy history and relevant data (CBC, other laboratory values, EKG if indicated).
  3. Review history of past experience with chemotherapy and related medications.
  4. Have knowledge of immediate and delayed side effects of the medication(s) being administered.
  5. Use proper procedure for identification of the patient.
  6. Identify yourself to the patient and family, and answer questions they may have concerning chemotherapy.
  7. Verify that informed consent has been completed (if medication administered is an investigational agent).
  8. Inform patient (or significant other if indicated) to report adverse effects.
  9. Administer antiemetics or other premedications as ordered in preparation for chemotherapy.
  10. Administer medication observing the 5 Rights.
      a. Right patient.
      b. Right drug.
      c. Right dose.
      d. Right route.
      e. Right time.
  11. Chart medication according to agency policy.

FOR INTRAVENOUS MEDICATIONS:
12. Assemble equipment required to perform venipuncture if necessary.
13. Select site for venipuncture with regard to:
    a. Location of proposed intravenous site.
    b. General condition of veins.
    c. Previous trauma to proposed intravenous site.
    d. Medication to be administered.
14. When vesicant medications are to be administered:
    a. Avoid sites where damage to underlying tendons and/or nerves may occur (e.g., veins in the antecubital fossa, near wrist, or dorsal surface of hand) (Fig. 31–3).
    b. Perform venipuncture and stabilize needle or catheter (Figs. 31–3 and 31–4).
    c. Assess for blood return.
    d. Instill 5–10 ml of normal saline solution or sterile water for injection and assess patency of the vein.
    e. Administer chemotherapeutic medication by proper I.V. route (direct I.V., I.V. drip, I.V. sidearm, or Y-site).
    f. Administer in sequence based on knowledge and hospital/agency policy:
       (1) Vesicant first.
       (2) Vesicant last.

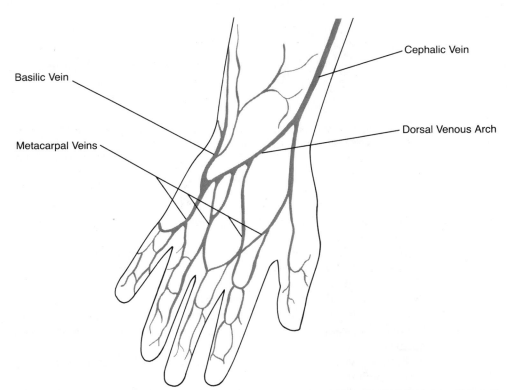

Figure 31–3. *Distal veins of the hand (metacarpal veins), suitable for infusion of non-vesicant chemotherapeutic agents. (Redrawn from Metheney, N. M., and Snively, W. D., Jr. Nurses' Handbook of Fluid Balance. 3rd ed. Philadelphia, JB Lippincott, 1979.)*

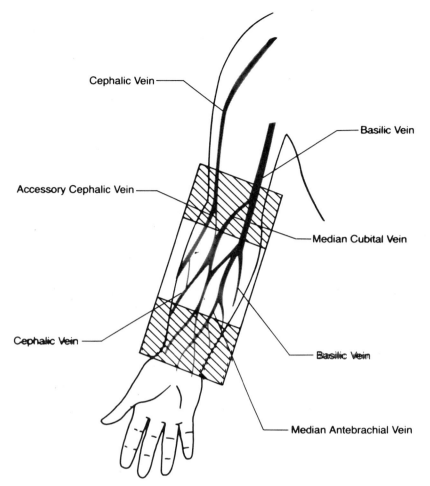

Cephalic Vein

Basilic Vein

Accessory Cephalic Vein

Median Cubital Vein

Cephalic Vein

Basilic Vein

Median Antebrachial Vein

Figure 31-4. *Superficial veins of the forearm: Shaded areas indicate antecubital veins, which should be avoided when administering vesicant chemotherapeutic agents. Region between shaded areas is the preferred administration site. (Adapted from Metheney, N. M., and Snively, W. D., Jr. Nurses' Handbook of Fluid Balance, 4th ed. Philadelphia, JB Lippincott, 1983.)*

    (3) Vesicant medication "sandwiched" between two nonvesicant medications.

  g. Administer medication slowly, and every 3–5 ml assess:

    (1) Adequate blood return.

    (2) Patency of the vein.

    (3) Signs of infiltration or extravasation.

  h. Flush tubing with 3–5 ml normal saline solution or sterile water for injection between medications and after the final medication has been administered.

  i. Be familiar with untoward side effects of medications and periodically assess patient for signs.

  j. Have patient report burning, stinging, or pain that may occur at the I.V. site.

NURSING MANAGEMENT OF EXTRAVASATION

A. Outcome
  1. The possible extravasation is detected and treated early.
  2. Undue harm to the patient is minimized or prevented due to early and knowledgeable intervention.
B. Definitions
  1. *Extravasation*—Infiltration or leakage of intravenous medication into the local subcutaneous tissue surrounding the administration site. May result in severe local tissue damage if agent infiltrated is a vesicant.
  2. *Irritant*—A medication that may produce pain and inflammation at the administration site or along the path of the vein by which it is administered.

Table 31–1. VESICANT/IRRITANT CHEMOTHERAPEUTIC MEDICATIONS

Generic Name	Trade Name	Description*	Local Antidote†
Carmustine	BiCNU, BCNU	I	Sodium bicarbonate +
Dacarbazine	DTIC-Dome	I, V	Sodium thiosulfate +
Dactinomycin	Actinomycin-D	V	Sodium thiosulfate +
Daunomycin	Daunorubicin	V	Hydrocotisone +
Doxorubicin	Adriamycin	V	Corticosteroid and normal saline by local subcutaneous instillation. (m) Apply cold to site
Etoposide	VePesid, VP-16	I, V (in large volume)	As for Vinblastine
Mechlorethamine (nitrogen mustard)	Mustargen	V	Sterile isotonic sodium thiosulfate (1/6 molar). Dilute 4 ml 10% sodium thiosulfate for injection with 6 ml sterile water for injection. Apply cold compress to site for 6–12 hours. (m)
Mithramycin	Mithracin (Plicamycin)	V	Apply cold compresses as tolerated × 24 hr +
Mitomycin C	Mutamycin	V	Sodium thiosulfate +
Streptozotocin	Zanosar	I	None
Vinblastine	Velban	V	Local injection of normal saline or hyaluronidase (Wydase) and application of moderate heat to site. (m)
Vincristine	Oncovin	V	As for vinblastine
Investigational Agents			
Amsacrine	M-AMSA	V	
Bisantrene		V	
Dihydrogalacticol	Galacticol, DAG	V	
Maytansine		V	
Mitoquazone	Methyl-GAG	I	
Teniposide	VM-26	I	Normal saline +
Neocarzinostatin	Vinostatin	V	
Vindesine	Eldisine	V	

* V = Vesicant, I = Irritant.
† + = Theoretical antidote, m = Manufacturer's recommended antidote.

Table 31–2. CONTROVERSIAL ISSUES IN CHEMOTHERAPY ADMINISTRATION

Issue	Solution	Rationale
Administration site	Use antecubital fossa	Larger veins, easier starts. More rapid infusion.
	Avoid antecubital region	Mobility of arm restricted. Extensive tissue damage can occur with extravasation.
Needle size	Larger gauge (#19–21 scalp vein needle)	Decreases administration time.
	Smaller gauge (#23–25)	Less likely to puncture wall of small vein, less scar tissue formed. Less pain on insertion. Reduced incidence of mechanical phlebiti. Slow infusion of agent may reduce side effects.
Sequencing of medications	Administer vesicant first	Vascular integrity decreases over time. Vein more stable and less irritated at the beginning of treatment. Irritating agent may cause venous spasm, pain.
	Administer vesicant last	Other medications can be administered before irritating effects of vesicant occur. Venous spasm may occur at beginning of IV push injection and may be misinterpreted as pain at IV site.
Thermal management of site after extravasation occurs	Apply heat	Increased blood flow to area promotes reabsorption of remaining vesicant. Facilitates dispersion of antidote in subcutaneous tissue.
	Do not apply heat	Increases metabolic demands and may increase cell destruction.
	Apply cold	Constricts peripheral veins, decreases absorption of extravasated medication. Slows metabolism and reduces ability of vesicant agent to cause cell destruction. Minimizes local pain.

3. *Vesicant*—A medication that has the potential to cause cellular damage or tissue destruction with leakage into subcutaneous tissue.

C. Medications that may be irritant or vesicant agents are listed in Table 31–1.

D. Nursing interventions:

1. Be familiar with vesicant medications and hospital or agency policy for reporting and intervention in the event leakage occurs.
2. Discontinue chemotherapy. Leave needle in place.
3. Aspirate residual medication and blood (total 3–5 ml) via I.V. tubing or needle.
4. Instill intravenous antidote if recommended (see Table 31–1). If not, proceed to step 5.
5. Remove needle.
6. If recommended, use a TB syringe and 25- to 27-gauge needles to inject the subcutaneous antidote into the area of infiltration. Use a new needle for each injection.
7. Avoid applying pressure to suspected area of infiltration.
8. Apply topical steroid ointment if ordered.
9. Apply a sterile occlusive dressing.
10. Apply heat or cold as indicated (Table 31–2).
11. Elevate the involved extremity.
12. Notify physician of extravasation.
13. Observe site regularly for pain, erythema, induration, swelling, necrosis, and functional ability of involved extremity.
14. Document incident. Extravasation record may be used (Fig. 31–5). If such a form is not available, document in nursing note and include:
    a. Date.

Extravasation Record

Chemotherapy Drug Extravasation Record

__________Diagnosis____________________Drug and/or Drug Regimen

Home Phone No.__________
Date:__________

Route of Administration
____I.V. Push
____Piggyback
____In Dilution amt. & sol.
____I.M. (location)
____Sub. Q. (location)
____Flush only
____Other

Needle Size
____Scalp Vein Butterfly
____#25
____#23
____#21
____#19
____Other

Condition of Veins
____Soft, Pliable
____Fragile, Thin-walled
____Thready
____Hard, Knotty
____Other (Specify)

Injection Site

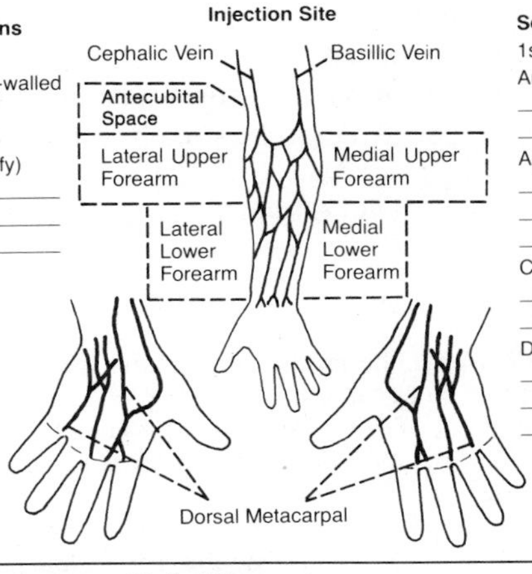

Sequence of Drugs
1st drug____
Amt./Name/Method of Flush

Approx. amt. infiltrate

Concentration

Doctor Notified:
____Time of extravasation
____Time M.D. called
____Time responded

Appearance of Infiltration Site:
Describe:

Color and Dimension of Infiltration Site:
Describe:

Agents and Amt. Used
____SoluCortef 25 mg. (I.V. Push)
____Xylocaine 1% (I.V. Push)
____Wydase (S.Q.)
____Decadron LA
____Na Bicarb. (I.V. Push)
____Na Bicarb (S.Q.)
____Na Thiosulfate (I.V. Push/S.Q.)
____Other

Nursing Assessment/Patient Comments:

Plan and Follow-up (Use reverse side if necessary):

____
Signature and Date

Figure 31–5. *Sample extravasation record. (Reproduced with permission of Stanford University Hospital and Clinics, Stanford Medical Center, Stanford, CA.)*

    b. Time.
    c. Needle size and type.
    d. Site of insertion.
    e. Medication(s) infiltrated.
    f. Sequence of medications.
    g. Approximate amount of drug extravasated.
    h. Subjective symptoms reported by patient.
    i. Nursing assessment of site.
    j. Nursing interventions.
    k. Effects of treatment.
    l. Physician notification and intervention.
    m. Instructions given to patient.
    n. Follow-up measures taken.
    o. Nurse's signature.

Note: Photograph of site may be required.

15. Provide clear, written and verbal instructions to the patient including:
    a. Application of steroid cream and/or dressing, change if indicated.
    b. Reporting of symptoms and status of site.
    c. Follow-up visit—time, date, place.
    d. Encouragement to use and move involved extremity as much as possible.
16. An extravasation tray or kit should be kept in an area accessible to the nurse administering chemotherapy. Contents of tray will vary according to agency policies.

STUDY QUESTIONS

1. Identify at least five (5) general safety measures to be used during preparation and administration of chemotherapeutic agents.
2. Describe safe procedures for priming or disposing of tubing when administering I.V. chemotherapy.
3. Describe technique for safe administration of parenteral chemotherapy.
4. Discuss three (3) controversial issues in the administration of vesicant chemotherapeutic agents.
5. Describe measures to be taken if extravasation of a vesicant should occur.

Bibliography

American Society of Hospital Pharmacists: Procedures for Handling Cytotoxic Drugs. Bethesda, MD, American Society of Hospital Pharmacists, 1983.

Anderson, R. W., Puckett, W. H., Dana, W. J., Nguyen, T. V., Theiss, J. C., and Matney, T. S.: Risk of handling injectable antineoplastic agents. American Journal of Hospital Pharmacy, 39:1881–1887, 1982.

Ballentine, R.: Nursing implications of cancer chemotherapy. Nursing '83, 13(7):55–56, 1983.

Barry, L. K. and Bair Booker, R.: Promoting the responsible handling of antineoplastic agents in the community. Oncology Nursing Forum, 12(5):41–46, 1985.

Benoliel, J. Q., Downs, F., and Notter, L. E.: Handling methotrexate—A safety problem? American Journal of Nursing, 82:1531, 1982.

Bergemann, D.: Handling antineoplastic agents. American Journal of Intravenous Therapy and Clinical Nutrition, 8(1):13—17, 1983.

Brager, B. L. and Yasko, J.: Care of the Client Receiving Chemotherapy. Reston, VA, Reston Publishing Company, 1984.

Cloak, M. M., Connor, T. H., Stevens, K. R., Theiss, J. C., Alt, J. M., Matney, T. S., and Anderson, R. W.: Occupational exposure of nursing personnel to antineoplastic agents. Oncology Nursing Forum, *12*(5):33–39, 1985.

Connor, T. H., Laidlaw, J. W., Theiss, J. C., Anderson, R. W., and Matney, T. S.: Permeability of latex and polyvinyl gloves to Carmustine. American Journal of Hospital Pharmacy, *41*:676–679, 1984.

Crudi, C.: A compounding dilemma: I've kept the drug sterile but have I contaminated myself? National IV Therapy Association Journal, *3*:77—78, 1980.

Crudi, C. and Stephens, M.: Antineoplastic agents: An occupational hazard? National IV Therapy Association Journal, *4*:233–234, 1981.

Cullen, M. L.: Issues in chemotherapy administration: II. Current interventions for Doxorubicin extravasations. Oncology Nursing Forum, *9*(1):52–53, 1982.

Frogge, M. H.: Issues in chemotherapy administration: III. Sequence of administering vesicant cytotoxic drugs, B. Give the vesicants last. Oncology Nursing Forum, *9*(1):54, 1982.

Fudge, R.: Working with Adriamycin—Preventing the "Blow-Back" Phenomenon—Handling Damaged Vials. Columbus OH, Adria Laboratories, 1981.

Govoni, L. E., and Hayes, J. E.: Drugs and Nursing Implications, 5th ed. Norwalk, CT, Appleton-Century-Crofts, 1985.

Guidelines for Handling Antineoplastic Drugs. University of Texas, M.D. Anderson Hospital Department of Pharmacy, 1982.

Gurwell, A.: Protect yourself from the hazards of anticancer drugs, RN, *46*(10):66–68, 1983.

Harrison, B. R.: Developing guidelines for working with antineoplastic drugs. American Journal of Hospital Pharmacy, *38*:1686–1693, 1981.

Hoffman, D. M.: The handling of antineoplastic drugs in a major cancer center. Hospital Pharmacy, *15*:302–304, 1980.

Jones, R. B., Frank, R., Mass, T.: Safe handling of chemotherapeutic agents: A report from the Mt. Sinai Medical Center. Ca-A Cancer Journal for Clinicians, *33*:258–263, 1983.

Knobf, T.: Intravenous therapy guidelines for oncology practice. Oncology Nursing Forum, *9*(2):30–34, 1982.

Laidlaw, J. L., Connor, T. H., Theiss, J. C., Anderson, R. W., and Matney, T. S.: Permeability of latex and polyvinyl chloride gloves to 20 antineoplastic drugs. American Journal of Hospital Pharmacy, *41*:2618–2623, 1984.

Lentner, C., Eds: Geigy Scientific Tables. 8th edition, Volume 1. Basel, Ciba-Geigy, 1981.

Miller, S. A., Dodd, M., Goodman, M. S., Pluth, N., Ryan, L. S., and Medvec, B. R.: Cancer Chemotherpay—Guidelines and Recommendations for Nursing Education and Practice. Pittsburgh, Oncology Nursing Society, 1984.

Miller, S.: Nursing actions in cancer chemotherapy administration. Oncology Nursing Forum, *7*(4):8–16, 1980.

Nursing update—Nursing implications of cancer chemotherapy. Nursing '83, *13*(7):57–58, 1983.

Physician's Desk Reference, 39th ed. Oradell, NJ, Medical Economics, 1985.

Power, L.: ASHP technical assistance bulletin on handling cytotoxic drugs in hospitals. American Journal of Hospital Pharmacy, *42*:131–137, 1985.

Puckett, W. H.: Online oncology—Computerized learning in the practices and procedures of oncology. (Computer program.) Syracuse, N.Y., Bristol Laboratories, 1984.

Recommendations for the safe handling of parenteral antineoplastic drugs. Bethesda, MD, U.S. Department of Health and Human Services, Public Health Service (Pub. No. 83-2621), 1982.

Satterwhite, B.: What to do when Adriamycin infiltrates. Nursing '80, *10*(2):37, 1980.

Sea-Lasley, K. and Ignoffo, R.: Manual of Oncology Therapeutics. St. Louis, C. V. Mosby, 1981.

Solimando, D. A., Jr.: Preparation of antineoplastic drugs: A review. American Journal of IV Therapy and Clinical Nutrition, *10*(16):18–21,24,26,27, 1983.

Spross, J.: Issues in chemotherapy administration. Oncology Nursing Forum, *9*(4):50–52, 1982.

Stolar, M. H., Power, L. A., and Viele, C. S.: Recommendations for handling cytotoxic drugs in hospitals. American Journal of Hospital Pharmacy, *40*:1163–1171, 1983.

Stuart, M.: Issues in chemotherapy administration: III. Sequence of administering vesicant cytotoxic drugs, A. Give the vesicants first. Oncology Nursing Forum, *9*(1):53–54, 1982.

Stuart, M.: Issues in chemotherapy administration: III. Sequence of administering vesicant cytotoxic drugs, B. Give the vesicants last. Oncology Nursing Forum, *9*(1):53–54, 1982.

Tenenbaum, L.: The Quick Reference Guide to Cancer Chemotherapy. Ft. Lauderdale, FL, L. Tenenbaum, 1984.

Troutman, J.: Step-by-step guide to trouble-free IV chemotherapy. RN, *48*(9):32–34, 1985.

Work practice guidelines for personnel dealing with cytotoxic (antineoplastic) drugs (draft). Washington, D.C. Office of Occupational Medicine, U.S. Department of Labor, 1985.

Yasko, J.: Guidelines for Cancer Care: Symptom Management. Reston, Va, Reston Publishing Company, 1983.

Yasko, J. M.: Nursing Management of Symptoms Associated With Chemotherapy. Columbus, OH, Adria Laboratories, 1984.

Zellmer, W. A.: Fear of handling anticancer drugs (editorial). American Journal of Hospital Pharmacy, *41*:665, 1984.

32

Communicating with the Patient and Family/Significant Others

ANNE E. BELCHER, RN, PhD

ASSESSMENT OF MEANING OF CANCER EXPERIENCE

A. Identification of patient's family and/or significant others.
   1. Operational definition of family: "a psychosocial group consisting of the patient and one or more persons (children or adults) in which there is a commitment for members to nurture each other."
   2. Nuclear versus extended family—members, physical proximity, roles.
   3. Nontraditional family, i.e. single parent or same sex partners.
   4. Significant others, i.e. friends, lover.
B. Determination of their myths and misconceptions about, past experiences with, and knowledge about the cancer experience.
   1. Cancer as a disease may still have a stigma attached, i.e., death, contagion, guilt, which affects family's or significant others' response to the patient's diagnosis.
   2. Cancer as a chronic disease may be seen as a threat to the integrity and continued functioning of the family system; this threat is perceived as greater than that posed by other diseases.
   3. Family or significant others may identify potential role changes based on past experience with cancer or other diseases, e.g., those of sexual partner, breadwinner, homemaker.
   4. Past experiences with cancer in an inpatient, outpatient, or home care setting may affect family's or significant others' response to the diagnosis and treatment plan.
   5. Family or significant others may blame the patient for developing cancer as a way of handling their own guilt and sense of responsibility for the diagnosis.
   6. The patient with cancer often gives the family or significant others an unpleasant sense of their own vulnerability and mortality.

ASSESSMENT OF THE FAMILY UNIT (NUCLEAR AND EXTENDED)

A. Description of group of interrelations and interdependence among individuals, which may include parents/stepparents, children, siblings, grandparents, extended family members.
  1. Cohesion—concern about and commitment to family members; degree to which family members are helpful to and supportive of one another.
  2. Expressiveness—degree to which individual family members are allowed and encouraged to act openly and express feelings directly.
  3. Conflict—degree to which there is open expression of anger and aggression.
  4. Independence—assertiveness, self-sufficiency, members making own decisions.
  5. Organization—structuring of family activities, financial planning, rules, and responsibilities.
B. Analysis of interpersonal relationships among patient and family members (based on interview and/or observation).
  1. Protectiveness—a natural, almost instinctual need to shelter the patient (and others) from the realities of cancer.
  2. Concealing emotions—the patient may hide his or her true feelings in order to avoid upsetting already overburdened family members.
      The family may feel the need to be cheerful and optimistic for the patient's benefit; they may also try to mask their aversion to or fear of changes in the patient's physical condition and behavior.
  3. Use of outside resources—the patient and family members base their requests for information and/or assistance on their previous experience in handling crises, the effectiveness of outside resources, and an assessment of the status of intrafamily resources.

ASSESSMENT OF EMOTIONAL IMPACT OF CANCER ON RELATIONSHIPS

A. Possible alterations in relationships among family members or significant others.
  1. Emotional responses, e.g., frustrations, helplessness, guilt, grieving.
  2. Shifting positions in family unit—independent versus dependent roles, reallocation of responsibilities.
  3. Altered sexual interaction between spouses or lovers.
  4. Modification of family traditions, i.e., holidays, recreational activities.
  5. Increased need for closeness, physical and/or psychological.
  6. Changes in children's behavior.
      a. Awareness of parent(s) repeated absences, preoccupation of well parent, changes in daily routine.
      b. Manifested by regression, behavioral problems at home (e.g., bedwetting, insomnia, eating disturbances, disobedience) or at school (e.g., decreased school performances, acting out or aggressive behavior).
  7. Disruption of family's objective future orientation and plans.
  8. Changes in constellation of external reference group(s), e.g., church, club(s), social friends, co-workers.

9. Conceptual themes.
   a. *Powerlessness*, a dominant theme throughout the patient's illness; family members or significant others want patient to be comforted but identify real or perceived lack of communication with patient and/or health care providers.
   b. *Ambivalence* often emerges after the diagnostic and/or treatment phases. It is particularly strong when family members or significant others expect a lengthy illness or recovery period or the development of irreversible disabilities.
   c. *Interdependence* of demands related to the superimposition of two worlds, one associated with the illness and the other with natural daily activities.
   d. *Uncertainty*, which initially relates to the patient's diagnosis and prognosis; during remission the focus is on a hope for cure versus the possibility of recurrence.
   e. *Role restructuring*, which occurs during each phase of illness, with the characteristics of realignment, reacquisition and legitimization.
   f. *Resiliency*, which is particularly noticeable when there are children in the family. It is natural for children to "self-right" in the face of a wide variety of difficulties.
B. Factors affecting relationships:
   1. Age and developmental status of family members, i.e., newlywed, first child, empty nest.
   2. Patient responsibilities within the family, e.g., source of income, homemaker.
   3. Pre-existing stresses or problems, as well as previous responses to and ability to cope with stressors.
      a. Poor relationship prior to cancer diagnosis may adversely affect patient support.
      b. Prior coping strategies may or may not be effective in this situation.

IDENTIFICATION OF IMPACT OF CANCER ON ROLES

A. Analysis of role changes.
   1. Roles influence functions, govern relationships, confer power.
   2. Crucial family roles.
      a. Provider of financial resources.
      b. Housekeeper/maintenance person.
      c. Caretaker/socializer of children.
      d. Sexual partner.
      e. Recreational planner.
      f. Therapeutic agent.
      g. Kinship maintainer.
   3. Changes may occur in role assignment based on patient status and family members' ability to increase or change responsibilities.
B. Evaluation of individual's reaction to role changes.
   1. Based on number and types of roles held.
   2. Affected by nature of role assignment.
      a. Ascribed—based on characteristic over which family member has no control, i.e., age, sex.

      b. Achieved—based on efforts and abilities, which result in greater cohesion, less role conflict and strain, more open communication.
3. Skills of other family members.
4. Presence of external resources, i.e., friends, social support systems.
5. Tasks to be accomplished by family of the patient with cancer.
      a. Living with cancer, which includes the phases of impact, functional description, search for meaning, informing others, and engaging emotions.
      b. Restructuring in the living-dying interval, which includes the phases of reorganization and framing memories.
      c. Bereavement, which includes the phases of separation and mourning.
      d. Reestablishment, with the emphasis on expansion of the social network.

ENHANCEMENT OF STRENGTHS THAT HELP FAMILIES COPE

A. Support systems, e.g., family ties, friendships, health care team, co-workers.
1. Need to interpret the cancer experience as a daily process of managing, coping, and supporting one another.
2. Need to know how to interpret what has happened, to anticipate and make sense of what might happen, to participate in and thus control what is happening.
B. Religious and philosophical beliefs.
C. Personal attitudes of family members toward illness, cancer, the patient, and the health care system.
D. Patient's response to cancer experience, i.e., coping strategies used, resources sought, perspective on family's role.

NURSING STRATEGIES FOR EFFECTIVE COMMUNICATION

A. Ongoing assessment of needs for communication.
1. Do not treat family members or significant others as bystanders; they may wish to be actively involved in patient's care.
2. Realize that family members or significant others share the strains and demands of the illness.
B. Provision of information.
1. Family members or significant others are seeking an honest, accurate report of the patient's condition, test results, and so forth.
2. The physician is seen by most family members or significant others as the primary resource; thus the nurse serves as mediator and advocate.
C. Use of therapeutic skills.
1. Focus on patient and family members or significant others as people, not victims.
2. Help all involved develop new defenses as well as strengthen existing ones.
D. Flexible visiting policies.
1. Special arrangements should be made for young children.
2. 24-hour privileges for parent or spouse or significant other may be of help.

E. Referral to appropriate resources.
  1. Support groups or programs, e.g., CanSurmount, I Can Cope.
  2. Living arrangements, e.g., Ronald McDonald House.
  3. Financial assistance.
  4. Home care/respite/hospice.
F. Nurse's personal behaviors, i.e., competence, caring, compassion, cooperation, collaboration, coordination.

STUDY QUESTIONS

1. What data would be most useful in your assessment of the following:
  a. The meaning of the cancer experience for the patient and family members or significant others.
  b. The status of the family unit.
  c. The emotional impact of cancer on the family's or significant others' relationships.
2. List at least three (3) nursing strategies for effective communication with the patient and family members on significant others.

Bibliography

Dyck, S. and Wright, K.: Family perceptions: The role of the nurse throughout an adult's cancer experience. Oncology Nursing Forum, *12*:53–56, 1985.

Edstrom, S. and Miller, M. W.: Preparing the family to care for the cancer patient at home: A home care course. Cancer Nursing, *4*:49–52, 1981.

Fisher, S. G.: The psychosexual effects of cancer and cancer treatment. Oncology Nursing Forum, *10*:63–68, 1983.

Frank-Stromberg, M., Wright, P. S., Segalla, M., and Diekmann, J.: Psychological impact of the "cancer" diagnosis. Oncology Nursing Forum, *11*:16–22, 1984.

Giacquinta, B.: Helping families face the crisis of cancer. American Journal of Nursing, *77*:1585–1588, 1977.

Lewis, F. M., Ellison, E. S., and Woods, N. F.: The impact of breast cancer on the family. Seminars in Oncology Nursing, *1*:206–213, 1985.

Moos, R. N. and Moos, B. S.: A typology of family social environments. Family Process, *15*:357–371, 1976.

Skorupka, P. and Bohnet, N.: Primary caregivers' perceptions of nursing behaviors that best meet their needs in a home care hospice setting. Cancer Nursing, *5*:371–374, 1982.

Smilkstein, G.: The family APGAR: A proposal for a family function test and its use by physicians. The Journal of Family Practice, *6*:1231–1239, 1978.

U.S. Department of Health and Human Services. Public Health Service. National Institutes of Health. Coping with Cancer. A Resource for the Health Professional. Bethesda, MD, National Cancer Institute, 1980.

Vess, J. D., Moreland, J. R., and Schwebel, A. I.: A follow-up study of role functioning and the psychological environment of families of cancer patients. Journal of Psychosocial Oncology, *3*:1–14, 1985.

Wegmann, J. A., and Ogrinc, M.: Oncology nursing conflict: A case presentation of holistic care and the family in crisis. Cancer Nursing, *4*:43–48, 1981.

Welch-McCaffrey, D.: When it comes to cancer, think family. Nursing '83, *17*:32–35, 1983.

Wellisch, D. K.: The psychologic impact of breast cancer on relationships. Seminars in Oncology Nursing, *1*:195–199, 1985.

33

Teaching the Patient and Family or Significant Other

BARBARA K. REDMAN, RN, PhD

A. Patient education—any combination of learning opportunities designed to affect the knowledge level, skills, attitudes, or other behaviors of patients and persons closely associated with them. The expected outcome is the enhancement of health practices by individuals and families experiencing cancer, including their ability to live with the disease.
B. Cancer patient education—focused on goals related to coping, rehabilitation, informed consent, adherence, and prevention. It has been documented to be effective in each of these realms. Nurses caring for persons at risk for cancer or living with it must incorporate in their practice responsibility for providing relevant education, as professional and legal standards require.

USE OF OUTCOME STANDARDS FOR PATIENT EDUCATION

A. Standards related to individual and family: nurses will provide the individual and family with knowledge and skills that will assist them to:
1. Identify accurate and current information about cancer and related treatment modalities.
2. Manage stress within their physical, psychological, and spiritual capacities.
3. Preserve a reasonable emotional balance.
4. Establish a positive self-image.
5. Strengthen relationships with family and friends.
6. Prepare to live a life of uncertainty.
7. Maintain, according to ability and desire, a sense of control and participation in their own health care.
8. Mobilize individual and family resources.
B. Standards related to health-illness continuum: nurses will provide the individual and family with knowledge and skills that assist them to:
1. Identify cancer warning signals that are unique to their cancer status.

353

2. Modify health behaviors and practices to prevent other cancers and to promote health.
3. Recognize the importance of diagnostic and staging procedures.
4. Determine their position on the health-illness continuum in order to maximize self-care for alterations in hydration, nutrition, ventilation, mobility, elimination, comfort, and sexuality.
5. Recognize signs, symptoms, and appropriate action for potential problems related to malignant disease.
6. Evaluate treatment options.
C. Standards related to the health care system: nurses have a responsibility to provide education about the health care system that assists the individual and family to:
   1. Identify the components of the health care system required and those that are available to them.
   2. Describe the roles of the various members of the health care team involved in cancer care.
   3. Use the appropriate components of the health care system.
   4. Assess financial factors related to utilization of the health care system.
D. Standards related to community and environment: nurses will assist the individual and family to:
   1. Identify cancer-related resources at the local, regional, and national levels.
   2. Describe their human rights for informed consent.
   3. Identify the effect of environmental pollutants on carcinogenesis.
   4. Recognize legislative actions that influence cancer prevention and management.
E. Standards related to the nursing process:
   1. Nursing process: used to develop an education program as follows:
      a. Assess educational needs.
      b. Set mutually acceptable educational goals and objectives.
      c. Select appropriate educational methods and materials.
      d. Implement an educational program.
      e. Formulate acceptable criteria for evaluation of learning behaviors.
   2. Research process: nurses providing educational opportunities will:
      a. Demonstrate knowledge of the status of viable cancer patient education programs.
      b. Identify current research that may apply to cancer patient education.
      c. Describe nursing problems that are amenable to educational intervention.
      d. Participate in cancer patient education research efforts by serving as data collector, observer, or facilitator of the teaching-learning situation.

PURPOSE AND IMPLEMENTATION

A. These standards reflect nursing's holistic philosophy and are developed to be congruent with the individuals' and families' estimate of their needs, their priorities, and their sense of well-being. The standards further aim to make the complex health care system, community resources, and the social and legal structure relevant to the disease and tools for the family's use.

B. The standards also require the use of nursing's full set of professional tools and functions to guide and evaluate the nursing process at several levels of aggregation:

1. The quality of the individual nurse's practice and rewards for the quality, such as advancement up clinical ladders.
2. The functioning of a service such as an oncology unit, often through formal quality assurance activities.
3. The degree to which organizational structures within an institution providing cancer care serve to support the delivery of patient education.
4. The adequacy of staff development activities regarding patient education in oncology nursing.
5. As measures of effectiveness of the health care institutions as a system, within a community.
6. As measures of quality in professional certification, accreditation, and licensing activities.
7. In a court of law as reflecting the profession's definition of quality care in oncology nursing.
8. In society, to measure the nursing profession's contribution to cancer patient care; thus, used to set social policy.

KEY COMPONENTS OF CANCER INTERVENTION

A. Goals and Objectives:

1. Prevention—Individuals at risk for cancer need knowledge about the risks and how to decrease them, skills to detect signs and symptoms and to take positive preventive actions such as adequate nutrition, and an attitude of caution toward being "at risk" without excessive fear.
2. Informed consent—An educational process that ethically should be obtained for all diagnostic and treatment activities. There is repeated evidence that many individuals do not understand that to which they "give consent." Active participation of the learner, repetition and reinforcement, and use of categorization of content should help. (See Chapter 37.)
3. Adherence—For that treatment to which the patient agrees, he or she needs skills to carry it out. This point is especially important today as more treatment is given on an outpatient basis and is self-administered. The patient also needs to recognize and control side effects. Tailoring the regimen, reducing complexity of the regimen, creating greater involvement, using incentives for the person and his or her social network that reinforce adherence, and improving satisfaction with the provider-patient relationship have been found to be useful.
4. Coping—Adjusting to the course of the disease while still retaining a sense of control, preventing medical crises and managing them if they occur, decreasing anxiety, preventing social isolation, normalizing life style, and learning to use community resources are important for patient and family well-being. Ineffective coping in individuals may affect those with limited resources, small social networks, or a sense of helplessness. Ineffective family coping often is precipitated by the impact of illness on lifestyle and family roles and relationships and shifting life goals. Education should include development of understanding of the relationship between coping and the perception of stressors, and skill in problem-solving behavior. Relaxation techniques can be of assistance.

5. Rehabilitation—This goal involves helping the person to obtain maximum physical, social, psychological, and vocational functioning within the limits imposed by the disease and its treatment. Treatable problems contributing to disability often include pain, general weakness, and psychological problems. Decrease in negative affect, realistic outlook and meaningfulness of life, and return to work or active time usage are goals of rehabilitation.

B. Assessment of readiness must take place repeatedly as the patient's needs change. *Readiness* may be defined as ability and proclivity to learn based on motivation and on present understanding, skills, and attitudes.
   1. Readiness may be affected by:
      a. Misconceptions and partial knowledge about cancer, its causes, treatments, and effects.
      b. Being in crisis, fear, pain, fever; experiencing side effects from drugs; or entering a new stage of the disease as for example, for persons with advanced disease, families become ready to develop skill in basic nursing care and in pain control.
   2. Readiness may be stimulated by:
      a. Placing needs as defined by the individual as highest priority.
      b. Creating supportive participative environments with clear expectations of responsibilities.
      c. Assisting the individual gain some measure of control.
   3. Readiness is assessed by gathering data and coming to a conclusion (diagnosis) about the individual's status in relation to the goals and objectives and his learning abilities.
      a. Assess subjective and objective information.
      b. Set mutual goals.
      c. Remember, teaching without assessment is like treatment without diagnosis.

TEACHING SERVICES

A. Formal teaching programs.
   1. Packaged programs such as "I Can Cope" or "Reach to Recovery," the former includes information on:
      a. Learning about the disease.
      b. Coping with daily health problems.
      c. Communication with others.
      d. Liking yourself.
      e. Living up to your limits.
      f. Resources that can help.
   2. Structured educational programs developed within an institution.
B. Informal teaching as a planned part of consumer-provider interaction.
C. Support groups with educational elements.
D. Topics in oncology education include: the experience of having cancer; the disease; treatment modalities that will be used such as surgery, radiation therapy, chemotherapy, immunotherapy; nutrition; infection; and pain control.
E. Educational approaches:
   1. Discussion.
   2. Role modeling or role playing.

3. Demonstration, redemonstration, practice.
4. Recitation.
5. Behavior modification.
6. Learning contracts.
7. Evaluation of learning by observation and testing and reteaching when necessary.

F. Educational tools include:
1. Books and brochures.
2. Tapes, filmstrips, audiotapes, visual aids, television.
3. Models of body parts such as breast lump simulator.
4. Games.
5. Drama/puppets/play.
6. Role models.
7. Telephone information services.
8. Computer-aided or -managed instruction.

G. Teaching and learning in most troubled health states require a relationship between provider and patient. In the coaching function, the nurse:
1. Interprets the unfamiliar diagnostic and treatment demands.
2. Supports the patient
3. Identifies changing relevance.
4. Ensures that cure is enhanced by care.

H. Organizational structures to support teaching:
1. Protocols or defined programs of patient education.
2. Teaching materials, teaching plans, consultation about teaching problems readily available.
3. Coordination of planning, training, implementation, monitoring, and evaluation functions for the program.
4. Expectations of and rewards to providers for good performance in education.
5. Continuity of patient education services between home and institutional care.

PRINCIPLES OF LEARNING AND TEACHING

A. Learning activities should promote movement toward the objectives.
B. Learning is more effective when undertaken in response to a felt need, usually problem-centered.
C. Learning is more effective when it relates to what the person already knows and what is meaningful to him or her.
D. Learning must be reinforced and used.
E. A learner's confidence in his or her ability to carry out actions (self efficacy) is essential to adequate coping and rehabilitation.
F. Learning is easier if the learner is aware that progress is being made and is rewarded internally and externally.
G. Tasks that are broken into units and use of structured protocols will not overwhelm learner's capabilities and help make the learning seem possible; they also provide points by which to measure progress and review learning.
H. Mutual planning of goals and participation in all parts of the teaching-learning process increases commitment and learning.
I. Individual models of thinking about cancer must be assessed and errors of fact corrected.

Table 33–1. ACTIVITIES INVOLVED IN TEACHING–LEARNING PROCESS

Development of desired objectives with the patient and family

Assessment of present learning against those objectives

Stimulating the patient's and family's readiness to learn

Choosing instructional approaches that will move the patient toward the objectives

Obtaining and screening teaching tools for accuracy and teaching effectiveness

Providing instruction and assisting the patient to learn and to master skills

Allowing the patient to practice using the learned material

Mutually evaluating progress toward the goals, including the patient's confidence

Note: Any of these steps may be repeated in sequences of teaching-learning. They should always be in the context of the demands of the illness and the patient's satisfaction at various stages of it

J. Behavior can change attitudes, as well as the reverse; frequently, persuading a person to change a behavior will lead to subsequent attitude change.
K. Interventions that provide descriptions of impending invasive procedures and/or instruction in coping strategies or behaviors have been shown to have a positive effect on reactions to and recovery from surgery.
  1. The nurse's judgement of the patient's ability to adequately learn a set of skills such as those required for home parenteral nutrition, or continuous chemotherapy infusion, may lock the person into or out of certain options for living.
  2. It is essential to clearly state those skills that must be learned and to be as flexible as possible in teaching approaches that help the patient to master those skills.
L. Activities in teaching-learning process (Table 33–1).

STUDY QUESTIONS

1. Define patient education.
2. Discuss the role of outcome standards for patient education.
3. State three (3) principles of learning that are relevant to patient education.
4. Discuss methods of teaching that may be relevant to various client situations.

Bibliography

Barofsky, I.: Therapeutic compliance and the cancer patient. Health Education Quarterly, *10*(Suppl):43–55, 1984.

Benner, P.: The oncology clinical nurse specialist: An expert coach. Oncology Nursing Forum, *12*(2):40–44, 1985.

Cromes, G.: Implementation of interdisciplinary cancer rehabilitation. Rehabilitation Counseling, *21*:2390–2397, 1978.

Doak, C., Doak, L., and Root, J.: Teaching Patients with Low Literacy Skills. Philadelphia, J.B. Lipincott, 1985.

Johnson, J.: Coping with elective surgery. Annual Review of Nursing Research, 2:107–132, 1984.

Johnson, J. and Flaherty, M.: The nurse and cancer patient education. Seminars in Oncology, 7:63–70, 1980.

Johnson, J. and Green, M.: Client education: An integral part of cancer nursing. *In* Marino, L.: Cancer Nursing. St. Louis, C.V. Mosby, pp. 79–97, 1981.

Long, J.: Teaching and learning strategies. *In* McIntire, S. and Cioppa, A. (eds.): Cancer Nursing: A Developmental Approach. New York, John Wiley & Sons, pp. 583–594, 1984.

McNally, J. C., Stair, J. C., Somerville, E. T., and ONS Clinical Practice Subcommittee on Guidelines (eds.): Guidelines for Cancer Nursing Practice. Orlando, Grune & Stratton, 1985.

Oncology Nursing Society Education Committee: Outcome Standards for Cancer Patient Education. Pittsburgh, The Oncology Nursing Society, 1982.

Redman, B. (ed.): The Process of Patient Education. St. Louis, C.V. Mosby, 1984.

34

Identification of and Referral to Resources

JODY BURNS, RN, MSN

CANCER NURSING PRACTICE

A. Outcome standards for cancer nursing practice.
   1. Oncology Nursing Society
      3111 Banksville Road
      Pittsburgh, PA 15216
      Telephone (412) 344-3899
      a. Provides support to oncology nurses. Promotes the highest professional standards of oncology nursing. Encourages study, research, and exchange of information.
      b. Helpful publications include:
         (1) Outcome Standards for Cancer Nursing.
         (2) Subject and Author Index to *Oncology Nursing Forum*.
         (3) Cancer Chemotherapy: Guidelines and Recommendations for Nursing Education and Practice.
   2. American Nurses Association
      2420 Pershing Road
      Kansas City, MO 64108
      Telephone (816) 494-5720
B. Nursing management of patient/family problems (Table 34–1)
   1. Oncology Nursing Society (see previous listing)
      a. Provides a recently published *Subject and Author Index*, which contains a summary of *Oncology Nursing Forum* articles (from Volume 3, 1976 to Volume 12, 1984) and addresses nursing management of patients.
   2. American Association of Cancer Education
      Dr. Stephen Stowe
      Building A-1020
      New Jersey Medical School
      100 Bergen Street
      Newark, NJ 07103
      Telephone (201) 456-5365

Table 34–1. COMMUNITY RESOURCES FOR PEOPLE
WITH CANCER*

Organization/Resource	Service/Location
Directory of Human Services	A primary and central point for locating assistance in any community is the directory of human services. Directories are published through the cooperative efforts of United Way and other community service groups and are available at a nominal cost. In many communities, a directory of human services can also be found in public libraries. The directories provide a listing of all human services available within a geographical area. In areas that have small populations, usually two or more counties join together to publish a directory. These directories are divided according to subject index, and service categories are listed alphabetically. Included are the names, addresses, telephone numbers, and descriptive narratives of services available, to whom they are available, and catchment areas that are served.
Community Organizations	Although not listed in directories of human services, civic organizations within a community often provide human services that may be of assistance to patients and their families. The local chamber of commerce can provide nurses with such a listing.
State and Local Departments of Health and Social Services	Departments of health and social services provide information and a variety of services for patients with cancer and their families. Listings are found in local telephone directories.
National Hospice Organization	This organization is a private, nonprofit, membership organization that is divided into 10 regions and state organizations. The National Hospice Organization is dedicated to promoting and maintaining quality care for terminally ill patients. Literature, films, and a directory of hospice programs are available through the organization at the following address: 1901 North Fort Meyer Drive, Arlington, Virginia 22209.
National Cancer Institute	The National Cancer Institute is a branch of the National Institutes of Health, which is part of the United States Department of Health and Human Resources. Its primary responsibility is to establish a structure for a systematic attack on cancer throughout the United States through a network of treatment centers. The address of the National Cancer Institute is: National Institutes of Health, Bethesda, Maryland 20014. The major activities of the institute's treatment centers are setting standards for research facilities, sharing information, and funding research studies.
American Cancer Society	The American Cancer Society is the largest national voluntary organization that is dedicated to fighting cancer. Its efforts include education, research, patient services, and rehabilitation programs. The society is composed of 59 chartered divisions and approximately 3,000 local county units. Division units are found in all states, the District of Columbia, Puerto Rico, and the Canal Zone. The address of the National Headquarters is: American Cancer Society, 777 Third Avenue, New York, New York 10017. State divisions and local county units can be found in local telephone directories. In addition to numerous pamphlets, films, and educational displays, a variety of direct patient services are available to assist patients and their families. Direct services include sickroom supplies and comfort items, transportation for medical care, dressings, nursing, and homemaker and home health aide services. Because the types and quantity

Table 34–1. COMMUNITY RESOURCES FOR PEOPLE
WITH CANCER* (*continued*)

Organization/Resource	Service/Location
	of direct patient services vary from one local unit to another, it is important to speak to personnel at the local American Cancer Society unit to determine what resources are available in the local community.
Comprehensive Cancer Center Network	The National Cancer Institute has designated comprehensive cancer centers throughout the United States. The cancer centers carry out basic and clinical medical research and also provide patient care and treatment. New methods and practices for diagnosis, treatment protocols, and drug therapies are investigated. For information concerning the comprehensive cancer center in your area, contact the Cancer Information Service.
Cancer Information Service	The Cancer Information Service is a nationwide, toll-free telephone inquiry system that provides information relating to cancer. It provides support, understanding, and rapid access to the latest information on cancer and local resources. Cancer Information Service units are located and associated with the major cancer centers throughout the country.
	The Cancer Information Service is funded by the National Cancer Institute through contracts with designated comprehensive cancer centers and, in many areas, with the cooperation of the American Cancer Society. Trained staff members provide information on:
	Causes of cancer
	How to help prevent cancer
	Methods used for detection, diagnosis, and treatment
	Availability of medical facilities, home care, and rehabilitative services
	Availability of financial assistance
	Emotional support and counseling services
	Appropriate referrals regarding investigational treatments
	Further information can be obtained by calling the Cancer Information Service listed in the local telephone directory.
	Cancer study groups are located throughout the country and in the comprehensive cancer centers. Nurses should write to the local comprehensive cancer center or make a telephone call to the National Cancer Institute to find out which comprehensive cancer centers have study groups investigating and conducting research on a given disease.
Support and Self-Help Groups	○ Reach to Recovery: a rehabilitation program for women who have undergone mastectomy. Volunteers who have undergone this operation visit such women and provide psychologic support, demonstrate rehabilitative exercises, and provide temporary prostheses.
	○ International Association of Laryngectomees: a rehabilitation program for persons who have undergone laryngectomy. Volunteers who have undergone this operation visit such persons and provide psychologic support, information, and teaching that enables persons who have had the operation to become self-sufficient in communicating and caring for a laryngectomy.
	○ I Can Cope: an educational program that provides psychologic support and information to patients.
	○ Can Surmount: a program that provides education, emo-

Table continued on following page

Table 34–1. COMMUNITY RESOURCES FOR PEOPLE
WITH CANCER* (*continued*)

Organization/Resource	Service/Location
	tional and psychologic support to patients with cancer and their families.

○ Candlelighters Foundation
Suite 1011
2025 I Street, NW
Washington, D.C. 20006
This international organization assists the parents of children who have cancer. Local groups serve as a forum for such parents, sponsoring 24-hour crisis lines, buddy systems, parent to parent contact, professional counseling, and self-help groups.
○ Cancer Care, Inc.
One Park Avenue
New York, NY 10016
This organization operates in the tristate metropolitan area of New York, New Jersey, and Connecticut. It is a voluntary social service agency that provides professional counseling, public education, and planning as well as home care services to patients with advanced cancer and their families.
○ Make Today Count
514 Tama Building
P.O. Box 303
Burlington, IA 52601
This national organization is divided into local chapters that provide mutual support to help patients who have serious illnesses live life in a positive, meaningful manner.
○ United Ostomy Association, Inc.
2001 West Beverly Boulevard
Los Angeles, CA 90057
This organization provides services throughout the United States and abroad. There are local chapters throughout the world. The overall goal of the association is to achieve complete rehabilitation for all ostomates. National, regional, state, and provincial conferences are held throughout the year.
○ After—ask a friend about reconstruction
99 Park Avenue
New York, NY. 10016
This volunteer group provides educational materials and personal support for the woman considering breast reconstruction.
○ Encore
A YWCA sponsored group for postoperative breast cancer patients, which combines exercise and discussion.
○ DES Action
Long Island Jewish Hillside Medical Center
New Hyde Park, NY. 11040
This group is active in education and legislation related to DES.
○ Leukemia Society of America, Inc.
211 E. 43rd St.,
New York, NY. 10017
Chapters located throughout the United States provide supplementary financial assistance to persons with leukemia, Hodgkin's disease, or lymphoma.

* Adapted from Morra, M. and Potts, E.: Choices: Realistic Alternatives in Cancer Care. New York, Avon Publishers, 1979.

a. Provides education and training programs for professionals involved with cancer care.

3. Nurse to nurse consultation—Provides nurse to nurse oncology consultation service for immediate and specific patient care problems.
   a. University of Texas
      Department of Nursing
      M.D. Anderson Hospital and Tumor Institute
      6723 Bertner Avenue
      Houston, TX 77030
      Telephone (713) 792-7100
   b. Johns Hopkins Cancer Information Service
      Nurse to Nurse Telephone Consultation
      550 N. Broadway
      Baltimore, MD 21205
      Telephone (301) 955-8638

4. Pharmaceutical companies provide self-paced learning computer programs that address treatment with and side effects of chemotherapeutic agents. These may be obtained by contacting sales representatives in your area.

C. Nursing management of oncologic emergencies.
   1. *Subject and Author Index* (Oncology Nursing Society).
   2. Current nursing textbooks.

D. Nursing administration of chemotherapy.
   1. Oncology Nursing Society (see previous listing)—provides *Cancer Chemotherapy Guidelines and Recommendations for Nursing Education and Practice*, 1984, which addresses preparation, handling, disposal, and administration of chemotherapy and extravasation techniques.
   2. National Institute of Occupational Safety and Health (NIOSH) publications
      Health and Human Service
      4676 Columbia Parkway
      Cincinnati, Ohio 45226
      Telephone (513) 841-4287
         Provides NIOSH Publications List, research materials, and guidelines pertinent for oncology nurses.
   3. Several pharmaceutical companies provide written guidelines for nursing management of extravasation based on company research.
   4. National Study Commission on cytotoxic exposure. *Recommendations for Handling Cytotoxic Agents*, September 1984.

E. Communicating with the patient and family/significant others.
   1. The American Cancer Society (see Table 34–1).
   2. National Cancer Institute (see Table 34–1).
   3. The National Cancer Information Clearing House
      Room 10A18 Building 31 NCI/NIH
      Bethesda, MD 20205
      Telephone (301) 496-4070
         Provides an exchange of information for patients.
   4. Cancer Information Service (CIS) (see Table 34–1).

F. Teaching the patient and family/significant others.
   1. Oncology Nursing Society (see previous listing)—provides published information in *Outcome Standards for Cancer Nursing* and *Subject and Author*

Index, which offer extensive information regarding patient and family education.
   2. Cancer nursing texts.
G. Identification of and referral to resources (see Table 34–1).
   1. Concern for Dying
      250 West 57th Street
      New York, NY 10107
      Telephone (212) 246-6962
         Provides information regarding the distribution of living wills, documents that record patient's wishes concerning treatments.
   2. Touch Cancer Control Program
      Earl Sanders
      Director of Hematology/Oncology
      Tinsley Harrison Tower
      Birmingham, AL 35294
      Telephone (205) 934-3814
         Touch provides assistance to cancer patients and families in forming realistic positive attitudes toward cancer and treatment.
   3. Psychosocial Counseling Service
      UCLA Jonsson Comprehensive Cancer Center
      10920 Wilshire Boulevard
      Suite 1106
      Los Angeles, CA 90024
      Telephone (213) 206-6017
         Provides telephone counseling services directed at the psychosocial needs of the patients and care givers.
   4. Ronald McDonald House
      Gloin/Harris Communications, Inc.
      500 Michigan Avenue
      Chicago, IL 60611
      Telephone: (312) 836-7129
         Provides information regarding the establishment of Ronald McDonald Houses and locations of homes.
H. Risk factors and coping skills for the oncology nurse.
   1. Nursing texts provide one of the best resources.
   2. Local chapters of the Oncology Nursing Society provide resources for dealing with risk factors and coping mechanisms for the oncology nurse.

TREATMENT OF CANCER

A. The topics are addressed in a variety of resources:
   1. Cancer nursing journals.
   2. Nursing texts.
   3. American Cancer Society publications (see Table 34–1).
   4. National Cancer Institute publications (see Table 34–1).
   5. Oncology Nursing Society's *Subject and Author Index* from the *Oncology Nursing Forum* focuses significantly upon treatment modalities (see Table 34–1).
   6. American Society of Clinical Oncology
      Suite 1717
      435 North Michigan Avenue

Chicago, IL 60611

Telephone (312) 644-0828

Provides and fosters the exchange of information relating to neo-plastic diseases with particular emphasis on human biology, diagnosis, and treatment.

ISSUES AND TRENDS AND CANCER CARE

A. The topics are addressed in a variety of resources.
  1. Concern for Dying (see previous listing).
  2. National Hospice Organization
     1901 North Fort Meyer Drive
     Suite 901
     Arlington, VA 22209
       Provides information for Hospice patients, a roster of Hospice pro-grams in the United States, and information for developing community Hospice programs.
B. Care settings (home care, ambulatory care, hospice), legal issues including cancer quackery and unproven methods, carcinogenesis legislation, and pa-tients' rights are addressed by the following:
  a. American Cancer Society (see previous listing).
  b. Nursing texts.
C. Information regarding cancer economics can be obtained from:
   Cancer Care, Inc.
   1180 Avenue of the Americas
   New York, NY 10036
   Telephone (212) 302-2400
     Provides planning and counseling services to cancer patients, including psychological counseling and supplemental financial assistance when appropriate.
D. The individual societies may provide financial resources and include such groups as:
  1. Leukemia Society of America
     733 Third Avenue
     New York, NY 10017
     Telephone (212) 573-8484
       Provides information and supportive materials for patients with leu-kemia and leukemia related diseases.
  2. International Association of Laryngectomees (see Table 34–1).
  3. United Ostomy Association (see Table 34–1).

CANCER PREVENTION AND DETECTION

A. American Cancer Society (see Table 34–1).
B. National Cancer Institute (see Table 34–1).
C. Cancer nursing textbooks.

DIAGNOSIS AND STAGING OF CANCER

Information about diagnosing cancer, staging, and grading is available in current general oncology textbooks.

PATHOPHYSIOLOGY OF CANCER

Alterations of cell biology, process of carcinogenesis, role of the immune system, and classification systems.
A. Cancer nursing texts, general oncology texts.
B. American Society of Clinical Oncology (see previous listing).
C. American Cancer Society (see Table 34–1).
D. Oncology Nursing Society (see previous listing) publishes *Subject and Author Index*, which addresses the pathophysiology of cancer.

CANCER EPIDEMIOLOGY

Information concerning appropriate terminology, cancer incidents, trends, patterns of occurrence, and cancer risk factors is available from:
A. American Cancer Society (see previous listing). Provides extensive information regarding cancer incidences, trends, patterns of occurrence, and risk factors.
B. Oncology texts should be referred to, since they also delineate detailed information regarding cancer epidemiology.
C. Historical perspectives in oncology nursing are most often described in cancer nursing texts.

STUDY QUESTIONS

1. Identify at least one resource for each of the following:
   a. Nursing management of the effects of disease, treatment, and complications.
   b. Communicating with the patient and family/significant others.
   c. Risk factors and coping skills for the oncology nurse.

35

Risk Factors and Coping Skills for the Oncology Nurse

MARY CUNNINGHAM, RN, BSN, OCN

STRESS AND BURNOUT CONCEPTS

A. Stress.
   1. Description:
      a. Is necessary for life.
      b. Demands adaptational change—physical, emotional, and intellectual.
   2. Discussion: Stress becomes a problem when the level of stress exceeds one's ability to effectively respond and when the adaptation is no longer growth-promoting but growth-inhibiting.
   3. Professional stress demands adaptational change in the performance of one's professional role.
   4. Stressor.
      a. Definition—a stressor is any stimulus that produces stress.
      b. Effect—the impact of a stressor is dependent upon these attributes:
         (1) Suddenness.
         (2) Chronicity.
         (3) Intensity.
         (4) Meaning of the stressor to the individual.
         (5) Occurrence as a single stressor or in addition to multiple stressors.
         (6) Vulnerability of the individual.
   5. Stress Response.
      a. Definition—stress response is the adaptational change made to stress (Stressor–Stress–Stress Response).
      b. Discussion—stress response has been described as a generalized response syndrome that occurs in three stages:
         (1) Alarm—mobilizes the body's defenses.
         (2) Resistance—serves to optimize one's adaptation to stress.
         (3) Exhaustion—depletes the individual's resources and renders the individual unable to resist stress.

369

B. Burnout.
  1. General.
    a. Burnout has been defined as exhaustion caused by excessive demands on energy, strength, or resources.
    b. Burnout is insidious, cumulative, and progressive.
  2. Professional Burnout is the deterioration of professional performance, which is directly related to the demand for adaptational change brought on by stressors in the work environment.

STRESSORS AFFECTING ONCOLOGY NURSES

A. Characteristics of the oncology nurse that contribute to burnout:
  1. Overly dedicated and committed.
  2. Authoritarian personality.
  3. Overidentification with patients.
  4. Strong dependency and achievement needs.
  5. Unrealistic goals and self-expectations.
B. Characteristics of the oncology patient and the nature of cancer care that contribute to burnout:
  1. Elusive etiology.
  2. Heterogeneity of malignancies.
  3. Variability of prognosis.
  4. Unpredictability of health-illness trajectory.
  5. Confrontation with disfigurement, disability, and death.
  6. Social stigma of working with people who have cancer.
  7. Knowledge base constantly in a state of flux.
  8. Repeated sense of failure if cure-oriented.
C. Factors within the work setting that contribute to burnout:
  1. Unbalanced staff-patient ratio.
  2. Inability to participate in decision making.
  3. Lack of recognition for good work.
  4. Lack of autonomy.
  5. Role ambiguity.
  6. Professional responsibilities versus bureaucratic conflicts.

STRESS RESPONSES

A. Physical responses:
  1. Constant state of fatigue.
  2. Sleep disturbances.
  3. Change in food, alcohol, drug, and cigarette consumption.
  4. Change in physical appearance.
  5. Repetitive accidents.
  6. Change in sexual behavior.
  7. Exacerbation of pre-existing medical problems.
  8. Muscular pain, particularly of neck and lower back muscles.
B. Emotional responses:
  1. Angry outbursts.
  2. Irritability.
  3. Feelings of worthlessness or a sense of failure.
  4. Depression.

5. Emotional distancing.
6. Paranoia.
7. Resistance to change.
8. Diminished initiative.
9. Critical of self and others.
C. Intellectual responses:
1. Forgetfulness.
2. Preoccupation.
3. Mathematical and grammatical errors.
4. Lack of concentration.
5. Lack of attention to details.
6. Past rather than present or future orientation.
7. Diminished productivity.
8. Impaired problem solving ability.
9. Inability to make decisions.
10. Change to abstract and analytical thinking.

STRESS PREVENTION AND MANAGEMENT STRATEGIES

A. Definition—any strategy for prevention and management of stress must include eliminating those stressors that can be eliminated, mastering those stressors that can not be eliminated, and developing mechanisms for prompt recognition and relief of stress responses.
B. Discussion:
1. A pivotal point in the prevention and management of stress is legitimization of one's own needs by pledging commitment to self care that begins with a self-assessment of these factors:
   a. Needs.
   b. Motivations.
   c. Long- and short-term goals.
   d. Support systems at work.
   e. Support systems away from work.
   f. Stress responses.
   g. Communication style.
   h. Time-management ability.
   i. Conflict-resolution skills.
2. Strategies for prevention and management of stress that are dependent upon this self-assessment may include:
   a. Physical activity.
   b. Social activity.
   c. Intellectual activity.
   d. Seeking professional counseling.
   e. Meditation or relaxation techniques.
   f. Assertiveness training.
   g. Time-management training.
   h. Practicing positive attitude.
   i. Establishing realistic goals and expectations and eliminating irrational beliefs.
   j. Advocating within the work environment the following:
      (1) Development of support groups.

(2) Balanced staff-patient ratios that support quality care.
(3) Employee benefit packages that provide for vacations, mental health days, payment for professional counseling.
(4) Recognition or merit systems that value quality performance.
(5) Physical space separate from the work environment.

STUDY QUESTIONS

1. Describe the nature of stress, including physical, emotional, and intellectual responses to it.
2. List at least three (3) strategies for managing burnout.

Bibliography

Calhoun, G. L., and Calhoun, J. G.: Occupational stress—implications for hospitals. *In* Selye, H. (ed.): Selye's Guide to Stress Research (Vol. 13). New York, Van Nostrand Reinhold, 1983.

Charlesworth, E. A. and Nathan, R. G.: Stress Management: A Comprehensive Guide to Wellness. New York, Antheneum, 1985.

Clark, C. C.: Burnout: Assessment and intervention. Journal of Nursing Administration, *10*(9):39–43, 1980.

Donovan, M.: Stress at work: Cancer nurses' report. Oncology Nursing Forum, *8*(2):22–25, 1981.

Ellis, A. and Harper, R.: A New Guide to Rational Living. Los Angeles, Wilshire, 1975.

Freudenberger, H.: The staff burnout syndrome. Journal of Social Issues, *30*(1):159–166, 1974.

Haber, J., Leach, A. M., Schudy, S. M., and Sideleau, B. F.: Comprehensive Psychiatric Nursing. New York, McGraw-Hill Book Co., 1982.

Jacobson, S. F. and McGrath, H. M.: Nurses Under Stress. New York, John Wiley & Sons, 1983.

Klagsburn, S.: Cancer, emotions and nurses. American Journal of Psychiatry, *126*(9):1237–1244, 1980.

McElroy, A.: Burnout: A review of the literature with application to cancer nursing. Cancer Nursing, *5*(3):211–217, 1982.

Newlin, N. and Wellisch, D.: The oncology nurse: Life on an emotional roller coaster. Cancer Nursing, *1*(6):447–449, 1978.

Ogle, M.: Stages of burnout among oncology nurses in the hospital setting. Oncology Nursing Forum, *10*(1):31–34, 1983.

Patrick, P.: Burnout: Antecedents, manifestations, and self-care strategies for nurses. *In* Marino, L. (ed.): Cancer Nursing. St. Louis, C. V. Mosby, 1981.

Rabkin, J. G. and Struening, E. L.: Life events, stress, and illness. Science, *194*:1013–1020, 1976.

Scott, D., Oberst, M., and Dropkin, M.: A stress-coping model. *In* Sutterley, D. and Donnelly, G. (eds.): Coping With Stress, A Nursing Perspective. Rockville, MD, Aspen Systems, 1982.

Selye, H.: The Stress of Life. New York, McGraw-Hill Book Co., 1956.

Storlie, F.: Burnout: The elaboration of a concept. American Journal of Nursing, *79*(12):2108–2111, 1979.

Vachon, M. L. S., Lyall, W. A. L., and Freeman, S. J. J.: Measurement and management of stress in health professionals working with advanced cancer patients. Death Education, *1*(4):365–375, 1978.

Wilson, H. S. and Kneisl, C. R.: Psychiatric Nursing. Menlo Park, CA, Addison-Wesley, 1983.

SECTION EIGHT

Issues and Trends in Cancer Care

Section Editor
JOANNE T. COSSMAN, RN, MPH

36

Historical Perspective

RUTH BOPE DANGEL, RN, MS, OCN
KATHLEEN FLYNN, RN, MS

CANCER: THE DISEASE

A. The earliest records.
   1. Cancer in man can be traced more than a million years. The oldest records are Egyptian (evidence of bone cancer identified in mummies in the Great Pyramid of Gizeh) and Indian (evidence of cancer found in an anthropoid in Java unearthed in 1891).
   2. Symptoms and primitive forms of treatment were described as early as 2500 B.C.
B. 460 B.C.–200 A.D.
   1. Hippocrates (c. 460–c. 370 B.C.).
      a. First described cancer using the Greek term *karkinos* (crab), which has evolved into the term carcinoma.
      b. Hippocrates described forms of the disease: breast, uterus, stomach, skin, and rectum; however, he erroneously described the etiology as an excess of black bile, thought to be produced by the spleen and stomach.
      c. Advocated no treatment for what he called "occult" cancer.
   2. Aurelius Cornelius Celsus (1st century A.D.) first operated on cancer.
   3. Galen (130–200 A.D.), the most prominent medical authority before the Renaissance, agreed with the black bile and non-treatment theories. His influence hindered the development of new knowledge until after the Renaissance.
      a. First correlated cancer with psychosomatic problems and emotions.
      b. Prescribed poppy seed infusions for pain relief.
      c. Middle ages provided no new discoveries significant to treatment.
C. 16th–18th Centuries.
   1. 16th and 17th Centuries.
      a. Fabricius Hildanus (1560–1634) began excising axillary lymph nodes as a treatment for breast cancer.
      b. Marcus Aurelius Severinus differentiated between benign and malignant tumors.

375

2. 18th Century.
   a. Prevailing public attitude was that cancer was contagious; persons with cancer were treated as lepers.
   b. The first cancer hospital was founded in Reims, France.
   c. The humoral theory of cancer was rejected by a French surgeon, Henri Ledran (1685–1770) who:
      (1) Demonstrated the path of spread along the lymphatics and the appearance of metastases.
      (2) Advocated surgery as only treatment and rejected the use of pastes and ointments.
   d. First cancer experiments on animals began.
   e. First occupational cancer was described by Percivall Pott—scrotal cancer in chimney sweeps.
   f. Advances were made in pathology:
      (1) John Hunter, Rene Laennec, and Marie Francois described cells as the basic unit of tumors. Bichet, even without a microscope, confirmed their finding.
      (2) Johannes Muller, with the use of a microscope, studied diseased tissues.

D. 19th Century.
   1. Rudolph Virchow, a pathologist and a student of Muller's, declared "every cell is born from another cell" (cellular theory) and dispelled belief in the humoral theory.
   2. Cancer surgery began to be more successful, and it was done on larger scale, partially as a result of the work of Louis Pasteur on infections and Joseph Lister on asepsis and antisepsis.
   3. Radiation therapy developed as a treatment for cancer.
      a. Wilhelm Roentgen discovered rays in 1895, now known as roentgen rays or x-rays.
      b. In 1898 Pierre and Marie Curie, two French scientists, found a new element, radium, in ore pitchblende.

E. 20th Century.
   1. In the early 1900's, individuals with cancer felt isolated and doomed; cancer was considered to be incurable, and few had any hope of surviving.
   2. During the 20th century modern cancer treatment evolved.
   3. Around 1940, chemotherapeutic agents with significant influence on cancer cells were discovered. Organized drug studies began in 1955.
   4. There were developments in radiation and surgical techniques and renewed interest in immunotherapy.
   5. Multimodality treatment approaches replaced the single treatment modality approach.
   6. In 1913, the American Cancer Society (ACS) opened as a voluntary organization dedicated to the control and eradication of cancer.
   7. In 1915, Hoffman, a statistician for the Prudential Insurance Company of America, compiled and published worldwide cancer statistics, which influenced the U.S. Census Bureau to analyze cancer mortality in registration areas of the U.S. for 1914 and led to the first field surveys of cancer incidence by Harold Dorn in 1937.
   8. 1930 cancer statistics revealed that fewer than 1 in 5 individuals with cancer were alive 5 years after diagnosis.

9. On August 5, 1937, President Franklin D. Roosevelt signed the first National Cancer Act, and on November 9, the National Advisory Cancer Council first met.

10. In 1940, cancer statistics reflected the trend that 1 in 4 individuals with cancer were alive 5 years after diagnosis. Early detection and prevention gained some recognition, and the ACS publicized the early warning signals of cancer.

11. In 1955 the National Cancer Institute's Cooperative Clinical Trials Program was initiated and described as the largest clinical treatment evaluation program in medicine.

12. In 1960 cancer statistics improved—1 in 3 individuals with cancer were alive 5 years after diagnosis.

13. In the 1970's diagnostic radiology increased the ability to diagnose and follow metastasis.
    a. Computed tomography (CT) was developed.
    b. Improvements in diagnostic ultrasound and radionuclide imaging were presented.
    c. Fine-needle percutaneous aspiration biopsy techniques were introduced.

14. In 1967 Dr. Cicely Saunders opened St. Christopher's Hospice in London. The influence of the European hospice movement began to have an impact in America.
    a. The first American Hospice, Hospice of New Haven (now called The Connecticut Hospice, Inc.), opened its doors in 1971. This program was modeled after the one at St. Christopher's and was influenced by Dr. Saunders.
    b. The National Hospice Organization was founded in 1978.

15. Two studies noted a change in attitudes with regard to informing individuals of a diagnosis of cancer: one in 1961 reported 90% of physicians withheld a confirmed diagnosis of cancer, and a 1977 study reported 98% did *not* withhold the diagnosis.

16. Pioneering work with terminally ill patients was published by Dr. Elisabeth Kübler-Ross in *On Death and Dying* in 1979.

17. On December 23, 1971, President Nixon signed the National Cancer Act of 1971.

18. In the 1980's, with advanced knowledge and treatments, statistics improved, showing that one out of two persons who develop cancer will be alive 5 years after diagnosis.

CANCER THERAPY

A. Surgery.
   1. In general, surgery was seldom used before the 18th century because of the black bile theory and the belief that cancer was not curable and should be left alone.
   2. 18th Century.
      a. Black bile theory was dispelled and surgeons began to develop a rationale for cancer surgery.
      b. Valsalva, in 1704, believed cancer spread by way of the lymphatics to regional lymph nodes and that cancer was inclined to recur.

    c. The assumption was formed that cancer was a local disease that was curable if found early enough.

3. 19th Century.

    a. Basic principles of cancer surgery were developed; William S. Halsted is thought to be the most influential person in this development. Halsted did not place significance on the blood stream as a mechanism for metastasis but advocated that cancer spread locally by contiguous growth from the original tumor, extending along the fascia and walls of lymphatic vessels.

    b. Virchow in 1860 advanced the precept that lymph nodes are barriers to passage of cancer cells. Based on these assumptions an anatomic basis developed for cancer surgery, en bloc dissection removing tumor lymphatics, lymph nodes, and a surrounding region of normal tissue in one large piece (Table 36–1).

4. 20th Century.

    a. Advances in surgery continued with new knowledge, surgical techniques, and advances in related fields such as anesthesia, antibiotics, and postoperative care.

    b. Despite advances, surgery provided a cure for only localized cancers; medical and radiation oncology developed.

    c. Surgery continued to contribute to diagnosis and staging, definitive treatment, palliative surgery, and neurologic control of cancer pain.

    d. Recent developments include; microsurgery for reconstruction, au-

Table 36–1. SELECTED HISTORICAL MILESTONES IN SURGICAL ONCOLOGY*

Year	Surgeon	Event
1809	Ephraim McDowell	Elective abdominal surgery (excised ovarian tumor)
1846	John Collins Warren	Use of ether anesthesia (excised submaxillary gland)
1867	Joseph Lister	Introduction of antisepsis
1850–1880	Albert Theodore Billroth	First gastrectomy, laryngectomy, and esophagectomy
1878	Richard von Volkmann	Excision of cancerous rectum
1880s	Theodore Kocher	Development of thyroid surgery
1890	William Stewart Halsted	Radical mastectomy
1896	G. T. Beatson	Oophorectomy for breast cancer
1904	Hugh H. Young	Radical prostatectomy
1906	Ernest Wertheim	Radical hysterectomy
1908	W. Ernest Miles	Abdomenoperineal resection for cancer of the rectum
1912	E. Martin	Cordotomy for the treatment of pain
1910–1930	Harvey Cushing	Development of surgery for brain tumors
1913	Franz Torek	Successful resection of cancer of the thoracic esophagus
1927	G. Divis	Successful resection of pulmonary metastases
1933	Evarts Graham	Pneumonectomy
1935	A. O. Whipple	Pancreaticoduodenectomy
1945	Charles B. Huggins	Adrenalectomy for prostate cancer

    * From Devita, V. T., Hellman, S., and Rosenberg, S. A. (eds.): Cancer Principles and Practice of Oncology (Vol. 1), 2nd ed. Philadelphia, J. B. Lippincott, 1985.

tomatic stapling devices, and advanced endoscopic equipment, which allows incision-free surgery.
B. Chemotherapy.
   1. The early years.
      a. In 1865, Lissauer demonstrated the anticancer effect of potassium arsenite (Fowler's solution).
      b. In 1898, Paul Erhlich, who is considered the father of chemotherapy, discovered the first alkylating agent. He coined the term chemotherapy to describe the use of a chemical that treated parasites but it was 50 years before chemotherapy was used to treat cancer in humans.
      c. In the early 1900's, inbred rodent lines that could carry transplanted rodent tumors were developed by George Clowes of Rosewell Park Memorial Institute and served as tests for potential anticancer agents.
   2. The modern era.
      a. In 1941, C. Huggins and C. V. Hodges reported that patients with prostatic cancer benefited from the administration of estrogen.
      b. During both World Wars, alkylating agents were developed as part of a secret gas warfare program. An explosion of nitrogen mustard gas in Naples harbor during World War II exposed seamen, who later were observed to have marrow and lymphoid hypoplasia. This led to the first human testing with alkylating agents for Hodgkin's disease at Yale University in 1943.
      c. During the late 1940's, Farber observed the effect of folic acid on leukemia cell growth in children with lymphoblastic leukemia, and the antifolates were developed as cancer drugs.
      d. In 1942 penicillin was discovered, and in the 1950's public use of the drug became common. In the 1950's the development of useful cancer chemotherapeutic agents accelerated with the support of the drug screening program of the NCI Cooperative Clinical Trials Program of 1955.
      e. In 1956 the first bone marrow transplant was performed and first Wilms' tumor was cured with chemotherapy.
      f. In the early 1960's, H. E. Skipper and colleagues established guiding principles of chemotherapy using as a model rodent leukemia (L 1210).
      g. During the 1960's single drug therapy proved to be ineffective with two exceptions, choriocarcinoma and Burkitt's lymphoma, and was replaced by combination chemotherapy. The first effective combination chemotherapy began with therapy of leukemia and lymphoma pioneered by Dr. Emil Frei and others. It has extended to virtually all cancers as an accepted addition to the multimodality approach to cancer.
      h. Currently, 2 out of every 3 patients who develop cancer are candidates for chemotherapy. In addition to oral, parenteral, and intravenous routes, chemotherapy may be instilled into spinal fluid, pleural and pericardial spaces, splenic, hepatic, and carotid arteries, and intraperitoneal spaces.
      i. Chemotherapy, once considered a last effort, is now responsible for long-term survival in a variety of cancers and an important part of cancer cure, prolongation of life, and palliation of symptoms (Tables 36–2, 36–3, and 36–4).

Table 36–2. DEVELOPMENT OF CHEMOTHERAPEUTIC AGENTS*

Approximate Date	Agent	Diseases Treated
1865	Potassium arsenite	Leukemias, various malignancies
1893	Coley's toxins	Various malignancies
1941	Estrogens	Carcinoma of prostate and breast
	Androgens	Carcinoma of breast
1945	Nitrogen mustard	Lymphomas, solid tumors
1948–1950	Adrenocorticosteroids	Leukemias, lymphomas, multiple myeloma
	Antifolates	Acute leukemia, choriocarcinoma
1950–1955	Busulfan	Chronic granulocytic leukemia
	6-Mercaptopurine	Acute leukemia
	Actinomycin D	Wilms' tumor, testicular tumors, choriocarcinoma
1955–1960	5-Fluorouracil	Carcinoma of breast and gastrointestinal tract
	Progestins	Endometrial carcinoma
	Cyclophosphamide	Lymphomas, solid tumors
	Miotane	Adrenal carcinoma
	Vinca alkaloids	Lymphomas, acute leukemia, miscellaneous tumors
	Mitomycin-C	Gastrointestinal tumors
1960–1965	Hydroxyurea	Chronic granulocytic leukemia
	Procarbazine	Hodgkin's disease
	Cytarabine	Acute leukemia
	Mithramycin	Testicular tumors
	Nitrosoureas	Lymphomas, brain tumors, solid tumors
	Daunorubicin	Acute leukemia
1965–1970	L-Asparaginase	Acute leukemia
	Dacarbazine	Melanoma
	Cisplatin	Testicular and ovarian tumors
1970–present	Doxorubicin	Sarcomas and a wide spectrum of other tumors
	Bleomycin	Lymphomas, head and neck cancer
	Antiestrogens	Breast cancer
	Etoposide (VP-16)	Small cell lung cancer, germ cell tumors
	Streptozocin	Islet-cell carcinoma

* From Haskell, C. M.: Cancer Treatment, 2nd ed. Philadelphia, W. B. Saunders, 1985.

Table 36–3. THIRTEEN CANCERS CURABLE
WITH CHEMOTHERAPY*†

Choriocarcinoma	Ovarian carcinoma
Acute lymphocytic leukemia in children	Acute myelogenous leukemia
	Wilms' tumor
Hodgkin's disease	Burkitt's lymphoma
Diffuse histiocytic lymphoma	Embryonal rhabdomyosarcoma
Nodular mixed lymphoma	Ewing's sarcoma
Testicular carcinoma	Small cell cancer of the lung

* A fraction of patients with advanced disease, the remainder often have useful prolongation of life. These 13 cancers accounted for about 75,000 new cases in 1984. About 15,000 of these patients are curable with current chemotherapy. These 13 cancers account for about 10% of all cancers per year and about 10% of all cancer deaths per year.

† From Haskell, C. M.: Cancer Treatment, 2nd ed. Philadelphia, W. B. Saunders, 1985.

Table 36–4. ADVANCED CANCERS RESPONDING
TO CHEMOTHERAPY*†

Breast carcinoma	Gastric carcinoma
Chronic myelogenous leukemia	Malignant insulinoma
Chronic lymphocytic leukemia	Endometrial carcinoma
Follicular lymphoma	Adrenal cortical carcinoma
Multiple myeloma	Medulloblastoma
Small cell carcinoma of the lung	Neuroblastoma
Soft tissue sarcomas	Polycythemia vera
	Prostatic carcinoma
	Glioblastoma
	Squamous carcinomas of the head and neck

* Improved survival is demonstrable. The cancers listed above account for about 40% of all new cancers per year and about 30% of all cancer deaths.
† From Haskell, C. M.: Cancer Treatment, 2nd ed. Philadelphia, W. B. Saunders, 1985.

C. Radiation Therapy.
  1. The early years.
    a. Radiation of cancer started with Roentgen's discovery of x-rays in 1895 and the Curies' discovery of radium in 1898. Following these discoveries, Einstein, Compton, and Fermi began exploring ionizing radiation.
    b. In 1932, H. Coutard developed the protracted application of radiation with dose fractionalization; his work was based on the 1922 work of C. Regaud who attempted to sterilize a ram's testicle.
    c. In the early years, methods of measuring tissue dosage were not available; the optimum dose-time relationship was also not understood. There were recurrences caused by under irradiation and necroses due to overirradiation.
    d. The first type treated was basal cell skin cancer.
    e. Delivery of irradiation by x-ray tubes was the method in widespread use; radiation was administered by radiologists.
  2. The modern era.
    a. Since 1950 great progress in radiation therapy has been possible owing to the development of sophisticated equipment capable of generating and delivering high energy radiations: telecobalt units, linear accelerators, cyclic accelerators.
    b. In the early 1950's Read and Gray made the scientific community aware of the importance of molecular oxygen as a modifier of the biologic effect of ionizing radiation.
    c. For decades, radiation doses in patients were extrapolated from measured exposure doses (i.e., the roentgen). More dependable methods of measuring dosage have become available, and current clinical use requires the measurement of radiations that are absorbed at the anatomic point of interest as implied by the dose unit, the rad (radiation absorbed dose).
    d. Dose-time relationship is better understood.
    e. Increased technology has enabled increased penetration, skin sparing, reduced bone absorption, and reduced lateral scattering.

    f. Radiation oncologists have replaced radiologists in this specialized field.

    g. By 1980, approximately ½ to ⅔ of all patients with cancer are treated with radiation therapy.

    h. Although current conventional use is limited to high-energy x-rays, high-energy electrons, gamma rays, and beta rays, other types of ionizing radiation such as protons, neutrons, and pi-mesons, and heavy ions are being studied. There is now a revived interest in interstitial use, intracavitary use, total body irradiation, and systemic use (e.g., phosphorus-32).

    i. Currently in use to cure, prolong, and palliate and is part of the multimodality approach.

D. Immunotherapy.

  1. From 1900 to 1930.

    a. Development of an immune response against cancer was a popular concept at the turn of the century when it was observed that a strong immunity against transplantable neoplasms could be induced in randomly bred laboratory rodents.

    b. Following this observation, intense laboratory and clinical investigation followed patients treated with a variety of agents including autogenous and autologous tumor vaccines, antitumor sera, bacterial adjuvants. For example, Coley's toxin, a mixture of killed bacteria vaccines, was developed at the turn of the century by Dr. Bradford Coley following his observation of a complete regression in a patient with recurrent inoperable sarcoma of the neck following an episode of erysipelas.

    c. Occasional regressions with immunotherapy were reported, but results were inconsistent.

  2. From 1930 to 1950.

    a. Interest in immunotherapy declined partly because of past inconsistent results and partly because of the use of genetically identical strains of animals and the recognition that acceptance or rejection of transplanted tumors was due not to tumor immunity but to the inability of foreign tissue to grow in a genetically deviant host.

    b. Many doubted the existence of tumor-specific antigens.

  3. From 1950 to present.

    a. The modern era began in 1953 when E. J. Foley reported conclusively on the existence of tumor-specific antigens in methylcholanthrene-induced sarcomas of mice.

    b. In 1964, fetal antigens were found in hepatomas by Y. S. Tatarinov, and in 1965, carcinoembryonic antigens were found in colonic carcinomas by P. Gold and S. O. Freedman. Until the 1970's there was little direct evidence of any human tumor-associated antigens capable of eliciting in immune response. Today tumor-associated antigens have been found in a variety of human neoplasms: Burkitt's lymphoma, malignant melanoma, neuroblastoma, skeletal and soft tissue sarcoma, and carcinoma of the colon, lung, breast, bladder, and kidney.

    c. In the late 1960's three studies revived interest in immunotherapy. E. Klein reported in 1969 that skin carcinomas regressed after the induction of local delayed cutaneous hypersensitivity with certain chemicals. G. Mathe and co-workers in 1969 reported disease free interval and survival could be prolonged for patients in remission from acute lymphoblastic leukemia by treatment with bacille Calmette-Guérin (BCG) or allogeneic leukemia cells or both. D. L. Morton and co-workers in 1970 reported dramatic regression of cutaneous nodules of malignant melanoma following intralesional injection with BCG.

    d. In 1978, human interferon studies were conducted, based on the discovery of interferons by A. Issacs and J. Lindenmann.

    e. In 1975, G. Kohler and C. Milstein produced a hybrid cell line (a hybridoma) by fusion of mouse myeloma cell line with mouse spleen cells, creating a clone of cells that retain ability to live indefinitely and an ability to produce a single antibody molecule.

    f. Bone marrow transplantation continues to be investigated at several centers.

    g. On March 4, 1981, a Biologic Response Modifiers Program was officially established as a part of the NCI. Despite the only moderate benefit from nonspecific immunotherapy there is still hope that other avenues of immunotherapy such as active vaccines, interferons, and monoclonal antibodies, which are currently being pursued, will produce significant advances in cancer treatment.

CANCER NURSING DEVELOPMENTS

A. Early Leaders.

    Cancer nursing, viewed from contributions of early leaders, influenced events in cancer patient care and linked a common interest in the care and in the profession of nursing.

    1. Virginia Derriks and Josephine Craytor were early clinical specialists in the care of persons with cancer.

    2. Katherine Nelson, an educator at Columbia University Teachers' College, developed and taught the first clinical specialty program at the Master's level.

    3. Renilda Helkemeyer who was in a nursing service setting at the M. D. Anderson Hospital, Texas, wrote of cancer nursing and of her concern for the occupational safety of nurses caring for patients receiving radiation therapy.

    4. Virginia Barkley, an American Cancer Society (ACS) consultant in nursing care, wrote and spoke of her experience in cancer nursing care, developing nursing roles and cancer nursing education.

B. Education and Research Leaders.

    1. Anayes Derdiarian, at UCLA, developed a graduate program in cancer nursing that became a model (funded by NIH).

    2. Rosalie Peterson at the National Institute of Health (NIH) and Elizabeth Walker and Susan Hubbard at the National Cancer Institute (NCI) were located in settings that participated in cancer patient care research and wrote about their experiences.

    3. Speciality Nursing Organizations.

    The Oncology Nursing Society (1974), and the Pediatric Oncology Nursing Society (1974) developed as responses to nurses' interest in and work with cancer patients.

C. The Early Years—1850 to 1900.
   1. Early Events and Developments.
     a. 1851—The Royal Marsden Hospital, London, England, was established exclusively to treat patients with cancer.
     b. 1890—Patients with incurable cancer were not wanted in hospitals and, at times, not permitted to remain at home. Cancer, as a euphemism and as a word, was avoided owing to the stigma assigned and ignorance.
   2. Hospice Care.
     a. 1890—First hospice for cancer patients in America: Rose Hawthorne (sister of Nathaniel Hawthorne) and Alice Huber opened St. Rose's Free Home for Incurable Cancer.
     b. 1900—House of Calvary for Chronic Illness cared for cancer patients; run by Dominican Sisters of the Sick Poor, Bronx, New York.
D. Turn of the Century—1900 to 1939.
   1. Nursing practices change.
     a. Public health nursing focuses on cancer because home was the primary care environment (because of the difficulty in supplying hospital beds for cancer care).
     b. There were isolated articles by nurses on care of the patient with cancer that focused on the disease and treatments. Of 16 articles on nursing and cancer only three were written by nurses.
     c. 1916—American Cancer Society published booklet: *How the Public Health Nurse Can Help to Control Cancer.*
   2. Research.
   A study by the Boston Community Health Association of Home Care for terminal cancer patients identified:
     a. Need for long-term home care for cancer patients because of the continued shortage of hospital beds.
     b. Nurses instructed unskilled attendants to give nursing care; the nurses' instruction to aides was more important than having the nurse as direct care giver.
     c. Nausea and incontinence were most common problems in terminal patients.
     d. Cost of care was expensive; those who could, paid $.85 a nursing visit.
E. World War II—1940 to 1950.
   Historic perspectives on cancer nursing viewed through this time frame saw a shortage of nurses. For the most part, nursing care was given by non-nurses. Private duty nursing was a popular professional nursing role. Student nurses in hospital diploma schools staffed many of the hospitals. Marriage and family led to early retirement for many nurses.
   Survivors of a bombed ship carrying mustard gas demonstrated a depression of leukocyte formation, which led to the use of nitrogen mustard in the treatment of leukopoetic tissue disorders and then to reports of remissions of selected cancers. These events opened a new era in nursing practice and nursing care of cancer patients in selected medical centers.
   1. Cancer nursing practice.
     a. Public health nursing now focused on cancer control and prevention.
     b. Recognition of the need to teach community nurses about cancer. Nurses did cervical pap smears and taught that early detection and

treatment of uterine cancer could lead to a cure. The importance of the six-week post-partum examination for detection of cervical cancer was presented in maternity nursing courses.

   c. Nurses had to adapt to what the patient had in the home; creative nursing care and supplies had to be on hand. Homemade equipment and dressings made by volunteers who met in homes in groups of four to six, were given to nurses for home care and to hospitals. Rental equipment and disposable supplies were not readily available.

   d. Surgery was the major mode of cancer treatment; patients often had long hospital stays. Nursing care focused on the disease and limited attention was given to the emotional effects of the disease or treatment.

2. Communication with patients about their disease and prognosis and truth-telling issues.

   a. Patients were *not* told their diagnosis, and the arguments "to tell or not to tell" were presented in the literature.

   b. Truth was withheld because it was believed that it would do more harm to know the diagnosis.

   c. Nurses referred patients to their doctor to answer all questions. Nurses were instructed to avoid discussions of the diagnosis with the patient.

3. Research.

   a. 1948—First published nursing research on the numbers of cancer patients cared for by the public health nurses.

   b. 1951—Study to identify the number of patients with cancer in the caseload of public health nurses.

4. Cost of Care—Nursing journals published studies that showed that 80% of patients discharged from hospitals would need nursing care, and the cost of cancer nursing care was expensive. The American Cancer Society reimbursed $1.00 of the cost.

5. Education for Nurses in Cancer Nursing.

   a. 1947—First Master's level college course in cancer nursing at Teachers' College, Columbia University, taught by Katherine Nelson.

   b. 1950—ACS published *A Cancer Source Book For Nurses.*

   c. 1952—NCI funds undergraduate cancer nursing education.

   d. 1956—Federal grants established for cancer nursing education.

F. Developments during the 1960's.

1. Nursing Developments.

   a. 1964—Protective isolation implemented at the NCI (Total Body Isolation for preventing infection secondary to chemotherapy; it was the forerunner of laminar flow).

   b. 1964—ACS published *Care of Your Colostomy—A Source Book of Information.*

   c. 1966—Graduate preparation for nurses at Boston University for advanced practice as clinical nurse specialists. Clinical experience with cancer patients, but no formal cancer nursing content was in the curriculum.

   d. 1967—First textbook, *Nursing Care of the Cancer Patient,* by Rosemary Bouchard. Second and third editions with Norma Owens in 1972 and 1976.

2. Nursing Practice.
   a. Home care was provided by visiting nurses, but service was available only Monday through Friday.
   b. Insurance covered long hospital stays of patients. Private duty nurses were available to patients with economic means.
   c. Pain is perceived as a common problem, but drugs were often used sparingly.
   d. Considerable focus on the care of the dying patient in the nursing literature.
   e. Occupational safety procedures for nurses caring for patients with radium implants emerged.
   f. The patient with breast cancer was treated with a radical mastectomy, and nurses cared for patients who were bandaged like mummies after surgery. The bandages prohibited arm and shoulder motion necessitating rehabilitation via exercises.
   g. Chemotherapy is administered by nurses in selected medical centers with strong pharmacology units. Skilled nurses shared the responsibility with physicians for giving chemotherapy. Chemotherapy nurse specialists emerged. Outside the major medical centers, physicians often mixed and administered the cancer drugs, while nurses observed patients for side effects.
   h. Skilled nurses wrote about specialized care as vital for bone marrow transplantation and for interarterial chemotherapy.
   i. As survival and remission rate reports began to offer hope, nurses began to think with some optimism about cancer patients being treatable. The majority of nurses were actually working with dying patients and those with long-term care needs.
   j. As patients discussed their concerns and difficulties, sexuality and sexual functioning in patients treated for cancer emerged as an interest to nurses who were in direct contact with patients.
3. Research.
   1963—Landmark clinical nursing research on the impact of mastectomy by Jeanne C. Quint (Benoliel). This study identified the psychological needs of women who had breast cancer and were treated with radical mastectomy. The women studied expressed fear of dying.
4. Communications with patients.
   a. Concerns about telling the truth about the cancer diagnosis and prognosis by caregivers continues. Cancer as a word was avoided by nurses in discussions with patients, often because nurses were not sure of what to say.
   b. Avoidance of talking with patients was common among families, patients, and professional staff. Patients would often talk with the nurse and be given hints of knowledge of their diagnosis, but nurses were not permitted to pursue the discussion even though the patient was asking to be told his or her diagnosis.
   c. Nurses began to write about how to talk to patients with cancer. In 1969, Elisabeth Kübler-Ross, M.D., published her clinical research in *On Death and Dying,* creating awareness that patients would talk, and wanted to talk, about dying and their feelings. Stages of behavior and the grieving process in the dying patient were identified.
G. 1970's—The rapidly developing years of cancer nursing as a specialty.

1. Selected nursing developments as specialization develops around treatments.
    a. 1970—Occupational safety for nurses exposed to radiation is addressed in the literature.
    b. 1971—National Cancer Act provides funds for cancer nursing education and research.
    c. 1971—Landmark nursing research study identifies that children ages 6 to 10 are aware of their cancer as a fatal illness.
    d. 1973—First National Conference on Cancer Nursing was sponsored by ACS with 2,500 nurses in attendance.
    e. 1974—Association of Pediatric Oncology Nurses (APON) formed.
    f. 1974—Oncology Nursing Society (ONS) incorporated, with Lisa Begg Marino elected the first president.
    g. 1975—First ONS Congress in Toronto, Canada.
    h. 1976—First issue of *Oncology Nursing Forum* published; Susan Baird was the editor.
    i. 1977—Foreign Exchange Nurse Visitors Program for Cancer Nursing at the NCI Clinical Center. Nurses visited from Great Britain, Belgium, and the Netherlands.
    j. 1978—The first edition of *Cancer Nursing: An International Journal for Cancer Care* was published. Rachael Ayers and Carol Reed Ash were the editors.
    k. 1978—Landmark clinical nursing research "Facilitating Home Care for Children Dying of Cancer," by Ida Martinson and co-workers.
    l. 1978—Ten national research priorities in cancer nursing identified.
    m. 1978—Nurses studying nutritional support for cancer patients determine that women with breast cancer gain weight, whereas other patients with cancer lose weight.
2. Cancer nursing practice.
    a. In 1978, there is recognition of the need to change attitudes of nurses about cancer nursing.
    b. Ethical issues involved in cancer nursing care are addressed by nurses in the literature.
    c. Patients' participation in decision making about treatment is a consideration and concern of nurses.
    d. 1979—Outcome Standards for Cancer Nursing Practice developed by the ONS.
    e. Nurses focus on the distress of treatments and attempt to reduce drug-induced alopecia.
    f. Disease and treatment related infections are major problems in patient care, presenting a challenge to nursing.
H. 1980—Period of Growth and Specialization.
    1. Nursing practice.
        a. Ambulatory treatment clinics make it necessary for patients to be involved in their care.
        b. Nurses routinely administer chemotherapy in all settings. There is increased demand for technically skilled nurses for chemotherapy administration.
        c. Master's program–prepared Clinical Nurse Specialists are sought after for professional positions.
        d. When cancer patients who have received chemotherapy and radiation

therapy survive, concern about the possible mutagenic effects on pro-creation leads to sperm banking and is addressed in nursing literature.

    e. Concern for potential carcinogens from antineoplastic agents voiced by nurses who are administering drugs daily.

    f. Cancer as a word is still linked closely with death, and provides on-going nursing consideration.

2. Education and Classification Events.

    a. 1982—Cancer nursing textbook *Care of Children With Cancer*.

    b. 1983—Survey of Master's program–prepared nurses working in cancer nursing.

    c. 1983—Outcome Standards for Public Cancer Education developed by the ONS.

    d. 1984—Journal of the American Pediatric Oncology Nurses published.

3. Focus of Cancer Nursing Research.

Because of limited funds to support research, the ACS and NCI are aided by product and pharmaceutical company grants.

    a. Increased visibility of clinical nursing research covers many aspects of care, e.g., home care, economics, quality of life, early detection, symptom distress, interrelatedness of aspects of care.

    b. Nurses conducting basic science research identify possible mechanisms for immunologic effects of psychological and emotional variables and interrelatedness between psychological and biologic factors.

STUDY QUESTIONS

1. Briefly describe the history of chemotherapy.
2. What medical discoveries led to improved success rates in cancer surgery?
3. What progress has been made in radiation therapy since 1950?
4. Trace the impact of home health nursing on cancer care from 1900 to the present.
5. Identify a nurse who made significant contributions to oncology care and list her contributions.
6. List contributions of the ONS to the care of cancer patients.

Bibliography

Alston, F., et al.: Perfusion. American Journal of Nursing, *60*:1603–1607, 1960.

American Cancer Society: Care of Your Colostomy: A Source Book of Information. New York, American Cancer Society, 1964.

American Cancer Society: How the Public Health Nurse Can Help to Control Cancer. New York, American Cancer Society, 1916.

Barkley, V.: A visiting nurse specializes in cancer nursing. American Journal of Nursing, *70*:1680–1683, 1970.

Barkley, V.: Enough time for good nursing. Nursing Outlook, *64*:4, 14–22, 1964.

Barkley, V.: The best of times and the worst of times: Historical reflections from the American Cancer Society National Consultant. Oncology Nursing Forum, *9*(3):54–56, 1982.

Barkley, V.: The crisis of cancer. American Journal of Nursing, *67*:278–280, 1967.

Barkley, V.: What can I say to the cancer patient? Nursing Outlook, *6*:316–318, 1958.

Barlock, A. L., Howser, D. M., and Hubbard, S. M.: Nursing management of Adriamycin extravasation. American Journal of Nursing, *79*:94–96, 1972.

Benoliel, J. Q. and McCorkle, R.: Ethical Considerations in Treatment. Proceedings of the Second National Conference on cancer nursing. New York, American Cancer Society, pp. 63–68, 1977.

Bergeron, J. H.: A patient's plea: "Tell me what I need to know." American Journal of Nursing, 71:1572–157, 1971.

Beihusen, I.: Cancer nursing is expensive. Nursing Outlook, 4:438–441, 1956.

Bouchard, R.: Nursing Care of the Cancer Patient. St. Louis, C. V. Mosby, 1967.

Bouchard, R. and Ownes, N. F.: Nursing Care of the Cancer Patient, 2nd ed. St. Louis, C. V. Mosby, 1972.

Cloak, M. M., Connor, T. H., Stevens, K. R., Theiss, J. C., Alt, J. M., Matney, T. S., and Anderson, R. W.: Occupational exposure of nursing personnel to antineoplastic agents. Oncology Nursing Forum, 12(5):33–39, 1985.

Craytor, J.: Talking with persons who have cancer. American Journal of Nursing, 69(4):744–748, 1969.

Craytor, J. K.: Highlights in nursing education for cancer nursing. Oncology Nursing Forum, 9(4):51–59, 1982.

Craytor, J. K., Brown, J. K., and Morrow, C. D.: Assessing learning needs of nurses who care for persons with cancer. Cancer Nursing, 1(3):211–220, 1978.

DeVita, V. T.: Principles of chemotherapy. In DeVita, V. J., Hellman, S., and Rosenberg, S. A. (eds.): Cancer Principles and Practice of Oncology. Vol. 1, 2nd ed. Philadelphia, J. B. Lippincott, pp. 257–285, 1985.

Dixon, J., Moritz, D. A., and Baker, F. L.: Breast cancer and weight gain: An unexpected finding. Oncology Nursing Forum, 5:5–7, 1978.

Dolan, J. A., Fitzpatrick, M. L., and Herrmann, E. K.: Nursing in Society: A Historical Perspective. Philadelphia, W. B. Saunders, 1983.

Donovan, C. T.: Protective isolation, Oncology Nursing Forum, 9:50–53, 1982.

Evans, L., et al.: Nursing cancer patients in their home. New England Journal of Medicine, 198:240–246, 1928.

Farber, S., et al.: Temporary remission in acute leukemia in children produced by folic acid antagonists and aminoplerayl glutamic acid. New England Journal of Medicine, 238:737–739, 1948.

Fochtman, D. and Foley, G. (eds.): Nursing Care of the Child in Cancer. Boston, Little, Brown and Co., 1982.

Glaser, B. and Strauss, A.: The social loss of dying patients. American Journal of Nursing, 64:119, 1964.

Golby, R.: Chemotherapy of cancer. American Journal of Nursing, 4:521–528, 1960.

Goodman, L. S., et al.: Nitrogen mustard therapy. Journal of the American Medical Association, 132:126–132, 1946.

Graham, E. A. and Singer, J.: Successful removal of an entire lung for carcinoma of the bronchus. Journal of the American Medical Association, 101:1371–1374, 1933.

Green, P. E.: The Association of Pediatric Oncology Nurses: The first ten years. Oncology Nursing Forum, 10(4):59–63, 1983.

Greenfield, L. D., Herman, M. W., and Patrick, J.: Radiation safety precautions with 131 iodine therapy. Cancer Nursing, 1(5):379–384, 1978.

Hammond, B.: Home care improvisations. Nursing Outlook, 64(4):49–51, 1964.

Haskell, C. M.: Principles of cancer chemotherapy. In Haskell, C. M. (ed.): Cancer Treatment, 2nd ed. Philadelphia, W.B. Saunders, pp. 21–106, 1985.

Helkemeyer, R. and Kinney, H. E.: Teaching cancer nursing. Nursing Outlook, 4:177–180, 1956.

Helkemeyer, R.: A historical perspective in cancer nursing. Oncology Nursing Forum, 9(2):47–56, 1982.

Hellman, S.: Principles of radiation therapy. In DeVita, V. J., Hellman, S., and Rosenberg, S. A. (eds.): Cancer Principles and Practice of Oncology (Vol. 1), 2nd ed. Philadelphia, J.B. Lippincott, pp. 227–255, 1985.

Higgenbothan, S.: Arm exercises after mastectomy. American Journal of Nursing, 12:1573–1574, 1957.

Hubbard, S.: The foreign exchange nurse visitors program: An international program for cancer nurses. Cancer Nursing, 24:351–352, 1979.

Hubbard,, S. P. and DeVita, V. T.: Medical oncology, drug development and the chemotherapy nurse. American Journal of Nursing, 76:560–565, 1976.

Hubbard, S. P.: The Practice of Cancer Nursing. Proceedings of the Second National Conference on Cancer Nursing. New York, American Cancer Society, pp. 23–29, 1977.

Kaempfer, S. H., Hoffman, D. J., and Wiley, F. M.: Sperm banking: A reproductive option in cancer therapy. Cancer Nursing, 6:31–38, 1983.

Kübler-Ross, E.: On Death and Dying. New York, Macmillan Company, 1969.

Lovejoy, N. C.: Preventing hair loss during adriamycin therapy. Cancer Nursing, 2(2):117–122, 1979.

Martinson, I. M., et al.: Facilitating home care for children dying of cancer. Cancer Nursing, 1(1):41–45, 1978.

Maxwell, M. B.: Scalp tourniquets for chemotherapy-induced alopecia. American Journal of Nursing, 900–902, 1980.

Morton, D. L.: Cancer immunotherapy: An overview. *In* Kruse, L. C., Reese, J. L., and Hart, L. K. (eds.): Cancer Pathophysiology, Etiology, and Management. St. Louis, C. V. Mosby, 1979.

Nelson, K. R. Cancer Nursing as a Specialty: Issues Problems, and Progress. Proceedings of the Second National Conference on Cancer Nursing, American Cancer Society, 1–5, 1977.

Oberst, M.: Priorities in cancer nursing research. Cancer Nursing, 1(4):281–290, 1978.

Oncology Nursing Society and American Nurses' Association Outcome Standards for Cancer Nursing Practice. Kansas City, MO, 1979.

Peterson, R. I.: Federal grants for education for cancer nursing. Nursing Outlook, 4:105, 1956.

Peterson, R. I.: Study of cancer caseload. Public Health Nursing, 45:566, 1951.

Peterson, R. I. and Soller, G. R.: Cancer nursing in the basic professional nursing curriculum. Government Printing Office, 49:43–45, 1951.

Quint, J. C.: Awareness of death and the nurse's composure. Nursing Research, 15(1):49–55, 1966.

Quint, J. C.: Improving nursing care of the dying. Nursing Forum, 14:368–378, 1967.

Quint, J. C.: The impact of the mastectomy. American Journal of Nursing, 63:88–92, 1963.

Rosenberg, S. A.: Principles of surgical oncology. *In* DeVita, V. J., Hellman, S., and Rosenberg, S. A. (eds.): Cancer Principles and Practice of Oncology (Vol. 1), 2nd ed. Philadelphia, J.B. Lippincott, pp. 215–225, 1985.

Rummerfield, P. S. and Rummerfield, M. J.: What you should know about radiation hazards. American Journal of Nursing, 70:780–786, 1970.

Stream, P., Harrington, E., and Clark, M.: Bone marrow transplantation: An option for children with acute leukemia. Cancer Nursing, 3(3):195–199, 1980.

Visintainer, M. A., Valpicelli, J. M., and Seligman, M. E. P.: The effects of inescapable shock in tumor rejection in rats. Science, April 23, 1982.

Waechter, E.: Children's awareness of fatal illness. American Journal of Nursing, 7:1168–1197, 1971.

Yasko, J. M.: A Survey of Oncology Clinical Nursing Specialists. Oncology Nursing Forum, 10(1):25–30, 1983.

37

Informed Consent

MINERVA APPLEGATE, RN, EdD

ETHICAL CONSIDERATIONS

A. Factors Supporting Consent (these factors will enhance the consent process):
  1. Authenticity—to promote and support genuine respect for another.
  2. Self-determination—to promote and support an individual's freedom to determine his or her destiny without intentional interference by others.
  3. Justice—to apply moral principles or laws without discriminating against individuals.
  4. Accountability—to be responsible for one's actions.
  5. Free choice—to promote and support the individual's opportunities to freely choose between alternatives without constraint or interference from others.
  6. Free action—to promote and support the individual's opportunities to freely act on his or her choices without constraint or interference from others.
  7. Autonomy—to support freedom to choose and act on one's choice without constraint or interference from others.
  8. Independence—to support independent decision making and action without constraint or interference from others.
  9. Control—to support the person's ability to control his or her own decisions and actions with a sense of having power in the decision making process.
  10. Beneficence—to do good.
  11. Nonmaleficence—to prevent harm.
  12. Advocacy—to stand up for and support another's rights.
  13. Veracity—to tell the truth.
  14. Respect—to respect the person's rights and obligations.
  15. Dignity—to support the person's dignity as an individual.
  16. Privacy—to respect the person's rights to privacy.
  17. Confidentiality—to respect confidentiality as an individual's right.
  18. Integrity—to support and promote an individual's needs for faith and accuracy.

19. Competence—to ensure that the person is mentally, physically, and legally capable of making informed choices.
20. Altruism—to respect the person's decision to consider the welfare of others and benefits to others.
21. Self-identity—to promote and support a sense of self as an autonomous, self-determining individual.
22. Uniqueness—to recognize each person as a unique individual.

B. Factors Negating Consent (these factors may inhibit the consent process):
  1. Vulnerability—the experiencing of feelings of loss of control and power, loss of autonomy and independence, loss of dignity, loss of privacy and confidentiality, and loss of uniqueness as an individual when receiving health care.
  2. Coercion—the ability of one individual to overtly or covertly influence the decision making ability, choices, and actions of another individual.
  3. Powerlessness—the experiencing of feelings of loss of power and control, loss of decision making abilities as an autonomous individual.
  4. Captivity—held under the control of another, such as when an individual is institutionalized or imprisoned.
  5. Paternalism—the protective paternal role assumed by some health care providers in which situation the patient is denied the freedom to exercise autonomous, independent choices and actions based on informed decision making.
  6. Incompetence—an individual may be mentally, physically, or legally unable to make informed choices.
  7. Oppression—the unjust exercise of authority or power that inhibits decision making.
  8. Depersonalization—the loss of sense of human dignity and uniqueness as an individual.
  9. Deception—the misrepresentation or false statements given to an individual for purposes of deceit.
  10. Mystique—the mystical attitudes and beliefs that some individuals believe surround the health profession, especially the practice of medicine.

STEPS IN THE CONSENT PROCESS (FOR INFORMED CONSENT, THESE STEPS ARE BASIC):

A. Explanation of medical condition.
B. Explanation of nature and purpose of the procedure.
C. Explanation of risks, alternatives, and consequences (severe consequences of risks with high probability of occurrence).

ELEMENTS ESSENTIAL TO DISCLOSURE (THESE ELEMENTS SHOULD BE PRESENT IF CONSENT IS TO BE INFORMED):

A. Legal Capacity—of legal age and sound mind; not requiring parent, surrogate, proxy, or guardian consent.
B. Mental Capability—capable of cognition and reason; no impairment due to chemical, physical, or psychological deficiencies.
C. Voluntariness—participation must be voluntary.

D. No Coercion, Deceit or Fraud—free of misrepresentation, free of deceit or fraud that would influence autonomous decision making.
E. Right to Refuse—participation is contingent upon the individual's right to refuse treatment or to withdraw from the procedure consented for at any time.
F. Language Comprehensible—language and terminology should be in lay terms that are readily comprehended by individuals.
G. Questions answered to individual's satisfaction—participants should demonstrate evidence of full understanding of all consent components.
H. Consideration of Privacy and Confidentiality—participants should be assured of confidentiality and anonymity; they should be informed of how data will be used and how it will be distributed.

EXCEPTIONS TO DISCLOSURE (FULL DISCLOSURE MAY NOT BE LEGALLY REQUIRED IN THESE SITUATIONS):

A. Emergencies—consent is usually implied.
B. Therapeutic privilege—a physician may withhold information related to risks if the physician judges that the individual might experience harm as a result of the disclosing of information.
C. Patient waiver—the individual may waive the right to be informed.
D. Prior knowledge—the person may have had previous knowledge of the risks, or the risks may be common knowledge.

FACTORS THAT MAY CONTRIBUTE TO INADEQUATE UNDERSTANDING (THESE FACTORS ARE PRIMARILY SOCIAL, CULTURAL, PSYCHOLOGICAL, AND PHYSIOLOGIC)

A. Social and Cultural:
   1. Coercion.
   2. Language barriers.
   3. Language not comprehensible.
   4. Lack of validation of understanding.
   5. Captive status.
   6. Illiteracy.
B. Psychological and Physiologic:
   1. Level of consciousness.
   2. Medication influences.
   3. Mental incompetence.
   4. Mental retardation.
   5. Age (i.e., infants, children, elderly).
   6. Sensory impairment.
   7. Cognitive impairment.
   8. Confusion or disorientation.
   9. Sensory deprivation.
   10. Toxic condition.
   11. Debilitating illness.
   12. Acute trauma.

NURSING'S ROLE IN INFORMED CONSENT— COMMUNICATION, COLLABORATION, AND ACCOUNTABILITY:

A. Physicians are responsible for medical procedures.

B. Nurses are responsible for nursing procedures.

C. Explain postoperative nursing procedures after informed medical consent is obtained to avoid confusion.

D. If comprehension is poor, reinforce information and notify physician.

E. Nurses may witness a consent signature.

F. Physicians may delegate consent procedures; without consent, physicians are liable.

G. If the person seems reluctant, notify physician.

H. Ascertain chart documentation of the consent process.

I. If the person seems confused or ambivalent, notify physician.

J. Encourage physician documentation on chart.

K. Make sure that consent is obtained before the person is sedated for procedures or treatments.

L. Encourage use of supplementary educational materials.

M. Respect the person's freedom to choose between alternatives.

N. Promote autonomy and independence in decision making.

STUDY QUESTIONS

1. Identify five (5) factors that enhance the consent process.

2. State an example of misrepresentation that could influence autonomous decision making in the informed consent process.

3. Identify five (5) social or cultural factors that may contribute to inadequate understanding during the consent process.

Bibliography

Curtin, L. L.: The nurse as advocate: A philosophical foundation for nursing. *In* Chinn, P. L. (ed.): Ethical Issues in Nursing. Rockville, MD, Aspen Systems Corp., pp. 11–20, 1986.

Fromer, M. I.: Solving ethical dilemmas in nursing practice. *In* Chinn, P. L. (ed.): Ethical Issues in Nursing. Rockville, MD, Aspen Systems Corp., pp. 81–87, 1986.

Ingelfinger, F. I.: Informed (but uneducated) consent. *In* Sarovity, S., et al. (eds.): Moral Problems in Medicine. Englewood Cliffs, NJ, Prentice-Hall, Inc., pp. 152–154, 1976.

Kilpatrick, K. Y.: Ethical issues and procedural dilemmas in measuring patient competence. *In* Chinn, P. L. (ed.): Ethical Issues in Nursing. Rockville, MD, Aspen Systems Corp., pp. 111–122, 1986.

Langen, E.: Human experimentation: New York verdict affirms patient's rights. *In* Sarovity, S., et al. (eds.): Moral Problems in Medicine. Englewood Cliffs, NJ, Prentice-Hall, Inc., pp. 142–150, 1976.

Nelson, M. J.: Authenticity: Fabric of ethical nursing practice. *In* Chinn, P. L. (ed.): Ethical Issues in Nursing. Rockville, MD, Aspen Systems Corp., pp. 89–94, 1986.

Rhodes, A. M. and Miller, R. D.: Nursing and the Law, 4th ed. Rockville, MD, Aspen Systems Corporation, pp. 200–229, 1984.

38

Care Settings

DEBORAH STEPHENS MILLS, RN, MSN

ROLE OF THE NURSE IN SELECTING AND RECOMMENDING CARE SETTINGS

A. Assessments must be made of patient, family and/or significant others, present care settings, and potential care settings in the community.
B. Collaborative planning should involve patient, family, and appropriate health team members (primary nurse, physician, community nurse or agency, social workers, dietitian, chaplain/minister, and so forth).
C. Evaluation within the chosen care setting should be ongoing; revisions should be made as changes occur and needs arise. Nursing must be sensitive, creative, and alert to the changing needs of patients and families within rapidly changing hospital or community health care systems.
D. Every effort must be made to allow the patients and families ultimate choice as to settings.
E. Assessment of the Patient.
　1. Assessment begins with the presenting nursing problem in any setting.
　2. Evaluate patient's physiologic needs:
　　a. Disease state.
　　b. Social needs (relating to family and community).
　　c. Emotional and spiritual needs (dealing with the sense of self and meaning).
　　d. Socioeconomic and vocational needs (involving work and financial responsibilities).
　3. Interventions must go beyond presenting problems to include anticipated needs.
F. Assessment of the Family and/or Significant Other:
　1. The family and/or significant others are affected by the diagnosis and treatment of the patient. The health care team must be sensitive to and address the needs of the patient/family unit. Open communication is foundational.
　2. A multidisciplinary approach to assess family coping is essential in identifying needs, strengths, and potential resources.

3. Identify, support, and evaluate the primary care given in the home as early as possible to minimize stress and maximize resource utilization. Personal and professional resources must be identified to both the family member and the patient.

4. The family must also have an opportunity to explore (with professional assistance) the meaning of the cancer diagnosis and treatment, and fears and sense of loss they may be experiencing, what role changes will be required, how they may participate in therapy logistics, and how finances and family life will be affected.

5. The follow-up needs of the family must be anticipated. Provide the appropriate phone number and instructions.

G. Assessment of the Present Care Setting:

1. Determine why the patient is in the present care setting. Also decide if this setting adequately meets the patient's needs.

2. Nursing care must reflect the needs of individuals in their care setting. Patients at home during gaps in therapy and between clinical appointments could benefit from a phone call or home visit from the nurse to provide ongoing support.

H. Assessment of Potential Care Settings within the Community:

1. Economic constraints require nurses to be highly innovative in their identification of resources and utilization of community agencies for patients and their families.

2. To develop a quick reference, nurses should catalogue resource people, supportive services, and health delivery agencies.

3. Assess the patient's/family's usual resources for skills, services, and funds.

4. Evaluate what is already available in the community. Home chemotherapy, antibiotic therapy, and parenteral nutrition may be available in the community, with reimbursement for services.

5. As people go through a health restorative process, they need professional assistance to maintain their adapted health status. Nurses can assess anew what is available to these individuals in the community, as well as what services need to be enhanced. As needs change, generating problem statements and need assessments assists in the development of other delivery systems.

IN-HOSPITAL CARE SETTINGS

A. The Oncology Unit.

1. An oncology unit is "a designated hospital area which facilitates the team approach to comprehensive cancer care by bringing into close proximity those personnel and facilities necessary for such care. The unit must provide not only for the physical needs of the cancer patient, but also for the ongoing emotional, social, and spiritual support of the patient and his or her family."

2. If cancer admissions to a hospital equal 15% or more of total medical-surgical admissions, an oncology unit should be organized.

3. Six tasks must be completed in opening an oncology unit:

a. A physical setting with ample room for nurses to work and conference together and room for patient and family comfort (including private space, kitchen facilities, and sleeping facilities for family members).

b. Adequate professional nursing staff to meet the specific needs of cancer patients. An oncology patient classification system can be quite helpful in substantiating patient acuity and required hours of nursing care.

c. Policies and procedures for unit operation using a multidisciplinary treatment approach.

d. A philosophy of nursing that recognizes the importance of participation, service, education, and research.

e. A nurturing work environment where staff is actively supported through orientation, staff development, stress management, and individualized reward systems.

f. An excellence of practice that is marked by continuous evaluation of quality of care.

4. Because of the continuous close contact with cancer patients, professional burnout is an issue of concern. Three major stressors contributing to burnout are staffing shortages, frustrating patient or family demands, and personal psychological strains. Nurses identified regular, scheduled support groups and one-on-one peer support as most helpful in combating burnout.

B. The Scattered-bed Unit.

1. In hospitals in which cancer admissions do not justify an organized oncology unit, cancer patients are treated on mixed medical-surgical units or specialty units.

2. Even with substantial numbers a scattered-bed approach may be necessary because of its cost-effectiveness. Cancer-specific skilled nursing care can be promoted by the presence of an oncology clinical nursing specialist and by ongoing continuing education programs to assist in providing continuity of care.

3. Families need special consideration when confronted by different nurses on every hospital admission. Family members' most frequent concerns are symptom management (patient suffering), fear of the future (unknown), waiting, and difficulty getting information (from physicians and "busy" nurses). The need for "family-centered" nursing is most critical when a child has cancer, and parents and well siblings require understanding and open, supportive communication.

4. The needs of persons with a life-threatening disease for technical proficiency combined with sensitivity requires the type of nursing described as "high touch in a high tech environment."

C. Oncology Transition Services.

1. Oncology transition services are a system of community-based, person-centered nursing services to assist patients with far advanced cancer and their families to cope with the progressive physical and social dependencies imposed by the disease and treatment, and the changing life goals associated with movement toward death.

2. The nurse assists in symptom and problem management and supports the patient and family and acts as a communication link between them and the larger hospital or community health care system. This facilitates personalized, cost-effective care planning and comfort for patient and family.

3. Coordination of care between in-patient and out-patient settings must be provided. Transition services enhance ease and accountability.

AMBULATORY CARE SETTINGS

A. Varied Settings for Cancer Care:
   1. Personnel assistance programs often provide routine examinations, follow-up laboratory studies, and even chemotherapy in the work place to assist patients to remain actively in the workforce.
   2. In rural settings with few physicians, the same physician who assessed the initial symptomatology may proceed with surgery and later oversee follow-up. This approach requires the office or clinic nurse to be both generalist and specialist. In order to assure the challenge of providing optimal cancer-related care, nurses must pursue resources such as professional cancer nursing journals, cancer nursing texts, and available oncology nursing seminars and workshops.
   3. In the private sector, care is provided by private practice physicians and specialists who participate in the workup and management of the presumed malignancy. Patients may get "lost" between services. Nurses involved in this dilemma can provide cross-service coordination of care.
B. Oncology Clinics.
   1. Speciality clinics that focus on surgical oncology, medical oncology (solid tumor and hematology), gynecologic oncology, pediatric oncology, and radiation therapy are frequently affiliated with regional cancer centers and other large hospitals.
   2. High patient volume-to-time ratios, time-consuming functional tasks, and inadequate staffing ratios are viewed as potential problems in an ambulatory care setting, and creativity in handling the responsibilities is a challenge to nurses.
   3. A primary nursing model promotes continuity and quality of care and may best be implemented through nurse-physician teams.
   4. Nursing research in ambulatory care could be potentially fortified by collaborating with physician colleagues who may already be doing research. Research skills added to a nursing knowledge base and experience, substantiate and validate clinical assumptions about the needs of patients with cancer.
   5. With expert care, patients can be spared unnecessary hospitalizations. Disease- and treatment-related sequelae are monitored so problems are anticipated and managed before becoming acute. Patients and families are encouraged to call their physicians or nurses when symptoms arise or to clarify instructions.
   6. Staff stress is a problem to be contended with in the ambulatory setting. Support for collaborative practice, with ample opportunities for interdisciplinary communication and involvement in the decision making related to therapeutic modalities, can lessen this problem.

HOME CARE SETTING

A. A Natural Setting for Care.
   1. All other care settings interface with home care. Health care professionals must not disregard or underestimate the commitment of family members providing care. Professionals must be sensitive to support the home care provider.

2. Patients or families choose institutional care over home care if there is a feeling of burden or an inability to provide patient comfort. Nurses must be aware of options available to support home care, build family confidence, and allay anxieties while offering appropriate resources.

3. The home is the patient's natural social environment. Most patients want to stay in their homes and to receive as much of their care as possible within the home.

B. Home Nursing Agencies and Home Health Care Agencies.

1. The Department of Health and Human Services defines home health care as "that component of a continuum of comprehensive health care whereby health services are provided to individuals and families in their places of residence for the purpose of promoting, maintaining or restoring health, or of maximizing the level of independence, while minimizing the effects of disability and illness, including terminal illness."

2. Home health agencies provide assistance for patients in dealing with such problems as pain, poor nutrition, elimination disturbances, sleeplessness, emotional strain, and so forth. Home care nurses can support the patient's choice to stay in the home and offer respite for primary care providers.

3. Ambulatory care and home care nurses must become cooperating partners to provide increased self-sufficiency. The specialty team approach to care has the following program objectives:
   a. Reduction of frequency and number of hospitalizations.
   b. Reduction in the incidence of infections (especially pulmonary).
   c. Prevention and/or recognition of potentially life-threatening complications and the implementation of appropriate actions.
   d. Restoration and maintenance of optimal performance of activities of daily living.
   e. Promotion of compliance with medical regimen.

4. Many skills and services offered in the hospital are now available in the home. The patient may contract for varied health care providers and services including home care nurses, home health aides, social workers, physical therapists, occupational therapists, respiratory therapists, dietitians.

5. Numerous "high tech" support services are now available in the home including I.V. therapy, parenteral nutrition, chemotherapy (I.V. arterial infusion pump, intrathecal), antibiotic therapy, analgesic infusion pump therapy, specimen drawing for laboratory studies. With a competent care provider in the home and appropriate reimbursement programs, there is no conceivable limit to what can be offered.

NURSING HOME OR CONVALESCENT CARE SETTING

A. Occasionally, patients or families respond to a home care crisis by initiating a hospitalization. These admissions may be painful because they are seen by families as a failure to meet the patient's needs at home.

B. If the patient and family still prefer home care, that option should be restored if at all possible. Temporary or permanent nursing home placement may be considered as an alternative if other resource avenues have been exhausted.

C. Future trends should align nursing homes and home health care agencies together as hospitals and home care agencies are today. Collaboration between the nursing home and home health staff provides continuity of care and individualized comprehensive care.

HOSPICE CARE SETTINGS

A. Hospice Care Concept.
  1. Hospice has come to mean a system of specialized care which provides support and assistance for the most difficult of journeys—facing one's own death. It is a concept of care that concentrates on rehumanizing the experience of dying and joins modern technologic methods of pain and symptom control and sensitive, respectful, noninvasive caring.
  2. Hospice care requires several unique properties:
     a. The patient and family are the unit of care.
     b. The care commitment is 24 hours per day, 7 days a week.
     c. An interdisciplinary team plans and provides care with family input.
     d. Volunteers are actively recruited and utilized as part of the care program.
     e. A physician is an integral part of the team, usually as the medical director.
     f. Pain or symptom control is highly emphasized, but psychosocial, emotional, and spiritual needs of patient and family are also addressed.
     g. Hospice care continues with the family after the patient's death, with bereavement follow-up.
  3. On November 1, 1983, legislation provided funding for certified hospices to care for Medicare-eligible patients. Operational and quality guidelines are specified.
  4. Hospice care provides many rewards for nurses and should include the same kind of support services to alleviate stress as are available to their patients and families.
B. Types of Hospice Care Settings.
  1. Community-based program—This hospice has no facility other than an office that houses a multidisciplinary team. Home care is the focus, with the goal of providing physical comfort, autonomy, and emotional and physical support to the patient and family. Patients may or may not be continuing in treatment regimens. The hospice team collaborates with cancer nurses or physicians to provide optional cross-coverage and continuity of care.
  2. Hospital-based program—This may be an in-patient program or a hospital-based home care program; the unit must meet the already described criteria. A patient might be admitted for a new symptom management protocol, for an emergency the family wasn't able to handle, or for respite care. The hospital-based home care program may have formal hospital backing or support, its own interdisciplinary team, or some of the team members may be available as consultants from the various hospital departments.
  3. Hospital-based hospice team (may also be called the palliative care team)—Receives patients through in-hospital referral or consultation. The team physician may become the patient's primary physician, or the referring physician may remain in that position and then work in concert

with the hospice team. The interdisciplinary approach is essential. Hospital beds may be allocated for hospice care, or patients may be seen throughout the hospital. Daily care is administered by the regular nursing staff and the hospice team rounds on the patients each day, making recommendations as needed.

4. Free-standing hospice—This type hospice is a free-standing facility, usually with a home care program. Should the family become unable to manage the patient's care at home, the patient or family may elect for an admission to the hospice facility. The transfer and transition can be facilitated by the same team member planning and implementing the patient's care. The hospice support continues if the patient returns home. The patient in this setting has usually stopped cancer therapy, so the primary physician may have relinquished all care responsibility to the hospice physician.

PRIVATE PRACTICE BY NURSES

A. Qualified nurses may choose to practice independently (for example, fee-for-service bereavement therapy through an American Cancer Society office) or in an associated practice (sharing the care of a patient population with a physician or other health care professional).

B. Margo Neal edited a textbook entitled *Nursing in Business* for nurses interested in initiating private practice. All the many factors that must be considered are outlined (securing a financial base, legal issues, physician relationships, marketing).

C. Holmes and Van Scoy-Mosher have both written about their personal experiences of starting private practices as oncology nursing specialists. They provide a wide range of services including physical examinations, family and patient education, family and patient counseling and psychotherapy, and coordinator of contracted services (social services, nutritional counseling, physical therapy, home nursing services).

D. Patients and families may contract with an oncology nurse in private practice when they perceive they have educational or service gaps and see the nurse as a "free agent" to help them sort out all the options available.

FUTURE TRENDS IN CARE SETTINGS RELATED TO LONG-TERM SURVIVAL

A. Ambulatory care—Ambulatory care settings are becoming the treatment site choice of patients. In planning care options for these patients, nurses must be proactive rather than reactive, exploring creative means of delivering care to patients who prefer the comfort of their own homes.

B. Cancer rehabilitation—Because of strong public education efforts, improved diagnostic testing, and multimodality treatment regimens patients with cancer are living longer and healthier lives. The goal of rehabilitation is to help the patient attain maximum function in all aspects of life within the limits imposed by disease and treatment. The nurse can assist in this through assessment, teaching, counseling, goal-setting, and coordinating support services.

C. Hospice care—The "continuous, comprehensive care" afforded through hospice is sorely lacking in today's cost-conscious episodic approach to health care. Hospice offers a model for holistic care for the dying, and "has demonstrated that it has a great deal to teach caregivers at other stages of the life cycle . . . (it offers) a pattern of team care that supports a continuum of needs—psychosocial and spiritual as well as physical/episodic."

STUDY QUESTIONS

1. Identify the components to consider in justification of the establishment of a cancer specialty unit.
2. List considerations the nurse has in preparation of discharge of a patient with cancer to a nursing home.
3. What components assist in the decision for a patient's transition from home care to hospice care?

Bibliography

Amenta, M. O.: Hospice USA 1984—steady and holding. Oncology Nursing Forum, 11(5):68–74, 1984.

Anderson, J. L. and Brown, M. L.: The cancer patient in the community: A nursing challenge. Nursing Clinics of North America, 15(2):373–388, 1980.

Arenth, L. M.: The development and validation of oncology patient classification system. Oncology Nursing Forum, 12(6):17–22, 1985.

Brown, J. K.: Ambulatory services: The mainstay of cancer nursing care. Oncology Nursing Forum, 12(1):57–59, 1985.

Connor, S. R.: Foreword: The hospice movement. Family & Community Health, 5(3):x–xi, 1982.

Cox, A. and Andrews, P.: The development of support systems on oncology units. Oncology Nursing Forum, 8(3):31–35, 1981.

Elpern, E. H., et al.: Associated practice: A case for professional collaboration. The Journal of Nursing Administration, November 27–31, 1983.

Fritz, W. S.: Maintaining wellness—yours and theirs. Nursing Clinics of North America, 19(2):263–269, 1984.

Geltman, R. L. and Paige, R. L.: Symptom management in hospice care. American Journal of Nursing, 83(1):78–85, 1983.

Germain, C.: The cancer unit—an ethnography. Massachusetts, Nursing Resources, 1979.

Googe, M. C. and Varricchio, C. G.: Pilot investigation of home health care needs of cancer patients and their families. Oncology Nursing Forum, 8(4):24–28, 1981.

Habeck, R. V., Romsaas, E. P., and Olsen, S. J.: Cancer rehabilitation and continuing care: A case study. Cancer Nursing, 7(8):315–319, 1984.

Henrick, R. L. and Schag, C. C.: A behavioral medicine approach to coping with cancer: A case report. Cancer Nursing, 7(6):243–247, 1984.

Holmes, B. C.: Private practice in oncology nursing. Oncology Nursing Forum, 12(3):65–67, 1985.

Hunter, G. and Johnson, S. H.: Physical support systems for the homebound oncology patient. Oncology Nursing Forum, 7(3):21–23, 1980.

Johnston, M.: Ambulatory health care in the 80's. American Journal of Nursing, 80(1):76–79, 1980.

Jones, L. S., Miller, N. J., and Wegmann, J.: Organizing cancer in-patient care: Scattered-bed versus oncology unit approach. Oncology Nursing Forum, 8(1):31–36, 1981.

Kramer, R. F.: Living with childhood cancer: Impact on the healthy siblings. Oncology Nursing Forum, 11(1):44–51, 1984.

Lewis, F. M.: Family level services for the cancer patient: Critical distinctions, fallacies, and assessment. Cancer Nursing, 6(6):193–200, 1983.

McCorkle, R., et al.: A new beginning: The opening of a multidisciplinary cancer unit. Part I. Cancer Nursing, 2(3):201–209, 1979.

McCorkle, R., et al.: A new beginning: The opening of a multidisciplinary cancer unit. Part II. Cancer Nursing, 2(4):269–278, 1979.

McCorkle, R. and Germino, B.: What nurses need to know about home care. Oncology Nursing Forum, 11(6):63–69, 1984.

McNally, J. C., Stair, J. C., and Somerville, E. T. (eds.): Guidelines for Cancer Nursing Practice. New York, Grune & Stratton, Inc., 1985.

Moseley, J. R. and Brown, J. S.: The organization and operation of oncology units. Oncology Nursing Forum, 12(5):17–24, 1985.

Munley, S. A.: Sources of hospice staff stress and how to cope with it. Nursing Clinics of North America, 20(2):343–355, 1985.

Neal, M. C.: Nurses in business. Pacific Palisades, California, Nurseco, 1982.

O'Donnell, M. and Ainsworth, T.: Health Promotion in the Workplace. New York, John Wiley & Sons, 1984.

Parkes, C. M.: Terminal care: Home hospital or hospice? The Lancet, 1(8421):155–157, 1985.

Paulen, A.: High touch in a high tech environment. Cancer Nursing, 7(6):201, 1984.

Putnam, S. T., et al.: Home as a place to die. American Journal of Nursing, 80(8):1451–1453, 1980.

Rodek, C. F. and Jacob, S.: Hospice legislation: A new trial. Cancer Nursing, 7(10):385–389, 1984.

Romsaas, E. P. and Juliani, L. M.: Resource utilization in an outpatient setting. Oncology Nursing Forum, 11(3):45–48, 1984.

Rothlis, J.: The effect of a self-help group on feelings of hopelessness and helplessness. Western Journal of Nursing Research, 6(2):157–173, 1984.

Shields, P.: Communication: A supportive bridge between cancer patient, family, and health care staff. Nursing Forum, 21(1):31–36, 1984.

Skorupka, P. and Bohnet, N.: Primary caregivers' perceptions of nursing behaviors that best meet their needs in a home care hospice setting. Cancer Nursing, 5(10):371–374, 1982.

Smith, S. N. and Bohent, N.: Organizational and administration of hospice care. The Journal of Nursing Administration, November 10–16, 1983.

Stephany, T. M.: Quality assurance for hospice programs. Oncology Nursing Forum, 12(3):33–40, 1985.

Stewart, B. E., et al.: Psychological stress associated with outpatient oncology nursing. Cancer Nursing, 5(10):383–387, 1982.

Tehan, C.: Hospice in an existing home care agency. Family & Community Health, 5(3):11–20, 1982.

Tighe, M. G., et al.: A study of the oncology nurse role in ambulatory care. Oncology Nursing Forum, 12(6), 23–27, 1985.

Tornberg, M. J., McGrath, B. B., and Benoliel, J. Q.: Oncology transition services: Partnerships of nurses and families. Cancer Nursing, 7(4):131–137, 1984.

Van Scoy-Mosher, C.: The oncology nurse in independent professional practice. Cancer Nursing, 1(2):21–28, 1978.

Wald, F. S., Foster, Z., and Wald, H. J.: The hospice movement as a health care reform. Nursing Outlook, March 173–178. 1980.

Weinstein, S. M.: Specialty teams in home care. American Journal of Nursing, 84(3):342–345, 1984.

Wright, K. and Dyck, S.: Expressed concerns of adult cancer patients' family members. Cancer Nursing, 7(10):371–374, 1984.

39

Legal Issues

MINERVA APPLEGATE, RN, EdD
REGINA M. SHANNON RN, MS

CANCER QUACKERY AND UNPROVEN TREATMENT METHODS

A. Definition—definitions of cancer quackery include the following key descriptors:
   1. Intentional.
   2. Deliberate.
   3. Impedes.
   4. Delays.
   5. Unproven.
   6. Unorthodox.
   7. Nonlegitimate.
B. Categories of cancer quackery:
   1. Machines or devices—ozone generators, color waves, vibrators.
   2. Nutrition or diet—raw foods, fasting, vitamins.
   3. Chemicals or drugs—Krebiozen, Laetrile, IAT.
   4. Psychic or occult—incantations, psychic surgery, injections.
C. Characteristics of caregivers and treatment promoters:
   1. Lack of regulation and control by government, professional organizations, and other regulatory agencies.
   2. Excessive fees.
   3. Cure is promised.
   4. Highly promoted.
   5. Poor record keeping.
   6. Caregivers lack appropriate credentials.
   7. Antagonistic attitudes toward traditional caregivers.
   8. Practice outside of mainstream of traditional health care setting.
D. Patient motivations—a variety of motivations for patients seeking cancer quackery have been identified:
   1. Fear.
   2. Frustration.

3. Hopelessness.
4. Ignorance.
5. Unmet needs.
6. Suspicion.
7. Lack of control.
8. Lack of involvement in decision making.

E. Nursing implications—in order to prevent cancer quackery and the patients seeking out unproven methods of treatment, the nurse should:
1. Keep abreast of national organization support systems and resources.
2. Inform patients and families.
3. Involve patients and families in decision making.
4. Meet patient's emotional, social, and physical needs.
5. Offer individualized care.
6. Maintain open communication.
7. Keep the public informed of misrepresentation, fraud, and deceit.
8. Assist the patient in coping and managing stress.
9. Promote positive nurse-patient relationships.
10. Be a patient advocate.

PATIENT ACCESS TO CARE

A. The "Gatekeeper" concept—an alternative to traditional health care delivery.
1. Primary care network; fee-for-service or per capita, specialty care limited; similar to Health Maintenance Organizations.
2. May result in less self-referral, fewer emergency room visits, assurance of access to health care services, and less freedom of choice.
3. Physician serves as case manager.
4. Differs from preferred provider organizations, which are characterized by economic incentives; patients are not "locked in" to a certain physician, and physicians are not at financial risk for patients.
5. Cost determines pattern for professional services. Care may be delayed and minimal; referrals specialists may be avoided.
6. Limits patients' choices.

B. Federal government is increasing its intervention in and concern about health care.
1. Increasing costs—1.2% of population consumes 20% of total national health expenditures.
2. Lack of access for patients in low socioeconomic groups.
3. More than 50% of all physicians are located in 10 states.
4. 129 counties in the United States have no active physician providing inpatient care.
5. Movement is toward promotion of increased efficiency.
6. Reforms are being promoted in reimbursement procedures, maldistribution of health care, consumer expectations, health planning, and implementation of technology.
7. Allocation of scarce resources.
8. Lack of continuity and coordination of care.

C. Impact on patients—contemporary alternatives to health care and increasing governmental regulation may lead to negative outcomes and increased access barriers for oncology patients.

1. Less coverage for preventive services.
2. Fewer annual physical examinations.
3. Decreased screening and early detection and treatment.
4. Access to services is dictated to patients.
5. Less opportunity for health teaching.
6. Lack of support services for psychosocial needs.
7. Insurance coverage may be contingent upon employment.
8. Lack of available primary care services.

D. Implications for nurses:
   1. Maintain awareness of social, economic, and political issues impacting upon health care delivery.
   2. Support reforms that will enhance health care delivery.
   3. Encourage primary and secondary preventive health-seeking patterns.
   4. Keep the public informed.
   5. Promote continuity and coordination of care.
   6. Support third-party reimbursement for nonphysician health care providers.
   7. Maintain an active role in community, state, and national health planning.
   8. Support patients' freedom to choose.

CARCINOGENESIS LEGISLATION

A. Priorities—the federal government's regulatory agencies have primarily focused on the following areas of carcinogen regulation and control:
   1. Hazardous waste exposure.
   2. Occupational exposure.
   3. Consumer product exposure.
   4. Environmental exposure.
   5. Food exposure.
   6. Air exposure.
   7. Water exposure.

B. Legislation—federal governmental agency regulation and control have led to the enactment of the following legislation which impacts on carcinogens:
   1. Resource Conservation and Recovery Act, 1976—hazardous waste exposure.
   2. Occupational Safety and Health Act, 1972—occupational exposure.
   3. Consumer Product Safety Act, 1972—consumer product exposure.
   4. Toxic Substances Control Act, 1976—environmental exposure.
   5. Federal Food, Drug, and Cosmetic Act, 1976—amended Delaney Clause Section 409 (c) (3) (A) and Sections 402 (a) (1); 706 (b) (5) (B); and 512 (d) (1) (H)—food additives, color additives, animal drugs, and adulteration of food.
   6. Clean Air Act, 1970—control of vinyl chloride and asbestos.
   7. Clean Water Act, 1972 and Safe Drinking Water Act, 1974—control of aldrin, dieldrin, benzedrine, and so forth.

C. Advantages for consumers and workers—the enactment of carcinogenesis legislation has afforded consumers and workers the following advantages:
   1. Participation in setting standards.
   2. Participation in enforcing standards.
   3. Potential for requiring regulatory agencies to exercise authority.

4. Participation in promoting decreases in carcinogenic exposure.
5. Potential for officially requesting inspections.
6. Participation in monitoring hazards.
7. Potential for collective bargaining to reduce carcinogen exposure.
8. Protection of consumers' and workers' rights.

PATIENT RIGHTS

A. American Hospital Association—Patients' Bill of Rights, 1973.
　　1. Right to care.
　　2. Information.
　　3. Informed consent.
　　4. Right to refuse treatment.
　　5. Privacy.
　　6. Confidentiality.
　　7. Reasonable response to request for service.
　　8. Information on hospital and professional relationships.
　　9. Information on human experimentation; right to refuse.
　 10. Reasonable continuity of care.
　 11. Examine and receive explanation of bill.
　 12. Knowledge of hospital rules and regulations applicable to conduct of patient.
B. Basic rights that should be afforded to all health care consumers include:
　　1. Adequate health care.
　　2. Full disclosure.
　　3. Self-determination.
　　4. Maintenance of integrity.
C. Issues pertinent to oncology—contemporary issues that have significant implications for oncology nurses include:
　　1. "Natural Death Act," 1976, California.
　　2. Living Wills.
　　3. Death with Dignity.
　　4. Euthanasia.
　　5. Right to Refuse Treatment.
　　6. Extraordinary vs. Ordinary Means of treatment.
　　7. Quality vs. Quantity of Life.
　　8. Individual vs. Society.
D. Treatment Decisions and the Right to Refuse Treatment—these decisions relate primarily to public interest positions or patient positions.
　　1. Public interest positions:
　　　　a. Preservation of society.
　　　　b. Sanctity of life.
　　　　c. Public morals.
　　　　d. Protection of the individual against himself.
　　　　e. Protection of third parties.
　　　　　　(1) Surviving adults.
　　　　　　(2) Fellow patients.
　　　　　　(3) Physicians.
　　　　　　(4) Surviving minors.
　　2. Patient positions.
　　　　a. Liberty and the right to choose freely.

    b. Loss of human dignity.
    c. Reduction of suffering.
E. Trends—contemporary trends that have evolved out of the Patients' Rights movement have implications for oncology nurses:
    1. States are recognizing Living Wills.
    2. States are selectively recognizing Refusals of Treatment, e.g., blood transfusions, renal dialysis.
    3. Informed consent is becoming more controlled.
    4. Human experimentation is becoming more controlled.
    5. Patients' rights are being protected.
    6. Health care providers' rights are being given more consideration.

EMPLOYMENT

A. Gainful employment generally symbolizes responsibility, independence, and other qualities of competence. The role work provides and the manner in which that role is filled are important indicators of an individual's success and ranking in society.
B. Discrimination.
    1. The American Cancer Society estimates a serious discrimination problem for approximately 90% of patients trying to return to work.
    2. Employment discrimination against the patient with a health history that lists cancer may be found in practices related to:
        a. Hiring.
        b. Promotion.
        c. Firing.
    3. Discrimination may be related to employers':
        a. Mistaken fear of contagion.
        b. Concern with continued illness and the higher absenteeism and prolonged sick leaves which may accompany this.
        c. Concern with potential increased cost of company health and life insurance.
        d. Fear of an increased risk of future injury.
        e. Concern of nonacceptance among co-workers.
C. Work performance.
    1. The work experiences of recovered cancer patients reveal reports of:
        a. Hostility expressed by fellow workers.
        b. Lack of salary advances.
        c. Reduction in health benefits.
        d. Ineligibility for newly available group life insurance.
    2. There is a strong need in recovered cancer patients, especially the very young, to prove that cancer has not impaired their ability to function adequately and to demonstrate their ability to perform stressful work and demanding tasks.
    3. Metropolitan Life Insurance Company in a study of their employees with a history of cancer, found work performance, absenteeism, and turnover rates comparable for persons both with and without cancer. They concluded:
        "selective hiring of persons who have been treated for cancer in positions for which they are physically qualified, is a second industrial practice."

4. American Telephone and Telegraph did not find "any impact of cancer on most work related criteria."
5. The Rehabilitation Act of 1973 defined a handicapped individual as "a person who has any impairment which substantially limits one or more of a patient's life activities."
   a. Section 501 required that all federal departments or agencies provide an affirmative action plan for the hiring, placement, and advancement of handicapped individuals.
   b. 1974 amendments to the Act expanded the definition of handicapped persons to include those individuals with a history of handicap and those perceived as having a handicap.
   c. Under the 1974 definition the Act may be construed to include cancer patients and persons with a history of cancer should the patient so desire to claim.

INSURANCE

A. Costs of Cancer.
   1. Direct (20–30%) include:
      a. Hospital and physician charges.
      b. Drugs.
      c. Professional services.
      d. Nursing home care.
   2. Indirect (70–80%) include:
      a. Costs related to special needs (e.g., diet, transportation).
      b. Losses of output due to mortality, morbidity, and disability.
      c. Loss of income from absence on the job due to clinic visits, treatment, and hospitalization.
      d. Costs related to inability to fulfill role (e.g., child care, home maintenance).
   3. Many direct costs such as hospitalization are covered by third party reimbursers such as:
      a. Medicare (for those over 65 or younger if disabled)—includes many restrictions.
      b. Medicaid—some state-specific limitations.
      c. Blue Cross/Blue Shield—varies according to plan.
      d. Other commercial insurance companies.
      e. The patient himself or herself may pay the complete costs or a deductable or copayment of one of the previously listed insurance plans.
   4. Indirect costs are rarely covered by insurance and can be the most costly to the person with cancer and his or her family.
   5. Costs may be compounded secondary to:
      a. Loss of employment, either temporarily or permanently.
      b. Increased premium rates of health and life insurance due to the cancer diagnosis.
B. Access and discrimination.
   1. Post diagnosis cancer patients may face insurance access barriers and discrimination including:
      a. Cancellations of existing coverage under health insurance policies.
      b. Reduction of health insurance benefits.

c. Increase in health insurance premiums.
d. Refusal of new insurance applications.
e. Extended waiting periods for coverage.
f. Exclusions of cancer-related coverage.
g. Loss of insurance owing to loss of employment.
h. The experience of being "locked into" one's current job for fear of losing insurance coverage.
2. In 1983, the American Cancer Society, California Division, estimated:
    a. 210,451 individuals would have a cancer health history.
    b. 16,200 insurance cancellations occurred after diagnosis or treatment.
    c. 8,100 cancellations were due to work termination and subsequent loss of group policy.
    d. 3,350 cancellations were due to cancer history.
3. Social Security Disability Insurance Program.
    To be eligible the applicant must demonstrate the inability to perform substantial gainful activity because of medically determinable physical or mental impairment. This limits coverage availability for those who lost coverage due to discrimination or situational problems.

INTERVENTIONS

A. Personal/individual goals should include:
    a. Increase the knowledge and awareness of our own health coverage.
    b. Increase understanding of fundamental insurance principles.
    c. Increase the understanding of types of insurance available and options, i.e., plans, benefits, dependent provisions, conversion provisions, cost.
    d. Increase understanding of local community opportunities, i.e., local HMO, guaranteed insurance plans with fraternal or professional associations, and one's rights as a consumer.
B. Administrative Interventions:
    1. Typically involve a formal complaint process to insurers.
    2. Complaints, petitions, and appeals should be filed to support the patient's legal rights.
    3. Regulation of insurance is difficult to effect since it is:
        a. Delegated by federal law at the state level.
        b. Responsible for the protection of rights of handicapped persons in terms of insurance.
        c. State insurance codes vary from state to state.
C. Community:
    1. Support and resource systems are needed for cancer patients and their families struggling with problems related to insurance.
    2. At the county level, information and referral services need further development.
    3. Consumer advocacy groups, disability law centers, and legal aid programs can be of assistance at the local community level.
D. Legal Interventions Available:
    1. Include court action, which is expensive and time consuming.
    2. Require consultation with legal aid society and/or a private attorney.

STUDY QUESTIONS

1. Identify four categories of cancer quackery and give at least one example of each.
2. Identify ways in which the nurse can prevent cancer quackery and assist persons to seek out appropriate health care.
3. Identify concerns related to carcinogen regulation and control, and employment discrimination due to a cancer diagnosis.

Bibliography

American Hospital Association Patients' Bill of Rights. Chicago, The American Association Hospital, 1973.

Anderson, J. L.: Insurability of cancer patients: A rehabilitation barrier. Oncology Nursing Forum, 11(2):42–45, 1984.

Ashford, N. A.: Legal implications of working with carcinogens. *In* Sontag, J. M. (ed.): Carcinogens in Industry and the Environment. New York, Marcel Dekker, Inc., pp. 47–76, 1981.

Bahamas government closes clinic "immediately and permanently" after AIDS contamination report. The Cancer Letter, 11(30):1–2, 1985.

Burkhalter, P. K.: Cancer quackery: What you need to know. *In* Burkhalter, P. K. and Donley, D. L. (eds.): Dynamics of Oncology Nursing. New York, McGraw Hill Book Company, pp. 428–442, 1978.

Cantor, N. L.: A patient's decision to decline life-saving medical treatment: Bodily integrity versus the preservation of life. *In* Beauchamp, T. L. and Perlin, S. (eds.): Ethical Issues in Death and Dying. Englewood Cliffs, NJ, Prentice-Hall, Inc., pp. 203–213, 1978.

CDC isolates HTLV-3 virus from Burton serum; patients warned of risks. The Cancer Letter, 11(33):5, 1985.

Chupack, N.: The "gatekeeper" concept. *In* Haug, J. N. and Sugar, R. (eds.): Socio-Economic Factbook for Surgery 1983–84. Chicago, American College of Surgeons, Surgical Practice Department, pp. 98–101, 1983.

Cohen, J. and Cordoba, C.: Psychologic, social and economic aspects of cancer. Surgery Annuals, 15:99–112, 1983.

Dietz, J. H.: Employment in Rehabilitation Oncology. New York, John Wiley & Son, 1981.

Donovan, M. I. and Girton, S. E.: Cancer Care Nursing, 2nd ed. Norwalk, CT, Appleton-Century-Crofts, pp. 58–90, 1984.

Eilter, M. A.: Physician Characteristics and Distribution in the U.S.: 1982 Edition. Chicago, American Medical Association, pp. 48–49, 1983.

Feldman, F. L.: Work and Cancer Health Histories: A Study of the Experiences of Recovered Blue-Collar Workers. San Francisco, American Cancer Society, California Division, Inc., 1978.

Feldman, F. L. Work and Cancer Health Histories: A Study of Recovered Patients (White Collar Study). San Francisco, American Cancer Society, California Division, Inc., 1976.

Goldhammer, G. S.: Evolution of the Delaney Clause. *In* Kessler, J. K. (ed.): Cancer Control: Contemporary Views on Screening, Diagnosis, and Therapy. Baltimore, University Park Press, pp. 209–213, 1980.

Hanken, J. C.: Patients' Rights. *In* Sorenson, K. C. and Luckmann, J. (eds.): Basic Nursing: A Psychophysiologic Approach. Philadelphia, W. B. Saunders Co., pp. 358–364, 1979.

Harkins, R. W.: The Delaney Clause and food safety. *In* Kessler, J. K. (ed.): Cancer Control: Contemporary Views on Screening, Diagnosis, and Therapy. Baltimore, University Park Press, pp. 223–241, 1980.

Johnson, A.: A healthy law for consumers. *In* Kessler, J. K. (ed.): Cancer Control: Contemporary Views on Screening, Diagnosis, and Therapy. Baltimore, University Park Press, 1980.

Kane, F. I.: Keeping Elizabeth Bouvia alive for the public good. Hastings Center Report, 15(6):5–8, 1985.

McCall, N.: Financing and delivery system research issues. *In* Cohen, J., Cullen, J. W., and Martin, L. R. (eds.): Psychosocial Aspects of Cancer. New York, Raven Press, pp. 91–101, 1982.

McCormick, R. A. and Hellegers, A. E.: Legislation and the living will. *In* Beauchamp, T. L. and Perlin, S. (eds.): Ethical Issues in Death and Dying. Englewood Cliffs, NJ, Prentice-Hall, Inc., pp. 305–310, 1978.

McNaull, F. W.: The costs of cancer: A challenge to health care providers. Cancer Nursing, 4(3):207–212, 1981.

Patrick, P. K. S.: Cancer quackery: Information, issues, responsibility, action. *In* Marino, L. (ed.): Cancer Nursing. St. Louis, C. V. Mosby Company, pp. 357–370, 1981.

Schweitzer, S. D.: Concepts and research issues in the economics of cancer prevention. *In* Cohen, J., Cullen, J. W., and Martin, L. R. (eds.): Psychosocial Aspects of Cancer. New York, Raven Press, pp. 81–90, 1982.

Sigel, C. J.: Legal recourse for the cancer patient-returnee: The rehabilitation act of 1973. American Journal of Law and Medicine, 10(3):309–321, 1973.

Stone, R. W.: Employing the recovered cancer patient. Cancer, 36:285–286, 1973.

Wheatley, G. M., Cunnick, W. R., Wright, B. P., and Van Keuren, D.: The employment of persons with a history of treatment for cancer. Cancer, 33(2):441–445, 1974.

40

Cancer Economics

MARCIA CLARK, RN, MS

OVERVIEW

A. Definition and Background.
   1. Economics of cancer care reflect the prevailing issues and trends on the contemporary health care scene and also embody unique concerns specific to this disease.
   2. After 20 years of expanding programs and escalating costs, the American health care system is undergoing revolutionary change. In 1982, the Federal government introduced Diagnostic Related Groups (DRG's), a form of prospective payment for in-hospital care provided to Medicare recipients. This reimbursement strategy promotes cost containment by:
      a. Discouraging proliferation or duplication of services.
      b. Financially rewarding institutions for efficient delivery of care.
   3. Health care providers recognize that further economic constraints, similar to those imposed by DRG's, are forthcoming:
      a. From the government for other federally financed health care.
      b. From commercial (nongovernmental, private) health care insurers.
   4. In the face of this economic constraint, the challenge to the contemporary health care system is two-fold:
      a. Maintain quality.
      b. Provide efficient, cost-effective care.
   5. Budget reductions, personnel cuts, and program cut-backs are inevitable. However, new programs are emerging to meet the challenge, a testimony to the creativity, ingenuity, and commitment of concerned health care providers.
B. It is essential that nurses have a clear understanding of the prevailing climate of economic constraint, because nursing has a key role to play in this new health care scene. In addition to an awareness of the patient's situation, the nurse understands the economic realities of the institution/agency providing health care. This understanding, experience, and clinical expertise is invaluable in the development and implementation of new programs. Nursing input is crucial to the emergence of new and better health care alternatives

on the cost-conscious American health care scene. As patient advocates and primary care-givers, nurses are in a unique position both requiring and enabling them to:

1. Recognize the economic needs of patients and families.
2. Identify existing and available financial resources.
3. Put patients and families in touch with appropriate resources.
4. Evaluate the effectiveness of existing resources.

C. In addition to these contemporary issues and trends, cancer care faces a set of disease-specific economic realities. Cancer is not one disease entity with a routine, circumscribed treatment regimen. Rather, it is a disease encompassing over 100 different conditions that are treated in a variety of ways. Manifestations of malignancy and associated treatment options characteristically fall on a continuum. Placement on this continuum can vary considerably among patients having a common diagnosis of "cancer." There is great diversity existing within this patient population:

FROM	TO
Local disease	Disseminated disease
Curable disease	Incurable disease
Treatable disease	Untreatable disease
Short-term illness	Long-term/chronic illness
(cure . . . death)	(remission . . . disability)
Routine therapy	Investigational therapy
Cost-effective therapy	Costly, ineffective therapy

In light of this diversity, it is evident that some cancer patients will experience little or no major economic hardship while others may be financially devastated by the diagnosis and its subsequent treatment.

D. Familiarity with cancer economics will assist the nurse caring for patients with cancer to implement the nursing process, addressing the patient's (family's) economic needs. Discussion of financial matters, a somewhat sensitive issue for many, is frequently avoided. However, experience indicates that:

1. Patients and families worry about finances and welcome assistance.
2. Resolution of financial worries enables the patient and family to focus energies on clinical aspects of the treatment program.

NURSING PROCESS

A. The degree of economic need experienced by an individual patient (or family) is significantly influenced by:

1. Disease and treatment parameters.
2. Source(s) of patient/family income.
3. Demands on patient/family income.
4. Availability of financial-aid resources.
5. Adequacy of existing resources.
6. Method of payment for health care.

B. Assessment:

1. What are anticipated costs of cancer care?
   a. *Direct costs* are incurred as a consequence of the disease and its treatment. Examples include charges made for:
      (1) Hospitalization.
      (2) Medical care (physician fees, office visits).

(3) Diagnostic tests.
(4) Cancer treatment.
  (a) Surgery.
  (b) Radiation.
  (c) Chemotherapy.
  (d) Immunotherapy.
(5) Ancillary therapies.
  (a) Physical therapy.
  (b) Occupational therapy.
  (c) Medications (analgesics, antiemetics, etc.).
  (d) Respiratory care.
  (e) Nutritional supplements.
(6) Home care.
(7) Transportation (for treatment, follow-up).

b. *Indirect costs* are incurred as a consequence of the disease, but not directly attributable to the diagnosis and/or treatment; they accrue when the diagnosis/treatment prompts an alteration in patient/family functioning. *Examples* of role or life style changes that influence indirect costs include:
  (1) Change in employment status of either the patient or of a family member (care-taker) which influences:
    (a) Income level.
    (b) Eligibility for health insurance.
  (2) Change in ability to perform usual role (household activity) creating a need for assistance with:
    (a) Housekeeping.
    (b) Meal preparation.
    (c) Shopping.
    (d) Child care.
    (e) Transportation.

c. *Social costs* are incurred by the *individual* patient and family experiencing the effects of the diagnosis/treatment of cancer and also by the larger *community* (professional, public, and voluntary sectors) striving to find the means to develop and provide the types of services required by this patient population. For *example*:
  (1) Individual patient/family costs include:
    (a) Isolation (disability, life style change, fear).
    (b) Discrimination (job, insurance, etc.).
  (2) Community social costs include:
    (a) Pressure to provide more services.
    (b) Shifting of limited resources, which results in a number of underserved areas.

2. What is the effect of prospective payment on the economics of cancer care?
  a. General experience to-date:
    (1) Applicable only to in-hospital care for Medicare recipients; patients are not held responsible for costs incurred beyond the prospective payment allowance.
    (2) Hospitals are motivated to provide cost-effective care, prompting:
      (a) Scrutiny of numbers or types of diagnostic tests done.
      (b) Earlier discharge of "sicker" patients.

        (c) Marketing for "favorable" DRG's.
        (d) Efforts to shift care from in-patient to out-patient settings.
    b. Special applicability to the cancer patient population:
        (1) Since cancer is a disease of aging, Medicare regulations have a significant impact on this group of patients and on those who provide care to cancer patients.
        (2) Diagnosis, treatment, and follow-up for the cancer patient entails extensive testing, making cancer care an expensive item for providers under the constraint of prospective (DRG) reimbursement.
        (3) Earlier discharge of "sicker" cancer patients has created problems because:
            (a) Patients now require more complex care and services in community (home and extended care) settings.
            (b) Medicare has begun tightening up regulations covering payment for services and equipment in the community setting.
        (4) The shift of cancer therapy from the in-patient to the out-patient setting requires:
            (a) More sophisticated outpatient treatment services.
            (b) More adequate patient transportation services.
            (c) Increased home care supervision.
    c. Projections:
        (1) Since DRG's have served to contain costs, it is anticipated that prospective payment in some form will:
            (a) Continue and expand into other areas of government-sponsored health care.
            (b) Be implemented by other health care insurers.
            (c) Extend beyond the in-hospital setting.
        (2) Other cost-containment approaches (i.e., HMO's, PPO's) will be introduced and implemented on a much wider scale.
        (3) Economics of cancer care will demand increased attention as cost-containment efforts intensify. Cancer treatment can accrue considerable expense due to:
            (a) The "high tech" approach used in both diagnosis and treatment.
            (b) Increased costs associated with investigational therapy.
            (c) The need for on-going monitoring of disease and treatment parameters, requiring numerous (often expensive) diagnostic procedures.
            (d) The "high touch" (labor-intensive) care needs of this patient population.
 3. Is this patient or family experiencing economic difficulty?
    a. What is this patient's disease, treatment plan, prognosis?
    b. What are the direct costs projected for this patient?
    c. How will this patient or family pay for care?
    d. Are any appropriate direct costs accruing that this patient or family is *not* able to meet?
    e. If the answer to d above is "yes," what would facilitate the patient's or family's ability to meet these expenses?
        (1) Revised payment plan (discounted care, free care, an installment plan for payment)?
        (2) An alternate insurance coverage?

(3) Supplemental financial assistance (governmental aid, voluntary agency funds)?

f. Is the patient or family incurring *inappropriate* direct expenses because of:

(1) Incorrect or incomplete use of insurance coverage?

(2) Inaccurate billing?

g. Is this patient or family likely to require assistance with indirect costs of care?

(1) Examine pertinent demographic data.

(a) Disease, treatment, prognosis.

(b) Age.

(c) Marital status.

(d) Position in family.

(e) Occupation (employment status).

(f) Socioeconomic status (financial security).

(2) Using demographic data, consider what effect this individual's illness will have on:

(a) The patient's own financial security.

(b) The family's financial well-being.

h. What indirect costs are actually accruing?

i. How is the patient or family meeting these demands?

C. Planning. The patient/family:

1. Knows what cancer care will cost.

2. Knows how health care providers will be paid for services rendered.

3. Receives necessary financial assistance.

4. Is able to seek help when financial concerns arise.

D. Implementation:

1. Interventions that assist patient/family to understand and anticipate the cost of cancer care:

a. Explanation of the treatment program:

(1) Therapy planned.

(2) Duration (number of treatments).

(3) Anticipated effects.

(a) Prognosis.

(b) Side effects (anticipated disability).

(4) Diagnostic tests (monitoring).

b. Itemization of anticipated direct costs:

(1) Project quantity of service and materials required to carry out proposed treatment plan.

(2) Calculate cost based on routine charges.

c. Estimation of indirect costs:

(1) Review individual demographic information.

(2) Correlate demographic information with disease and treatment parameters.

2. Interventions that assist patient and family to understand how health care providers will be paid for services rendered.

a. Review usual sources of payment:

(1) Self-pay.

(a) Full fee.

(b) Discounted charge.

(c) Installment payment plan.

      (2) Third-party insurers:
        (a) Blue Cross/Blue Shield.
        (b) Commercial insurance carriers.
        (c) Medicare.
        (d) Medicaid.
  b. Ensure that patient and family know which payment plan applies.
  c. Review extent of coverage available under the payment program used by patient and family:
      (1) List services and items covered and those that are NOT covered.
      (2) Identify anticipated out-of-pocket expenses.
        (a) For partially covered services and items.
        (b) For services and items that are *not* covered.
  d. Assist patient and family to provide appropriate financial reimbursement information to health care providers.
  e. Explain providers' expectations and policies regarding payment:
      (1) Accepts assignment.
      (2) Processes third-party claims for patients.
      (3) Provides forms, but does not process claims.
      (4) Expects payment at time of visit or treatment.
      (5) Bills for service.
        (a) Total amount due on receipt of bill; patient and family must seek reimbursement from third-party payor.
        (b) Submits claim to third-party payor; bills only for unpaid balance.
3. Interventions that assist patient and family to receive needed financial assistance:
  a. Identify appropriate sources of help (referrals):
      (1) Hospital/agency social service department.
      (2) Hospital/agency/office accounting department/person.
      (3) Third-party payor subscriber assistance department.
      (4) Government agencies:
        (a) Medicare office.
        (b) Medicaid office.
        (c) National Cancer Institute (NCI).
          i. Limited financial assistance available from NCI.
          ii. Accepts patients for investigational treatment *if* patient qualifies for inclusion in a study being conducted by the NCI.
          iii. Provides clinical departments in institutions with *investigational* drugs for use in approved clinical trials; no drug charges assessed to patients treated with these drugs.
      (5) Voluntary agencies: services offered vary from one local chapter/division to another; these agencies offer a wealth of services, including financial aid, transportation, counselling, information, and referral to other agencies as appropriate.
        (a) Leukemia Society serves patients having hematologic malignancies.
          i. Leukemia.
          ii. Lymphoma.
          iii. Hodgkin's disease.

(b) American Cancer Society—each division has some type of emergency financial aid program designed to assist patients and families confronted with the economic realities of cancer care.

  (6) Other resources—several pharmaceutical companies marketing cancer chemotherapeutic agents offer patient assistance programs; patients who meet a company's financial need guidelines are eligible to receive drug(s) at no charge. Medication is sent to the patient's physician directly from the company.

  b. Assist patient and family member to make contact with source(s) of help.

    (1) Make the referral for the patient and family.

    (2) Provide patient and family member with information necessary to make the referral:

      (a) Name of appropriate agency or contact person.

      (b) Telephone number.

      (c) Address.

  c. Provide guidance and direction as to:

    (1) Presentation of need or request.

    (2) Information required by agency.

    (3) Questions to ask of agency personnel.

E. Evaluation. The patient and family:

  1. Are incurring appropriate and accurate direct costs for cancer care.

  2. Are able to handle costs incurred.

  3. Are able to seek out financial assistance.

    a. Recognize when help is needed.

    b. Know where to seek assistance.

    c. Know how to seek assistance.

  4. Have a contact person in the health care system to facilitate requests for financial assistance.

  5. Are relieved of financial worries and thus able to concentrate energies on clinical concerns.

STUDY QUESTIONS

1. What assessment data do you need in order to anticipate the economic impact of a cancer diagnosis and treatment plan on an individual patient and family?
2. What is the most usual method of paying for health care in this country?
3. Describe the impact of prospective payment on:
   a. The American health care system.
   b. The individual and family facing cancer.
4. What additional or supplemental financial resources are available to help the patient and family meet costs associated with cancer care?

Bibliography

Bloch, H. and Pupp, R.: Supply, demand and rising health care costs. Nursing Economics, 3:119–123, 1985.

Brown, J. K.: Ambulatory services: Mainstay of cancer nursing care. Oncology Nursing Forum, 12:57–59, 1985.

Coleman, J. R. and Smith, D. S.: DRG's and the growth of home health care. Nursing Economics, 2:391–395, 1984.

Collins, J. and McDonald, J.: Health care for Medicare beneficiaries: The HMO option. Nursing Economics, 2:259–265, 1984.

Curtin, L.: Strategies for operating effectively in today's environment. Nursing Management, 15:7–8, 1984.

Davis, C.: Health care economic issues: Projections for oncology nurses. Oncology Nursing Forum, 12:17–22, 1985.

Davis, C.: The federal role in changing health care financing. Part I. National programs and health financing problems. Nursing Economics, 1:10–17, 1983.

Davis, C.: The federal role in changing health care financing. Part II. Prospective payment and its impact on nursing. Nursing Economics, 1:98–106, 1983.

Donley, S. R.: The effect of changing health care policy on cancer nursing. Oncology Nursing Forum, 11:64–66, 1984.

Franz, J.: Challenge for nursing: Hiking productivity without lowering quality of care. Modern Healthcare, 60–68, September 1984.

Fry, S.: Rationing health care: The ethics of cost-containment. Nursing Economics, 1:165–169, 1983.

Grimaldi, P. L.: Public law 97–248: The implications of prospective payment schedules. Nursing Management, 14:25–27, 1983.

Grimaldi, P. L.: Recent changes in Medicare payments for ambulatory clinical diagnostic tests. Nursing Management, 16:16–18, 1985.

Grimaldi, P. L.: Relying on HMO's to trim Medicare and Medicaid spending. Nursing Management, 15:74–77, 1984.

Hicks, L. and Boles, K.: Why health economics? Nursing Economics, 2:175–180, 1984.

Kanter, R. M.: Innovation—The only hope for times ahead? Nursing Economics, 3:178–182, 1985.

Lee, A. A.: How DRG's will affect your hospital and you. RN, 71–81, May 1984.

McNaull, J. and Wheeler, K. E.: The cancer patient's financial concerns. Oncology Nursing Forum, 5:1–4, 1978.

Micheletti, J. and Toth, R.: Diagnosis related groups: Impact and implications. Nursing Management, 12:33–39, 1981.

Spitzer, R. B.: Legislation and new regulations. Nursing Management, 14:13–21, 1983.

Tonges, M. C.: Quality with economy: Doing the right things for less. Nursing Economics, 3:205–211, 1985.

Yasko, J. M. and Fleck, A.: Prospective payment (DRG's): What will be the impact on cancer care? Oncology Nursing Forum, 11:63–72, 1984.

Index

Note: Numbers in *italics* refer to illustrations; numbers followed by (t) refer to tables.

423

Elspar. *See* L-Asparaginase.
Emergencies, 321–332
  cardiac tamponade as, 321–322
  disseminated intravascular coagulation as,
    322–323
  hypercalcemia as, 323–325
  informed consent and, 393
  sepsis as, 326–327
  spinal cord compression as, 327–328
  superior vena cava syndrome as, 328–330,
    329
  syndrome of inappropriate antidiuretic
    hormone as, 325–326
  tumor lysis syndrome as, 330–331
Emesis. *See* Vomiting.
Emotional impact of cancer, 348–349
Employment, 409–410
En bloc dissection, 200
Encore, 364(t)
Endoderm, 27
Endometrial cancer, 149–151
Endoscopy, 201
Endothelial tumors, 25(t)
Endotoxin, as biologic response modifier,
    239(t)
  sepsis and, 326
Enema(s), constipation and, 277
  steroid, in mucositis, 315
Enteral nutritional support, 253–255
Enteritis, radiation and, 249(t)
Entrapment, mechanical, 16
Environment, 32
  head and neck cancer and, 153
  patient education and, 354
Enzyme, 76–77(t)
Eosinophil, 78(t)
Epichlorohydrin, 46(t)
Epidemiologists, 31
Epidemiology, 29–51
  incidence and trends in, 35–39
  patterns of occurrence in, 41–43
  resources and, 368
  risk factors in, 45–51
  terminology in, 31–33
Epithelial tissue tumor, 25(t)
Epsilon–aminocaproic acid, 323, 324(t)
Epstein-Barr virus, 45, 153
Esophageal speech, 159
Esophagectomy, 249
Esophagitis, 313–315
  radiation and, 248(t)
Esophagus, dysphagia and, 279
  nutrition and tumors of, 247, 249
  staging and, 91
Estradiol, 74(t)
Estrogen(s), carcinogenesis and, 48, 49(t)
  development of, 380(t)
  in breast cancer, 113
  thrombocytopenia and, 275
  total, 74(t)
  use of, 60
Estrogen receptor assay, 74(t), 111, 113
Ethical considerations, 391–392
Ethnic differences, 42
Ethoxyquin, 13
Ethylene oxide, 47(t)

Etoposide, as vesicant irritant, 341(t)
  classification of, 233(t)
  development of, 380(t)
  in lung cancer, 100, 101, 102(t)
Ex vivo treatment, 239(t)
Excision biopsy, 123, 199
Exercise, aerobic, 61
Exercise pattern, 61
Experimental study, 32
Extended family, 347, 348
External radiation therapy, 212–217
  cervical cancer and, 143
  for prostate cancer, 134
  problems with, 104
Extradural block, 201
Extravasation, 16, *17*
  nursing management of, 341–344
Extravasation record, *343*
Eye contact by chemotherapeutic agent, 337

Familial polyposis, 163
Family, assessment of, 348
  care setting selection and, 395–396
  communication with, 347–351
  patient education and, 353
  teaching of, 353–359
Farber, S., 379
Fast-acting cancer virus, 11
Fat, 48
  in diet, 55
  metabolism of, 246
Fatigue, 288–290
  radiation and, 248(t)
Fecal impaction, 277
Fecal occult blood, 164
Fecal stoma, 145
Federal Food, Drug, and Cosmetic Act of 1976,
    407
Federal government, health care and, 406, 407
Feeding tube, 281
Female reproductive organs and bladder, *138*
  examinations of, 82–83
Ferritin, 76(t)
Fetal antigen(s), 19–20
  discovery of, 382
Fever, 287–288
  total parenteral nutrition and, 254(t)
Fiber, 48
  in diet, 56
Fibrinolytic system, 322
Fibrocystic disease of breast, 107
Financial assistance, 420
Fistula, after pelvic radiation, 145
  after tracheotomy or laryngectomy, 158
  hypokalemia and, 286
  radiation and, 249(t)
Fletcher's applicator, 144
Floxuridine, 233(t)
Fluid overload, 254(t)
Fluid replacement, in diarrhea, 279
  in mucositis, 314
  in nausea and vomiting, 304
  in sepsis, 327
Fluid shift to interstitial spaces, 283–284
Fluoride treatment, 317